Study Guide to

Accompany Introductory Clinical Pharmacology

Twelfth Edition

Susan M. Ford, MN, RN, CNE ret
Professor Emeritus, Former Associate Dean for Nursing
Tacoma Community College
Tacoma, Washington

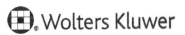 . Wolters Kluwer

Philadelphia • Baltimore • New York • London
Buenos Aires • Hong Kong • Sydney • Tokyo

Vice President, Nursing Segment: Julie K. Stegman
Director, Nursing Education and Practice Content: Jamie Blum
Senior Acquisitions Editor: Jonathan Joyce
Senior Development Editor: Julie M. Vitale
Editorial Coordinator: Vino Varadharajalu
Marketing Manager: Brittany K. Riney
Editorial Assistant: Molly Kennedy
Production Project Manager: David Saltzberg
Design Coordinator: Stephen Druding
Art Director: Jennifer Clements
Manufacturing Coordinator: Margie Orzech-Zeranko
Prepress Vendor: TNQ Technologies

Twelfth Edition

Preface

The *Study Guide to Accompany Introductory Clinical Pharmacology* is designed to help you get the greatest benefit from the twelfth edition of *Introductory Clinical Pharmacology*. Active learning strategies are used to give you the opportunity to become engaged in learning pharmacology. Used with your textbook, this guide is an important tool in helping you strengthen and build upon your reading and study habits, allowing you to clearly understand the most important ideas in each chapter. To help you learn, the following types of exercises are provided in this *Study Guide*.

ASSESSING YOUR UNDERSTANDING

This mix of *Study Guide* activities helps you become an engaged learner and gain better understanding of the information in the textbook.

- **Fill-in-the-Blanks**—Lead you to the important information in each chapter.
- **Dosage Calculations**—Strengthen your math skills and help you remember drug names, typical doses, and routes of administration.
- **Sequencing and Labeling**—Build your clinical judgment skills with logical progressions.
- **Matching Exercises**—Help you make key linkages between terms, drugs, and adverse reactions.
- **Short Answer Questions**—Help you reflect on the concepts in the book and how they are used in clinical practice situations.
- **Out in the Community Exercises**—Help you relate to drugs in the real world and give you the opportunity for

meaningful discussions with fellow learners and instructors.
- **Puzzles**—Help you recall important key terms, actions, and adverse reactions from the textbook in a fun way.

APPLYING YOUR KNOWLEDGE

Case studies feature the clients from the textbook. As their health care issues evolve in this *Study Guide*, you become engaged in the clinical situations that require clinical reasoning for positive outcomes. Use their stories to blend concepts learned in your classroom to gain the result—a stronger sense of clinical judgment skills!

Now Map It Out is an activity using concept mapping templates for each of the seven case study clients featured in the textbook and study guide are provided in the back of this guide. Your task is to map out the story of the client as you read about their individual drug use in both the textbook and study guide. As you add to your maps you will have the opportunity to discover drug–drug interactions, adverse reactions from medications, and much more. This visualizes the information you read and gives you added learning opportunities.

PRACTICING FOR NCLEX

Practice is the key to NCLEX success. Multiple-choice and multiple-response questions presented in NCLEX exam format help you analyze and apply pharmacology concepts. Rationales for answers are provided in the back of the *Study Guide*, thus solidifying the knowledge learned in the textbook.

Acknowledgment

Thanks go to everyone and anyone who has had a question about a drug and turned to me for an easy explanation, and then said, "I now understand and will take that medicine as prescribed." Any hard subject can be broken down into smaller, learnable pieces, and that is what I hope to have done in this edition of the study guide, then you too will be thanked for your expertise and understanding. Enjoy your studies, and know that this *Study Guide* is a tool that will help you better understand the sometimes complicated world of pharmacology.

—Sue

Contents

Nursing Foundation of Clinical Pharmacology

CHAPTER 1

General Principles of Pharmacology

Learning Objectives

- Define the term *pharmacology*.
- Compare and contrast the different names assigned to drugs.
- Distinguish between prescription drugs, nonprescription drugs, and controlled substances.
- Discuss drug development in the United States.
- Compare and contrast the various types of drug activity and reactions produced in the body.
- Identify factors that influence drug action.
- Explain drug tolerance, cumulative drug effect, and drug idiosyncrasy.
- Discuss the types of drug interactions that may be seen with drug administration.
- Examine the nursing implications associated with drug actions, interactions, and effects.
- Discuss the use of herbal medicines.

SECTION I: ASSESSING YOUR UNDERSTANDING

Activity A FILL IN THE BLANKS

1. Pharmacology is the study of drugs and their action on _____ _____.

2. Medications are derived from _____ _____, such as plants and minerals, or synthetically produced in a laboratory.

3. Prescription drugs are designated by the federal government as _____ _____ unless their use is supervised by a licensed health care provider.

4. _____ drugs are safe (when taken as directed) and obtainable without a prescription.

5. Controlled substances are carefully monitored and have a high potential for _____ and dependency.

Activity B LABELING

Label the different phases of drug activity in the body.

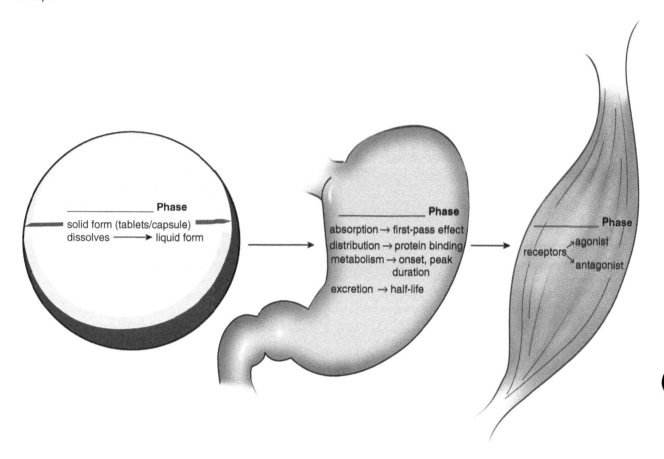

_____ Phase
solid form (tablets/capsule)
dissolves ───────→ liquid form

_____ Phase
absorption → first-pass effect
distribution → protein binding
metabolism → onset, peak
                      duration
excretion → half-life

_____ Phase
receptors ↗agonist
              ↘antagonist

Activity C MATCHING

1. Match the drug reactions given in Column A with their actions in Column B.

Column A

_____ **1.** Additive drug reaction

_____ **2.** Synergistic drug reaction

_____ **3.** Antagonistic drug reaction

Column B

a. One drug interferes with the action of another, causing neutralization or a decrease in the effect of one drug

b. Combined effect of two drugs is equal to the sum of each drug given alone

c. Drugs interact with each other and produce an effect, i.e., greater than the sum of their separate actions

2. Match the terms given in Column A with their process in Column B.

Column A

_____ **1.** Absorption

_____ **2.** Distribution

_____ **3.** Metabolism

_____ **4.** Excretion

Column B

a. Changes a drug to a more or less active form

b. Eliminates drugs from the body

c. Moves drug particles within the gastrointestinal tract

d. Dispenses drugs to various body tissues or target sites

Activity D SHORT ANSWERS

Briefly answer the following.

1. Explain the difference between drug tolerance and drug dependency in your own words.

_____

_____

_____

2. Which organization is responsible for approving new drugs? How long does it take for a drug to go from discovery to market?

_____

_____

_____

Activity E CROSSWORD PUZZLE

Across

1. An immediate hypersensitive reaction by the immune system
4. Drug with the potential for abuse and dependency
8. An undesirable reaction produced by a normal immune system

Down

2. Drug buildup when the body is unable to metabolize and excrete the drug
3. An undesirable drug effect
5. Poisonous or harmful
6. The inactive form of the original drug
7. A drug that causes abnormal development of the fetus leading to deformities
8. The time required for the body to eliminate 50% of a drug

SECTION II: APPLYING YOUR KNOWLEDGE

Activity F CASE STUDY

 You meet Mr. Park during your long-term care rotation. He tells you about growing comfrey in his garden, and he is thinking about ways to use it for digestion problems.

1. What are some of the health issues that can occur from consuming botanicals that the nurse can discuss with the client?

_____

_____

_____

2. Using Box 1.2 Teaching Points When Discussing Herbal Therapy, from the textbook, describe how to discuss the safety of herbs and natural supplements?

_____

_____

_____

SECTION III: PRACTICING FOR NCLEX

Activity G NCLEX-STYLE QUESTIONS

Answer the following questions.

1. At times it is very confusing for the client to recognize a drug by its name because there are different categories of drug names. To avoid confusion, which of the following categories of drug names should the nurse use when discussing drugs with the client?
   1. Brand name
   2. Scientific name
   3. Trade name
   4. Generic name

2. What is the purpose of the Controlled Substances Act of 1970? **Select all that apply.**
   1. Report adverse effects of drugs
   2. Regulate manufacture of drugs
   3. Organize distribution of drugs
   4. Control dispensing of drugs
   5. Encourage drug development

3. A client is seen at the urgent care center with severe dehydration. Which is the best route of fluid administration to quickly rehydrate the client?
   1. Oral route
   2. Subcutaneous route
   3. Intravenous route
   4. Intramuscular route

4. When a drug alters cellular function, which of the following symptoms might the client experience? **Select all that apply.**
   1. Decreased blood pressure
   2. Impaired vision
   3. Increased urine output
   4. Slurred speech
   5. Increased heart rate

5. Certain cancer drugs work by altering the cellular environment. If a client asks the nurse how cancer drugs work, which of the following should the nurse reply as the method of action of cancer drugs?
   1. Weaken the cell membrane
   2. Attach to the cell receptor
   3. Neutralize gastric acid
   4. Block receptor attachment

6. When assessing a client, the nurse takes note of certain factors that influence drug response. Which of the following factors will influence how a drug responds? **Select all that apply.**
   1. Client's age
   2. Existing disease
   3. Client's weight
   4. Client's appetite
   5. Client's income

7. A client is to undergo frequent serum diagnostic testing during the course of treatment at the health care facility. In which of the following conditions should the nurse expect to see frequent serum diagnostic tests?
   1. Impaired vision
   2. Impaired speech
   3. Impaired liver function
   4. Impaired hearing

8. Administration of a drug is primarily the responsibility of which health care provider?
   1. Nurse
   2. Physician
   3. Pharmacist
   4. Physician's assistant

9. The study of drugs and their action on living organisms is known as which of the following?
   1. Microbiology
   2. Pharmacology
   3. Biology
   4. Immunology

10. Which of the following agencies is responsible for the approval of new drugs in the United States?
    1. Food and Drug Administration
    2. National Formulary
    3. U.S. Pharmacopeia
    4. American Medical Association

11. Legend drugs refer to which of the following?
    1. Nonprescription drugs
    2. Nutraceuticals
    3. Prescription drugs
    4. Vitamin supplements

12. When the clinical pharmacist looks up information about a drug in the *U.S. Pharmacopeia*, the pharmacist would need to know which type of drug name?
    1. Generic name
    2. Trade name
    3. Chemical name
    4. Brand name

13. Which type of dependence is the habitual use of a drug, where negative physical withdrawal symptoms result from abrupt discontinuation?
    1. Physical dependence
    2. Psychological dependence
    3. Pleasurable dependence
    4. Abuse dependence

Administration of Drugs

Learning Objectives

- Discuss the five + 1 rights of drug administration.
- Examine general principles of drug administration.
- Identify the different types of medication orders.
- Designate general guidelines that should be followed when preparing a drug for administration.
- Describe methods used to help nurses reduce medication-related errors.
- Define the various types of medication-dispensing systems.
- Distinguish the administration of enteral and parenteral drugs.
- Discuss the administration of drugs through the skin and mucous membranes.
- Explain nursing responsibilities before, during, and after a drug is administered.

SECTION I: ASSESSING YOUR UNDERSTANDING

Activity A FILL IN THE BLANKS

1. Two drugs often associated with errors are _____ and _____.

2. The Z-track method of intramuscular injection is used when a drug is highly irritating to _____ tissues.

3. In the _____ dose system of dispensing medications, the pharmacist dispenses each dose in a package that is labeled with the drug name and dosage.

4. Nitroglycerin is commonly given by the _____ route.

5. Before giving any drug for the first time, ask the client about any known _____.

6. _____ distractions are one of the biggest issues being addressed by nurses to reduce medication errors.

Activity B SEQUENCING

Write the correct sequence of checking the drug label against the MAR during medication administration in the boxes provided.

1. Before administering the drug to the client

2. When documenting administration on the MAR

3. Immediately before removing the drug from the container

4. When the drug is taken from its storage area

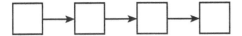

Activity C MATCHING

Match the item of accuracy in Column A with the statement made by the nurse to validate the item in Column B.

Column A

____ 1. Right client (patient)

____ 2. Right drug

____ 3. Right dose

____ 4. Right route

____ 5. Right time

____ 6. Right documentation

Column B

a. "BID can mean 8 a.m. and 6 p.m."

b. "IM injection is given on the deltoid muscle."

c. "Please tell me your name."

d. "The drug is Zyrtec, not Zyprexa."

e. "Chart the drug immediately after giving."

f. "0.25 mg, not 25 mg."

Activity D SHORT ANSWERS

The administration of a drug is a fundamental responsibility of the nurse. An understanding of the basic concepts of administering drugs is critical if the nurse is to perform this task safely and accurately. Briefly answer the following questions, which involve the nurse's role in the administration of drugs.

1. Correct identification of a client is important before a medication is given. List some different identifiers discussed in the textbook for proper client identification.

_____

_____

2. When discussing the reporting and reduction of medication errors, what does the term *Just Culture* mean?

_____

_____

Activity E **CROSSWORD PUZZLE**

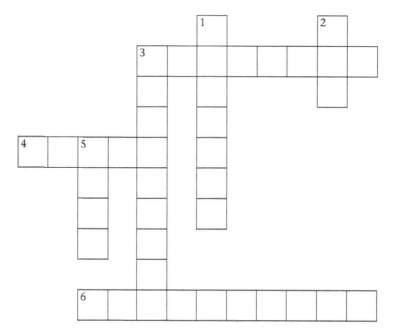

Across

3. Precaution recommendation that gloves and/or other protective gear is worn when touching any blood or body fluids, mucous membranes, or any broken skin area

4. The commission that determines yearly national client safety goals for health care institutions

6. Type of administration of a substance, such as a drug, by any route other than through the gastrointestinal system

Down

1. The medication system that is the most effective way to reduce administration errors

2. Type of order when a drug is administered as needed

3. A drug is given once, as soon as possible

5. Abbreviation for the nonprofit organization devoted to studying medication errors and prevention

SECTION II: APPLYING YOUR KNOWLEDGE

Activity F **CASE STUDY**

1. A nurse is caring for a group of clients in long-term care. When looking at the MAR, the nurse is confused by some drug names that sound similar, and a few spelled almost similarly. How can the nurse ensure that the right drug is administered to the right client?

_____

_____

_____

2. After administering a drug to a client, the nurse records the process immediately. Why is it important to document the drugs given immediately after administration?

_____

_____

_____

SECTION III: PRACTICING FOR NCLEX

Activity G NCLEX-STYLE QUESTIONS

Answer the following questions.

1. What nursing intervention should be performed to minimize risk of medication overdose when administering drugs by the transdermal route?
   1. Shave the area before applying the patch.
   2. Always apply patches on the same site.
   3. Moisten skin before applying patches.
   4. Remove the old patch before next dose.

2. A nurse is caring for a client with a superficial skin infection. What information should the nurse obtain from the primary health care provider before administering the prescribed topical drug to the client?
   1. Cause of the skin infection
   2. Instructions for drug application
   3. Reasons for selecting the drug
   4. Composition of the drug

3. While admitting a client to the long-term care facility, a nurse is required to perform the tuberculin skin test. The drug is to be administered by an intradermal injection. Which of the following sites is ideal for administering the intradermal injection to the client?
   1. Thigh
   2. Hairy areas
   3. Inner forearm
   4. Upper arm

4. A nurse has given a client an injection. A "sharps" container is not located in the room. Which of the following steps should the nurse perform in this situation?
   1. Recap the needle on the syringe.
   2. Take off the needle, and throw away the syringe.
   3. Slide the plastic guard over the needle and take it to the appropriate container.
   4. Bend the needle over and dispose in a waste container.

5. A nurse is required to administer 5 mL of a drug intramuscularly to an adult client. Which of the following is an appropriate step in preparing to administer the drug?
   1. Divide the drug and give it as two separate injections.
   2. Use a ½-inch-long needle for the injection.
   3. Administer the drug at the upper back.
   4. Insert the needle at a 45-degree angle.

6. A nurse is caring for a client with a nasogastric feeding tube. The nurse is required to administer a drug in tablet form to the client. Which of the following steps should the nurse perform during the administration of the drug? **Select all that apply.**
   1. Ensure that the tablet is completely dissolved.
   2. Put the tablets in water without crushing them.
   3. Flush the tube with water to clear the tubing.
   4. Flush the tube after the drug is given.
   5. Check the tube for placement.

7. A nurse should use how many methods to identify the client before administering the medication?
   1. 1
   2. 2
   3. 3
   4. 4

8. A primary health care provider writes an order for a client to use a Proventil HFA inhaler with the directions to inhale two puffs every 4–6 hours as need for wheezing. What type of order does this represent?
   1. STAT order
   2. Standing order
   3. PRN order
   4. Single order

9. Which of the following is an approved abbreviation? Select all that apply.
   1. U
   2. QD
   3. mL
   4. cc
   5. µg

10. Nurses need to be aware of the Joint Commission's National Patient Safety Goals (NPSG). How frequently does the Joint Commission update the NPSG?
    1. Semiannually
    2. Annually
    3. Quarterly
    4. Monthly

11. Which of the following organizations have medication safety and error reporting programs? **Select all that apply.**
    1. The Institute for Safe Medication Practices
    2. The Joint Commission
    3. The National Patient Safety Institute
    4. The Food and Drug Administration

12. Nurses are responsible for which part of the drug distribution process?
    1. Dispensing
    2. Ordering
    3. Dosing
    4. Administering

Making Drug Dosing Safer

Learning Objectives

- Explain how safety is provided by the use of systematic processes in drug administration.
- Identify information on a drug label used for calculating drug dosages.
- Describe the importance of labeling numbers during the calculation process.
- Accurately perform mathematical calculations when they are necessary to compute drug dosages.

SECTION I: ASSESSING YOUR UNDERSTANDING

Activity A FILL IN THE BLANKS

1. One in 10,000 hospital deaths occurs each year in the United States due to mistakes made specifically when _____ a drug dosage.

2. The manual redundancy system involves each person in the process of medication prescription and delivery to check the drug dosage for _____.

3. The _____ system is the preferred system of measuring medication doses.

4. The terms *basic, dimensional analysis,* and *ratio/proportion* are all names of the types of _____ used to calculate drug doses.

5. For safety purposes, _____ before decimal points (0.25) should be used as well as the abbreviation _____ for milliliters when calculating drug doses.

6. When working with solutions, _____ should be dated when opened, and unused solution in _____ discarded.

Activity B LABELING

Label the different sections of the drug package label.

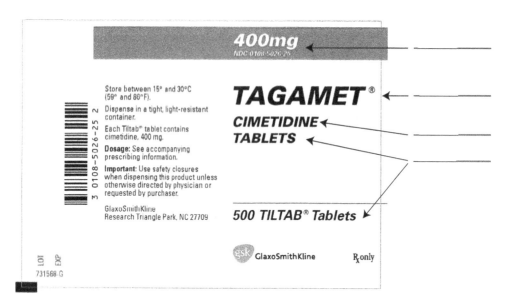

Store between 15° and 30°C
(59° and 86°F).

Dispense in a tight, light-resistant
container.

Each Tiltab® tablet contains
cimetidine, 400 mg.

Dosage: See accompanying
prescribing information.

Important: Use safety closures
when dispensing this product unless
otherwise directed by physician or
requested by purchaser.

GlaxoSmithKline
Research Triangle Park, NC 27709

400mg
NDC 0108-5026-25

TAGAMET®
CIMETIDINE
TABLETS

500 TILTAB® Tablets

gsk GlaxoSmithKline   R only

LOT EXP
731568-G

Activity C MATCHING

Match the terms in Column A with the descriptions given in Column B.

Column A

_____ **1.** Gram

_____ **2.** Liter

_____ **3.** Meter

_____ **4.** Kilogram

Column B

a. Measure of distance in the metric system

b. Measure of mass in the metric system

c. Measure of mass in the metric system, typically used to weigh clients

d. Measure of volume (liquid) in the metric system

Activity D SHORT ANSWERS

One of the nurses on your unit states the following: "Because we use the new computer system, we don't need to do the 5 rights and 3 checks anymore." Describe how you would respond to this nurse.

_____

_____

Activity E MEASUREMENT SUDOKU PUZZLE

mL				lb				mcg
	lb			F	mg	kg	C	mL
mcg		F			m	g	lb	mg
C	m	g		mcg	kg	lb		
kg				mL				g
		mL	C	g		mcg	kg	m
lb	g		F			mL		kg
m		mcg	kg	C			g	lb
F				m				C

SECTION II: APPLYING YOUR KNOWLEDGE

Activity F CASE STUDY

 Alfredo Garcia has a respiratory infection. An antibiotic is ordered, and the clinical pharmacist requests information about the client to prepare the drug. He weighs 215 lb and his temperature was 37°C.

1. The antibiotic is being prepared according to the mg/kg basis. How many kilograms does the client weigh?

   _____

   _____

2. Mrs. Garcia asks what her husband's temperature is on the Fahrenheit scale. Convert the client's temperature.

   _____

   _____

SECTION III: PRACTICING FOR NCLEX

Activity G NCLEX-STYLE QUESTIONS

1. Which of the following is the best method of error detection?
   1. Manual redundancy system
   2. Bar-coding system
   3. Computerized order entry system
   4. Manual order entry system

2. Clients may refuse a medication if they do not recognize which of the following?
   1. Brand name
   2. Nonproprietary name
   3. Generic name
   4. Chemical name

3. Which of the following measurement systems is most appropriate for drug dosing?
   1. Metric system
   2. Apothecary system
   3. Hospital measurements
   4. Household measurements

4. Which of the following represents correct placement of a zero in a decimal?
   1. 0.75
   2. 750.0
   3. 750
   4. 075

5. How many pounds are in 1 kg?
   1. 5.5 lb
   2. 1.2 lb
   3. 2.2 lb
   4. 3.4 lb

6. Arrange the following measurements from the smallest to the largest.
   1. Deciliter
   2. Milliliter
   3. Liter

7. In the metric measurement system, how many micrograms are in 1 mg?
   1. 0.1
   2. 10
   3. 100
   4. 1000

8. In the household measurement system how many teaspoons are in 1 tablespoon?
   1. 2
   2. 1
   3. 0.5
   4. 3

9. Which of the following drug forms is least likely to be a liquid?
   1. Single-use syringe
   2. Ampule
   3. Tablet
   4. Vial

10. How many milligrams are in 1 g?
    1. 100
    2. 10
    3. 1000
    4. 0.1

11. Which of the following are the steps associated with using dimensional analysis to calculate dosage problems?
    1. Express the dosage strength as a fraction with the numerator having the same unit.
    2. Write the next fraction with the numerator having the same unit of measure as the denominator.
    3. Write dosage strength with the numerator always expressed in the same unit that was identified before.
    4. Expand the equation by filling in the missing numbers using the appropriate equivalent.

12. Which of the following client characteristics are used to measure body surface area? **Select all that apply.**
    1. Age
    2. Height
    3. Race
    4. Weight

13. Which of the following are included on most drug labels? **Select all that apply.**
    1. Generic name
    2. Brand name
    3. Drug use
    4. Drug form
    5. Drug strength

14. Which of the following is characteristic of a generic name of the drug as mentioned on the label?
    1. Appears in capitalized style
    2. Written first on the label
    3. Identified by the registration symbol
    4. Written in smaller print

15. Which of the following represents a unit of weight?
    1. Liter
    2. Meter
    3. Gram
    4. Deciliter

CHAPTER 4

The Nursing Process

Learning Objectives

■ List the five phases of the nursing process.
■ Discuss assessment, analysis, nursing diagnosis, planning, implementation, and evaluation as they apply to the administration of drugs.
■ Differentiate between objective and subjective data.
■ Identify common nursing diagnoses used in the administration of drugs and nursing interventions related to each diagnosis.

SECTION I: ASSESSING YOUR UNDERSTANDING

Activity A FILL IN THE BLANKS

1. _____ data are facts obtained by means of a physical assessment or physical examination.

2. An _____ assessment is one that is made at the time of each client contact and may include the collection of objective data, subjective data, or both.

3. A nursing _____ is a description of the client's problems and their probable or actual related causes based on the subjective and objective data in the database.

4. Planning anticipates the _____ phase or the carrying out of nursing actions that are specific for the drug being administered.

5. The nursing care must be planned on an _____ basis after a careful collection and analysis of the subjective and objective data.

Activity B SEQUENCING

Using the nursing process, write the correct sequence of purchasing a new vehicle in the boxes provided.

1. Decide exactly which vehicle to buy and how to pay for the vehicle.

2. After purchase and use, decide how long to keep the vehicle before buying another one.

3. Make a chart and determine what each vehicle has to offer.

4. Purchase the vehicle.

5. Look at several different dealerships to find out more about vehicle types and brands.

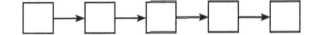

Activity C MATCHING

1. Match the phases of the nursing process in Column A with their functions in Column B.

Column A

_____ **1.** Assessment

_____ **2.** Analysis

_____ **3.** Planning

_____ **4.** Implementation

_____ **5.** Evaluation

Column B

a. Select steps for carrying out nursing activities or interventions that are specific and will meet the expected outcomes

b. Carry out a plan of action

c. Collect objective and subjective data

d. Determine the effectiveness of the nursing interventions in meeting the expected outcomes

e. Identify problems that can be solved or prevented by independent nursing actions

2. Match the nursing diagnoses in Column A with their definitions related to medication administration in Column B.

Column A

_____ **1.** Altered Health Seeking Behavior

_____ **2.** Altered Health Maintenance

_____ **3.** Knowledge deficiency

_____ **4.** Anxiety

Column B

a. Client may not take the medication correctly or follow the medication plan prescribed by the primary health care provider

b. Client is willing to incorporate the treatment plan into daily living

c. Client lacks sufficient understanding to take the drug correctly

d. Client is unable to focus on details

Activity D SHORT ANSWERS

A nurse's role in assisting clients to become well involves using the nursing process. This includes helping clients to understand and effectively manage the treatment plan. Using the nursing process requires practice, experience, and a constant updating of knowledge. Answer the following questions related to the nursing process.

1. a. What is the nursing process?

_____

_____

b. What are the five phases of the nursing process?

_____

_____

2. What is the difference between the initial and the ongoing types of assessment?

_____

_____

Activity E WORD FIND PUZZLE

Find the seven words about nursing process hidden in the puzzle.

O	N	G	O	I	N	G	A	R	L	I
K	W	P	U	F	Z	L	Q	A	E	N
X	J	A	T	G	R	Y	N	V	A	D
P	R	O	C	E	S	S	I	G	W	E
S	A	L	O	W	P	T	N	Z	D	P
Q	Y	Z	M	A	C	D	I	X	F	E
D	R	G	E	E	F	L	T	P	L	N
S	U	B	J	E	C	T	I	V	E	D
L	W	B	A	N	K	Q	A	Y	R	E
N	O	K	Y	J	Z	F	L	D	X	N
G	X	Y	R	W	A	L	P	Z	Q	T

SECTION II: APPLYING YOUR KNOWLEDGE

Activity F CASE STUDY

 Mrs. Moore will be starting three drugs for the treatment of difficulty breathing and swelling of her legs. The primary health care provider is concerned that she will not remain adherent to the medication plan. Using the information from Box 4.1 (in textbook), discuss what subjective data will give you information about Mrs. Moore's ability to adhere to the treatment plan.

_____

_____

SECTION III: PRACTICING FOR NCLEX

Activity G NCLEX-STYLE QUESTIONS

Answer the following questions.

1. A nurse is assigned to care for a client with a respiratory problem. During assessment, what question should the nurse ask to obtain subjective data from the client?
   1. Inquire about the number of cigarettes smoked per day
   2. Monitor the client's pulse rate and rhythm
   3. Monitor the client's blood pressure
   4. Assess the client's body temperature

2. What should a nurse focus on when developing expected outcomes for a client?
   1. The type of drug administered
   2. The client's ability to carry out a plan
   3. Dosage pattern administered to the client
   4. The client's ability to recuperate

3. A nurse is assigned to care for a client in a health care facility. Which of the following should the nurse include in selecting a nursing diagnosis?
   1. Problems that can be solved by independent nursing actions
   2. Problems that have a treatment marking a definite cure
   3. Identification of the client's condition and criticality
   4. Problems that cannot be prevented by nursing actions

4. A nurse is assigned to care for a client who has just been admitted to an acute care facility. What is the significance of planning for nursing actions specific to the drug to be administered? **Select all that apply.**
   1. It allows greater accuracy in drug administration.
   2. It allows absolute prevention of relapse.
   3. It allows client understanding of the drug treatment plan.
   4. It promotes an optimal response to therapy in minimum time.
   5. It promotes client adherence with prescribed drug therapy.

5. The following elements of the nursing process are given in random order. Reorder them.
   1. Analyze the data collected during assessment
   2. Formulate one or more nursing diagnoses
   3. Collect the objective and subjective data
   4. Identify the client's needs or problems
   5. Develop expected outcomes for the client

6. Select the answer that best illustrates the terminology to describe facts obtained by means of a physical assessment or physical examination.
   1. Objective data
   2. Subjective data
   3. Initial assessment
   4. Ongoing assessment

7. Facts supplied by the client or the client's family are considered which of the following?
   1. Objective data
   2. Initial assessment
   3. Subjective data
   4. Ongoing assessment

8. Which of the following is the first of the five steps in the nursing process?
   1. Analysis
   2. Implementation
   3. Assessment
   4. Planning
   5. Evaluation

9. The collection of subjective and objective data is completed during which step of the nursing process?
   1. Analysis
   2. Implementation
   3. Assessment
   4. Planning

10. Identification of problems that can be solved or prevented by the nurse without involvement of the physician is known as which of the following?
    1. Nursing diagnosis
    2. Nursing assessment
    3. Nursing documentation
    4. Nursing evaluation

11. Which of the following organizations is responsible for the continuation of defining, explaining, classifying, and researching summary statements about health problems related to nursing?
    1. The Joint Commission
    2. The National Council of State Boards of Nursing
    3. The individual states' nursing boards
    4. The North American Nursing Diagnosis Association-International (NANDA-I)

12. After the formulation of nursing diagnoses, what is the next step in the nursing process?
    1. Planning
    2. Implementation
    3. Evaluation
    4. Assessment

13. Which of the following nursing steps refers to the preparation and administration of one or more drugs to a specific client?
    1. Assessment
    2. Implementation
    3. Evaluation
    4. Analysis

CHAPTER 5

Client and Family Teaching

Learning Objectives

- Describe the steps of client teaching about drug therapy.
- Identify important aspects of the client–nurse relationship.
- Explain the three components of good health communication.
- Identify important aspects of the teaching/ learning process.
- Describe how to use information about relationship and communication with the nursing process.
- Discuss suggestions to make to the client for adapting drug administration in the home.

SECTION I: ASSESSING YOUR UNDERSTANDING

Activity A FILL IN THE BLANKS

1. The intervention of client _____ is an essential nursing task.

2. The relationship between a nurse and a client is built on _____ and _____.

3. Clients with _____ _____ literacy often try to hide their literacy issues.

4. _____ depends on the client's perception of the need to learn.

5. The _____ domain includes the client's and the caregiver's attitudes, feelings, beliefs, and opinions.

Activity B SEQUENCING

Write the correct sequence of providing educational instruction to your client in the boxes provided.

1. Present the information according to your client's learning style

2. Identify the health literacy level of your client

3. Gather up-to-date information about the drugs prescribed

4. Ask for a return demonstration or explanation

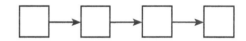

Activity C MATCHING

1. Match the learning domains in Column A with the corresponding client activities in Column B.

Column A	Column B
____ 1. Psychomotor domain	a. Decision making and drawing conclusions
____ 2. Affective domain	b. Learning physical skills
____ 3. Cognitive domain	c. Attitudes, feelings, and beliefs

2. Match the health communication concepts in Column A with their corresponding characteristics in Column B.

Column A

____ **1.** Cultural competency

____ **2.** Health literacy

____ **3.** Limited English proficiency

Column B

a. The ability to understand information about health and disease

b. 20% of the nation's population speak a language other than English at home

c. Respect of the traditions, norms, and traits of others

Activity D SHORT ANSWERS

1. *A nurse's role in determining the effectiveness of client teaching involves evaluating clients' knowledge of information presented. The nurse also helps clients answer their queries by interacting with them. Answer the following questions, which involve the nurse's role in evaluating the effectiveness of client teaching.*

a. A client has been taught exercises for strengthening eye muscles. How should the nurse ensure that the client remembers all the exercises that were taught?

_____
_____
_____

b. A client's relative has been instructed on how to measure the client's temperature using an ear thermometer. How does the nurse ensure that the client's relative has understood the procedure?

_____
_____
_____

2. *The nursing process can be used as a framework for client teaching, as well as for client care. Answer the following questions, using elements of the nursing process, learning styles, and domains of learning in the preparation for client teaching.*

a. A client admitted to an acute care facility is to be trained in the administration of antidiabetic drugs, specifically insulin, when discharged. The client is newly diagnosed with type 2 diabetes and has never taken insulin injections before.

What *nursing* diagnosis would the nurse use for this client?

_____
_____
_____

b. An asthma client is at the clinic for health teaching. You are to teach the client how to use and document readings of a peak flow meter.

What learning style are you addressing by using the equipment to teach this skill?

_____
_____
_____

c. A client with diabetes visits the clinic to join a weight loss program. The weight loss program recommends specific dietary control and regular physical exercise. However, the client states she is a dietician herself and expects her opinions to be respected as well.

What learning domain comes into the picture when the client makes this statement?

_____
_____
_____

Activity E CROSSWORD PUZZLE (*health care then and now*)

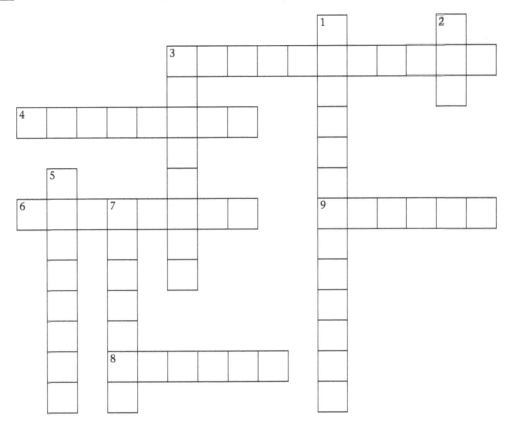

Across

3. Type of relationship in which the doctor would give the nurse an order to follow

4. Type of competency with the ability to understand, appreciate, and interact with persons different from yourself

6. The goal of clients with regard to their health

8. When clients had #3 across relationship, they viewed the doctor as this regarding their own health

9. These individuals learn when they have strong inner motivation

Down

1. As clients manage their own care, this item is an inexpensive yet effective means for tracking drug administration

2. How clients were labeled if they questioned care provided

3. What client and provider become when they work together in the decision-making process

5. Shared responsibility by the client and the providers

7. This type of health literacy leads to poor client outcomes

SECTION II: APPLYING YOUR KNOWLEDGE

Activity F CASE STUDY

 Alfredo Garcia is a Hispanic male who speaks very little English. He lives with his wife. His past medical history includes hypertension. Mr. Garcia has just been recently diagnosed with diabetes. He and his wife are seeing you for instruction on proper use of the glucometer.

1. What factors make them at risk for limited health literacy and what are ways you can assess the health literacy of Mr. and Mrs. Garcia?

_____

_____

_____

2. Mr. Garcia has been identified with both LEP and limited health literacy. What should be the focus of this teaching session?

_____

_____

_____

SECTION III: PRACTICING FOR NCLEX

Activity G NCLEX-STYLE QUESTIONS

Answer the following questions.

1. A client admitted to a rehabilitation care facility for diabetes is administered insulin injections. The client is improving and is expected to be discharged in a couple of days. The nurse assigned to the client needs to teach him how to administer his own doses of insulin. The client feels that administering insulin at home could be a bit too complicated for him. For which of the following reasons should the nurse use the Ineffective Health Management nursing diagnosis for this client? **Select all that apply.**

1. Useful in discharge teaching
2. Manages complicated medication regimen
3. Helps clients in achieving positive results
4. Informs the client about drug reactions
5. Teaches management of adverse effects of the drug

2. A 32-year-old client is admitted to an ambulatory surgical center for minor knee surgery and is prescribed a number of drugs. The nurse in charge of the client wants to teach him how to administer the prescribed drugs and has formulated a teaching plan. When and how should the teaching plan be implemented? **Select all that apply.**

1. After medication for pain
2. When the client is alert, and not sedated
3. When the client is admitted
4. Should involve a family member or friend
5. Wait and have home health nurse teach after discharge

3. A nurse caring for a client with pain needs to formulate a teaching plan to instruct the client on drug administration. Which of the following reasons are most important for a nurse to perform a client assessment before formulating a teaching plan? **Select all that apply.**

1. To determine barriers in the learning process
2. To improve client motivation
3. To improve client participation
4. To choose the best teaching methods
5. To select effective teaching tools

4. A nurse is assigned to care for a client with an infection on his toes. The nurse needs to teach the client how to bandage the wound at home. What learning domain should the nurse employ to teach the client?

1. Cognitive domain
2. Psychomotor domain
3. Affective domain
4. Intellectual domain

5. Which of the following statements indicates the client has good health literacy?

1. "They still don't know if smoking hurts you."
2. "Carbohydrates are an important dietary concept for diabetics."
3. "Pain medicine will make you an addict."
4. "Vaccines are bad."

6. A client with LEP admitted to an urgent care facility for bronchial asthma is prescribed drugs in the form of spray inhalers. The client needs to be taught how to administer the drugs. Which of the following is an example of translation?
   1. A professional interpreter is called to talk with the client.
   2. Staff member of the same nationality teaches the client.
   3. Pamphlet in the familiar language is provided.
   4. The nurse asks if a family member can speak English.

7. A group of nurses are at a conference. One member of the group pulls out a set of knitting needles and starts working on a hat. Another nurse asks, "Why do you come if you aren't going to pay attention?" The knitting nurse replies, "I learn best this way." What type of learner is the "knitting nurse"?
   1. Kinesthetic
   2. Visual
   3. Auditory
   4. Psychomotor

8. Which of the following is true of client teaching?
   1. It is an ongoing process.
   2. Nurses feel it is a tedious process.
   3. Clients view it as an unnecessary process.
   4. Client teaching is only a discharge process.

9. The hospital is developing Cambodian language materials for its ambulatory surgical center. Which group should review the materials for accuracy?
   1. Lay persons from the local Cambodian community
   2. Cambodian embassy staff members
   3. Cambodian-speaking nurses and doctors at the hospital
   4. Focus group of Cambodian clients

10. Which of the following conditions may prevent the client from learning? **Select all that apply.**
    1. Pain
    2. Tachycardia
    3. Hyperglycemia
    4. Hypotension

11. A young Hispanic client has now missed two follow-up appointments in the family planning clinic. The nurse plans to call her home. Questions asked should assess for which of the following issues?
    1. Marital relationship issues or abuse
    2. Indifference about family planning needs
    3. Chronically ill grandparents in the home
    4. Limited health literacy

12. The nurses working in long-term care received grant money to educate families about hospice care. Which educational materials would best educate the majority of adult learners?
    1. Pamphlets from the local hospice organization
    2. DVD about hospice care
    3. Cassette tapes explaining hospice care
    4. Newspaper ad about hospice services provided

13. In what way does developing a therapeutic relationship enhance client learning?
    1. Gives the client confidence in the nurse's knowledge
    2. Supports the client's ability to understand medical terms
    3. Makes the written materials easier to comprehend
    4. Helps the nurse talk the client into doing the correct treatments

Drugs Used to Fight Infections

Antibacterial Drugs: Sulfonamides

- Describe the concept of bacterial sensitivity.
- Explain the uses, general drug actions, and general adverse reactions, contraindications, precautions, and interactions for the sulfonamides.
- Distinguish important preadministration and ongoing assessment activities the nurse should perform on the client taking sulfonamides.
- List nursing diagnoses particular to a client taking sulfonamides.
- Examine ways to promote an optimal response to therapy, how to manage adverse reactions, and important points to keep in mind when educating clients about the use of sulfonamides.
- Identify the rationale for increasing fluid intake when taking sulfonamides.
- Describe the objective signs indicating that a severe skin reaction, such as Stevens–Johnson syndrome, is present.

SECTION I: ASSESSING YOUR UNDERSTANDING

Activity A FILL IN THE BLANKS

1. The sulfonamides are contraindicated in clients with hypersensitivity to the sulfonamides, during lactation, and in children younger than _____ years old.

2. The sulfonamides are primarily _____ due to their ability to inhibit (not destroy) the activity of folic acid in bacterial cell metabolism.

3. To avoid the adverse effects of _____ during sulfonamide therapy, clients should be cautioned to wear protective clothing or sunscreen when outside.

4. _____ juice is a commonly used remedy for preventing and relieving symptoms of urinary tract infections (UTIs).

5. The rare adverse reaction of _____ is manifested by easy bruising and unusual bleeding after moderate to slight trauma to the skin or mucous membranes.

Activity B DOSAGE CALCULATION

1. The primary health care provider has prescribed oral sulfadiazine, 3 g/day as maintenance dose to be divided and given in two equal doses. The drug is available in the form of a 500-mg tablet. How many tablets will the nurse administer to the client in each dose?

2. A client has been prescribed 2 g of Azulfidine per day, in four equal doses. The drug is available in a 500-mg tablet. How many tablets will the nurse administer to the client in each dose?

3. The primary health care provider has prescribed 4 g of erythromycin–sulfisoxazole per day, to be given orally four times a day in equal doses. After reconstitution, the concentration of the drug in the solution is 250 mg/5 mL. How many mg are to be given in each dose and how many mL of the solution should the nurse administer to the client for each dose?

_____

4. The primary health care provider has prescribed 1500 mg sulfasalazine per day. The drug is available in the form of 500-mg tablets. How many tablets should be administered to the client in a day?

_____

5. The primary health care provider has prescribed sulfamethoxazole–trimethoprim tablets, 2 g initially. The drug is available in 400-mg tablets. How many tablets should the nurse administer to the client in this initial dose?

_____

Activity C MATCHING

1. *Match the conditions caused by sulfonamides in Column A with their symptoms in Column B.*

Column A
_____ 1. Stomatitis
_____ 2. Anorexia
_____ 3. Crystalluria
_____ 4. Pruritus

Column B
a. Crystals in the urine
b. Itching
c. Inflammation of the mouth
d. Loss of appetite

2. *Match the conditions in Column A with their symptoms in Column B.*

Column A
_____ 1. Thrombocytopenia
_____ 2. Aplastic anemia
_____ 3. Leukopenia
_____ 4. Calculi

Column B
a. Decrease in red blood cells in the bone marrow
b. Decrease in number of white blood cells
c. Formation of stone in genitourinary tract
d. Decrease in platelet count

Activity D SHORT ANSWERS

A nurse's role in managing clients involves assisting clients in answering any queries regarding the treatment that is being provided. The nurse also helps clients by educating them about the precautions to be taken. Answer the following questions, which involve the nurse's role in management of such situations.

1. A client is being seen at the health care clinic regarding a UTI. What are the activities the nurse would perform as part of the preadministration assessment before the client is seen by the primary health care provider?

_____
_____
_____

2. The client has been examined and prescribed sulfonamide therapy. What should the nurse include in the teaching plan for the client and his family?

_____
_____
_____

Activity E CROSSWORD PUZZLE

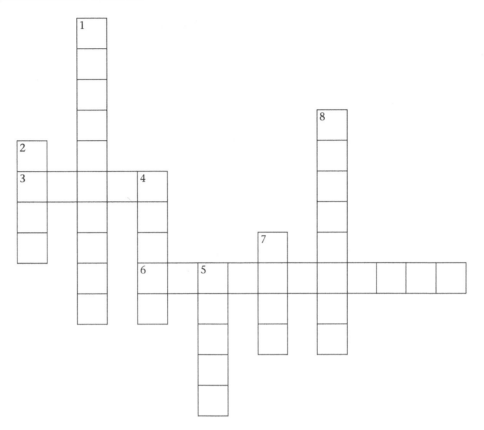

Across

3. Body fluid that may turn orange-yellow on these drugs
6. A term for constant blood level of a drug

Down

1. This may occur, limiting tasks requiring mental alertness
2. This easily happens when the skin is photosensitive
4. State of the stomach, means 1 hour before or 2 hours after meals
5. The number of 8-ounce glasses the client should drink daily when taking sulfa drugs
7. How to contact the primary health care provider if not better in 5–7 days
8. Amount of pills that should be taken when an anti-infective is prescribed

SECTION II: APPLYING YOUR KNOWLEDGE

Activity F CASE STUDY

 Mrs. Moore is an 85-year-old woman. She is diagnosed with an acute UTI. The primary health care provider would like to give Mrs. Moore a sulfonamide to treat her infection.

1. What information should the nurse obtain from Mrs. Moore before the primary health care provider sees her?

   _____

   _____

   _____

2. After the diagnosis of acute UTI, the primary health care provider prescribes Bactrim DS, one tablet every 12 hr for 14 days. What should the nurse tell Mrs. Moore about the prescription before letting her leave the primary health care provider's office?

   _____

   _____

   _____

Now Map It Out! Use the templates provided in the appendix to add information and make client connections on a concept map.

In the appendix, you will find instructions on how to use concept (or mind) mapping for this activity section. Use the template maps to complete and answer these questions found in this section of each chapter. What information do you have about Mrs. Moore from the chapter on Sulfonamides (Chapter 6)? She is 85 years old, sometimes confused, and forgetful. She had a urinalysis done and 3+ bacteria is the finding. Using the concept map template for Mrs. Moore, draw out the possible medical problems from your readings in Chapter 6 of the textbook and study guide that cause confusion. Do these connect with her current symptoms discussed here? (Hint: read the Nursing Process preassessment section of Chapter 6.)

SECTION III: PRACTICING FOR NCLEX

Activity G NCLEX-STYLE QUESTIONS

Answer the following questions.

1. A client with second-degree burns is seen at the urgent care center. Which of the following interventions should the nurse perform first as part of the client's treatment?
   1. Clean the surface of the skin.
   2. Apply a ½-inch layer of cream.
   3. Apply the drug with bare hands.
   4. Apply cream over debris on skin surface.

2. A client on sulfonamide therapy is at risk to develop thrombocytopenia. Which of the following interventions should the nurse perform to monitor the client's condition?
   1. Prevent the client from being moved until therapy is over.
   2. Instruct the client to avoid brushing teeth.
   3. Palpate the client's skin to assess for trauma.
   4. Inspect the client's skin daily.

3. A nurse is teaching a client about the measures to reduce the effects of photosensitivity. Which of the following precautions should the nurse instruct the client to follow regarding the effects of photosensitivity while on sulfadiazine therapy? **Select all that apply.**
   1. Stop using contact lenses during the treatment.
   2. Apply sunscreen to exposed areas when outdoors.
   3. Avoid lights while indoors.
   4. Wear protective clothing while outdoors.

4. Which of the following would be a serious adverse reaction that the nurse should assess for in a client during or after the application of mafenide?
   1. Orange-yellow urine
   2. Crystals in urine
   3. Facial edema
   4. Burning sensation in skin

5. A client is being discharged from the urgent care center with a prescription for sulfasalazine. As the nurse prepares to give discharge instructions, it is noted that the client wears soft contact lenses. Which of the following information should the nurse provide to the client about the use of contact lenses during the treatment?
   1. Burning sensation in eyes
   2. Headache and dizziness
   3. Permanent yellow stain in lenses
   4. Impaired vision

6. A client diagnosed with ulcerative colitis is being prescribed sulfasalazine. Which of the following interventions should the nurse perform while caring for the client? **Select all that apply.**
   1. Check the number and appearance of stool samples.
   2. Administer drug during meals or immediately afterward.
   3. Check appearance of urine and measure output.
   4. Assess for a mild loss of appetite.
   5. Monitor client for relief or intensification of the symptoms.

7. Sulfonamide therapy has been prescribed for a client with a UTI. Which of the following information should the nurse give to the client who asks about the use of cranberry juice during the treatment?
   1. Prevents bacteria from attaching to walls of the urinary tract.
   2. Prevents crystals from forming in the urine.
   3. Prevents effect of photosensitivity.
   4. Prevents formation of clots.

8. The physician has prescribed sulfonamide therapy for a client with a UTI residing at a long-term care facility. Which of the following is an advantage of sulfonamide therapy?
   1. Is easily absorbed by the GI system
   2. Kills bacteria cells to fight infection
   3. Decreases the number of white blood cells
   4. Does not have life-threatening adverse reactions

9. A client is on sulfonamide therapy. Which of the following symptoms should the nurse teach the client to be aware of that would indicate Stevens–Johnson syndrome (SJS)?
   1. Inflammation of the mouth
   2. Lesions on mucous membranes
   3. Crystals in urine
   4. Diarrhea

10. The body is equipped with a natural defense system that includes which of the following? **Select all that apply.**
    1. Saliva
    2. Tears
    3. Skin
    4. Sweat

11. Which of the following are ways in which microbes enter the body? **Select all that apply.**
    1. Break in the skin
    2. Ingestion
    3. Breathing
    4. Mucous membrane contact

12. Sulfonamides are classified as which of the following?
    1. Antibacterial
    2. Antifungal
    3. Antiviral
    4. Antiprotozoal

13. Drugs that slow or retard the multiplication of bacteria are known as which of the following?
    1. Bactericidal
    2. Bacteriostatic
    3. Bacteriostationary
    4. Bacteriophage

14. Drugs that destroy bacteria are known as which of the following?
    1. Bactericidal
    2. Bacteriostatic
    3. Bacteriostationary
    4. Bacteriophage

CHAPTER 7

Antibacterial Drugs That Disrupt the Bacterial Cell Wall

Learning Objectives

- Explain the uses, general drug actions, and general adverse reactions, contraindications, precautions, and interactions of antibacterial drugs that disrupt bacterial cell walls.
- Distinguish important preadministration and ongoing assessment activities the nurse should perform on the client taking an antibacterial drug that disrupts bacterial cell walls.
- List nursing diagnoses particular to a client taking an antibacterial drug that disrupts bacterial cell walls.
- Discuss hypersensitivity reactions as they relate to antibiotic therapy.
- Examine ways to promote optimal response to therapy, nursing actions to minimize adverse effects, and important points to keep in mind when educating clients about the use of antibacterial drugs that disrupt bacterial cell walls.

SECTION I: ASSESSING YOUR UNDERSTANDING

Activity A FILL IN THE BLANKS

1. Unlike the human cell, a bacterial cell has a _____, not a membrane.

2. The nurse should validate the administration of cephalosporins if the client has a history of allergies to cephalosporins or _____ with the primary health care provider.

3. Chronic use of cephalosporins may result in damage to the _____.

4. Penicillins and cephalosporins have a _____ _____, which breaks the bacterial cell wall and the bacterial cell dies.

5. An example of bacterial resistance is the ability of certain bacteria to produce _____, an enzyme that inactivates penicillin.

Activity B DOSAGE CALCULATION

1. A client has been prescribed 1 g of penicillin V. Available are penicillin V 500-mg tablets. How many tablets will the nurse administer to the client?

   _____

   _____

2. A client has been prescribed 500 mg of oxacillin intramuscularly. After reconstitution, the vial contains 250 mg of active drug per 1.5 mL of solution. How much of the reconstituted solution will be administered to the client?

   _____

   _____

3. A primary health care provider prescribes 250 mg nafcillin every 4 hours for a client. After reconstitution, the concentration of the drug is 500 mg/2 mL. How many mL of the reconstituted solution should be administered to the client in each dose?

_____

_____

4. A client undergoing hemodialysis has been prescribed a single 400-mg dose of cefpodoxime orally two times weekly. Cefpodoxime is available in a 400-mg capsule. How many tablets will the nurse administer to the client?

_____

_____

5. A client has been prescribed 500 mg of cefaclor every 12 hours for an infection due to a susceptible microorganism. The available drug is in the form of a 250-mg capsule. How many capsules should the nurse administer to the client each time?

_____

_____

6. A client with a bacterial infection is prescribed 2000 mg of aztreonam to be taken intravenously. The drug is available in the form of 1 g/50 mL. How much of the drug solution should the nurse prepare for IV administration in the client?

_____

_____

Activity C OUT IN THE COMMUNITY

Question 1. *Ways to reduce antibacterial resistance to drugs include taking all the medication, disposing of unused drugs, and never taking another person's prescribed drugs. For different reasons, we may find that we have a number of unused, expired drugs in our medicine storage. To be good client educators, we need to practice what we tell our clients to do. In this activity, you will look to see if you store unused and expired drugs in your own home.*

Class question: *Over time drugs lose their effectiveness. Is it a good idea to keep medications past their expiration dates? If we choose to get rid of them, how do we do it safely?*

Activity

1. Go to your medicine cupboard and check both your prescription and over-the-counter drugs for expired medications. Write down the number and type of drugs you find.

2. Contact the pharmacy that you typically use to get your medications; ask the pharmacist what they instruct consumers to do with their unused medications. Write that down now.

3. Now clean out your extra medications and safely dispose of the medications, too!

Report the following in your class discussion:

1. What types of medications do we keep that are outdated?

2. What did your pharmacist instruct you to do?

Activity D SHORT ANSWERS

A nurse's role in managing clients who are being administered penicillin and cephalosporins involves monitoring them and implementing interventions that aid in their recovery. Answer the following questions, which involve the nurse's role in management of such situations.

1. A client with pneumonia has been prescribed penicillin. What should a nurse assess for in the client before administering the first dose of penicillin?

_____

_____

_____

2. An elderly client has been prescribed cephalosporin. What nursing interventions are important when the client is to be administered cephalosporin IV?

_____

_____

_____

Activity E **CROSSWORD PUZZLE**

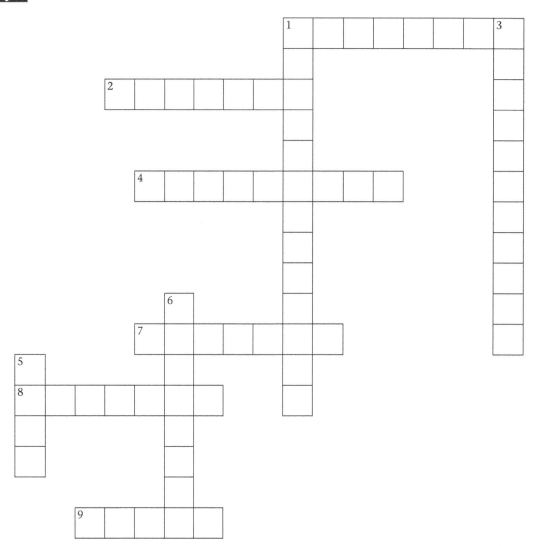

Across

1. A disease-producing microorganism
2. Brand name for a second-generation cephalosporin
4. Term meaning inflammation of the tongue
7. First class of penicillin used to combat infections
8. Brand name for a third-generation cephalosporin
9. Brand name for a first-generation cephalosporin

Down

1. The enzyme produced by bacteria against penicillin
3. Harmful and damaging to the kidneys
5. Abbreviation for the bacteria resistant to methicillin
6. Brand name for a fourth-generation cephalosporin

SECTION II: APPLYING YOUR KNOWLEDGE

Activity F CASE STUDY

 Janna Wong is a 16-year-old girl. She presents to the ambulatory clinic today with bilateral ear pain, nasal congestion, cough, and a low-grade fever. Her mother reports she is not taking any medications and has no drug allergies that she is aware of at this point. The primary health care provider writes a prescription for amoxicillin 250 mg/5 mL, 500 mg BID for 10 days.

1. Janna's mother is concerned that Janna may have an allergic reaction to the amoxicillin because she is allergic to bees. What signs or symptoms should the nurse tell Janna's mother to look for that may indicate an allergic reaction has occurred?

_____

2. What should the nurse tell Janna's mother about oral suspensions?

_____

Now Map It Out! Use the templates provided in the appendix to add information and make client connections on a concept map.

You will find that the case study clients from the textbook and the study guide may be the same for a given unit. Sometimes the study guide example will be a different client—such is the case in this chapter. Now you are working with two clients! Using the concept map template for Janna Wong, map out the possible infection you learned above. Draw out the possible medical problem, and maybe a client education need, based upon the 10 Commandments of Antibiotic Use from the textbook.

SECTION III: PRACTICING FOR NCLEX

Activity G NCLEX-STYLE QUESTIONS

Answer the following questions.

1. The nurse has administered cephalosporin intravenously to an older adult client. What specific condition should the nurse monitor for when this drug is given intravenously?
   1. Phlebitis
   2. Angina
   3. Fever
   4. Tenderness

2. The laboratory test report of a client on ampicillin therapy show a deficient production of RBCs. Which of the following adverse effects has the client developed?
   1. Nephrotoxicity
   2. Anorexia
   3. Anemia
   4. Toxic epidermal necrolysis

3. A nurse is caring for a client who is receiving penicillin. Which of the following assessments will a nurse perform as part of the ongoing assessment process? **Select all that apply.**
   1. Obtain client's general health history.
   2. Save sample of stool for tests.
   3. Evaluate client daily for response to therapy.
   4. Document improvement on client's chart.
   5. Perform additional culture and sensitivity tests.

4. A client who is receiving a carbapenem complains of diarrhea. Arrange the interventions a nurse will perform in the most likely sequence.
   1. If the stool tests positive for blood, save the sample.
   2. Notify primary health care provider if diarrhea is confirmed.
   3. Inspect all stools for signs of diarrhea.
   4. Save a sample of the stool to test for occult blood.

5. A nurse has just administered penicillin intramuscularly to a client as prescribed. The nurse suspects that the client is developing signs of anaphylactic shock. If the nurse is correct, which of the following symptoms would the nurse expect to see in this client? **Select all that apply.**
   1. Severe hypotension
   2. Nausea and vomiting
   3. Loss of consciousness
   4. Acute respiratory distress
   5. Pain at injection site

6. Which of the following interventions should a nurse perform in the event of increased fever in a client after being administered penicillin? **Select all that apply.**
   1. Discontinue administering the drug immediately.
   2. Take vital signs every 4 hours or more.
   3. Report the rise in temperature to the primary health care provider.
   4. Change the client's diet to a soft, nonirritating diet.
   5. Administer antipyretic drug as per primary health provider's instructions.

7. Which of the following is true of fourth-generation cephalosporins? **Select all that apply.**
   1. A broader spectrum of action
   2. A longer duration of resistance to beta (β)-lactamase
   3. A narrower spectrum of action
   4. The ability to treat viral infections

8. Natural penicillins exert what types of effects on microorganisms?
   1. Bactericidal
   2. Bacteriostatic
   3. Fungicidal
   4. Fungistatic

9. Penicillinase causes bacterial resistance by which of the following mechanisms?
   1. Enzymatic inactivation of the penicillin
   2. Destruction of the β-lactam ring of the penicillin
   3. Destruction of the penicillin cell wall
   4. Rupture of the penicillin membrane

10. Which of the following are ways that penicillins can be modified to broaden their spectrum of action? **Select all that apply.**
    1. Addition of a chemical compound to inhibit β-lactamase inhibitors
    2. Chemical modification of the penicillins to increase GI absorption
    3. Chemical modification to slow excretion of penicillins from the kidneys
    4. Chemical modification of the penicillin to increase tissue penetration

11. A nurse is caring for a client with a gram-negative bacterial infection. The client has to be administered aztreonam. As the nurse checks the client's medical history, which of the following items should the nurse report to the primary health care provider before giving the medication?
    1. History of GI distress with medications
    2. Hearing problems
    3. Ongoing fever
    4. Penicillin allergy

12. A nurse is caring for a client with a bacterial infection. The nurse has to administer vancomycin to the client through the parenteral route. The nurse ensures that every dose of vancomycin is administered over 60 min. The nurse should remain alert for which of the following conditions when caring for this client?
    1. Shock
    2. Severe hypertension
    3. Sudden increase in blood pressure
    4. Ringing in the ears

Antibacterial Drugs That Interfere With Protein Synthesis

Learning Objectives

- Explain the uses, general drug actions, adverse reactions, contraindications, precautions, and interactions of antibacterial drugs that interfere with protein synthesis.
- Distinguish important preadministration and ongoing assessment activities the nurse should perform on the client taking an antibacterial drug that interferes with protein synthesis.
- List nursing diagnoses particular to a client taking an antibacterial drug that interferes with protein synthesis.
- Examine ways to promote an optimal response to therapy, how to manage adverse reactions, and important points to keep in mind when educating clients about the use of antibacterial drugs that interfere with protein synthesis.

SECTION I: ASSESSING YOUR UNDERSTANDING

Activity A FILL IN THE BLANKS

1. Tetracyclines are primarily _____.

2. Aminoglycosides, macrolides, and lincosamides are primarily _____.

3. These drugs are used to treat a wide range of both gram-_____ and gram-_____ microorganisms.

4. Foods or drugs containing calcium, magnesium, aluminum, or iron prevent the absorption of the _____ if ingested concurrently.

5. _____ is a very serious adverse reaction affecting hearing that may occur when aminoglycosides are taken.

6. Neomycin and paromomycin are used orally in the management of _____ coma.

Activity B DOSAGE CALCULATION

1. A primary health care provider has prescribed 600 mg of demeclocycline per day for an adult client. The primary health care provider has ordered four separate doses of 150 mg each. Demeclocycline 150-mg tablets are available. How many tablets should the nurse administer per dose?

_____

_____

2. Doxycycline is prescribed by the primary health care provider for a 7-year-old client who weighs 75 lb. The medication is ordered in mg/kg. How much does the child weigh in kilograms?

_____

_____

3. For the child in the previous question, doxycycline is available in an oral solution of 17 mg/mL. How many mL of solution should the nurse administer if the child is prescribed 2 mg/kg?

_____

_____

4. A client has been prescribed 500 mg of clarithromycin, twice a day. Each tablet of clarithromycin contains 250 mg. How many tablets should the nurse administer to the client in each dose?

_____

_____

5. The primary health care provider has prescribed 300 mg of erythromycin to be given every 12 hours for a client. How many tablets should the nurse administer every 12 hours if they are available in tablets of 150 mg?

_____

_____

6. The primary health care provider has prescribed 600 mg of lincomycin for a client, which is to be administered intramuscularly every 24 hours. Lincocin for injection is available in lincomycin 300 mg/mL. How many mL should the nurse give to the client?

_____

_____

Activity C MATCHING

1. Match the drugs in Column A with their interaction with macrolides in Column B.

Column A

____ **1.** Antacids

____ **2.** Digoxin

____ **3.** Anticoagulants

____ **4.** Lincomycin

Column B

a. Increased serum levels

b. Decreased therapeutic activity of macrolide

c. Decreased absorption and effectiveness of macrolide

d. Increased risk of bleeding

2. Match the toxic reactions given in Column A with their signs and symptoms in Column B.

Column A

____ **1.** Nephrotoxicity

____ **2.** Ototoxicity

____ **3.** Neurotoxicity

Column B

a. Numbness, skin tingling, circumoral paresthesia

b. Proteinuria, hematuria, increase in BUN level

c. Tinnitus, dizziness, roaring in the ears

Activity D SHORT ANSWERS

A nurse's role in managing clients involves assisting the clients in answering inquiries regarding the treatment being provided. The nurse also helps clients by educating them about precautions to take. Answer the following questions, which involve the nurse's role in management of such situations.

1. A client with an upper respiratory infection caused by *Haemophilus influenzae* is prescribed azithromycin. What is the role of the nurse in monitoring and managing the client's needs?

_____

_____

2. A client is to be discharged from the urgent care facility. They has been prescribed demeclocycline for 10 days. What should the nurse include in the teaching plan to educate the client regarding the medication?

_____

_____

Activity E WORD FIND PUZZLE

Find the five nursing diagnoses hidden in the puzzle.

C	Z	L	I	B	A	X	Q	K	R
C	O	N	F	U	S	I	O	N	P
R	U	M	V	F	P	B	L	O	F
L	Q	B	F	J	K	D	E	I	V
Y	D	E	L	O	X	T	L	S	B
J	I	N	J	U	R	Y	D	U	Q
P	A	Y	K	T	A	T	F	F	I
X	R	U	M	Y	L	N	M	R	P
F	R	A	B	E	V	J	Z	E	L
M	H	D	P	Q	U	N	B	P	T
K	E	V	X	Z	N	R	N	K	U
B	A	R	D	I	E	T	A	J	M

SECTION II: APPLYING YOUR KNOWLEDGE

Activity F CASE STUDY

 Lillian Chase is a 36-year-old woman. She presents to the primary health care provider's office today seeking treatment for her acne. As you review medications in her health record, you see she is taking Ortho Tri-Cyclen Lo, a pill for birth control. The primary health care provider writes Ms. Chase a prescription for doxycycline 150 mg once daily.

1. What should the nurse tell Ms. Chase about taking oral contraception with doxycycline?

_____

_____

2. What adverse reactions should the nurse discuss with Ms. Chase?

_____

_____

Now Map It Out! Use the templates provided in the appendix to add information and make client connections on a concept map.

Here is where your nursing care becomes more complex—you have two clients to map: one from the textbook and a different client here in the study guide. Using the concept map template for Lillian Chase, map out the situation above. Draw out the possible medical problem and teaching needs of the client. See the prescribed medication above; are you alerted to a drug–drug interaction that you need to discuss with Lillian? Now look at your map for Mrs. Moore that you created for Chapter 6. Do you have to make changes based upon the new information in Chapter 8?

SECTION III: PRACTICING FOR NCLEX

Activity G NCLEX-STYLE QUESTIONS

Answer the following questions.

1. Lincosamides are contraindicated for which of the following clients?
    1. Clients with viral infections
    2. Clients younger than 13 years
    3. Clients who are lactating
    4. Clients with cardiac disease

2. A client being treated with lincosamides is to undergo an operation under general anesthesia. If a neuromuscular blocking drug is to be administered for anesthesia, what is the possible complication?
    1. Increased risk for bleeding
    2. Severe and profound respiratory depression
    3. Decreased absorption of the lincosamide
    4. Increased risk for digitalis toxicity

3. A nurse is assigned to take care of a client with an arm infection. The nurse will identify and document signs and symptoms of the infection. Which of the following items may be part of the infection documentation? **Select all that apply.**
    1. General malaise
    2. Diabetes
    3. Blood dyscrasias
    4. Chills and fever
    5. Redness

4. A client with high fever has been prescribed doxycycline. Which of the following tests should be performed before the first dose of drug is given? **Select all that apply.**
   1. Stress test
   2. Culture and sensitivity test
   3. Glucose tolerance test
   4. Renal function test
   5. Urinalysis

5. A nurse is caring for a 6-year-old client who has been prescribed an antibacterial drug. The client's father inquires about the risks of tooth discoloration. When the nurse checks the MAR, which of these drugs are they looking for that would cause this adverse reaction?
   1. Aminoglycosides
   2. Cephalosporins
   3. Macrolides
   4. Tetracyclines

6. A client in a long-term care facility is being seen for diarrhea. The primary health care provider suspects a GI superinfection. What nursing intervention should follow this observation?
   1. Save urine sample for tests.
   2. Measure and record vital signs.
   3. Check client's blood pressure.
   4. Save stool sample for *Clostridium difficile* test.

7. A primary health care provider has prescribed lincomycin to a client. What is the best way for the nurse to describe how the drug is to be administered?
   1. Administer the drug on an empty stomach.
   2. Administer 1–2 hours before and after food.
   3. Administer the drug 4 hours after food in between meals.
   4. Administer the drug with fruit juice.

8. If a client taking aminoglycosides presents with hematuria, proteinuria, and an elevated BUN, these are all indications of which of the following adverse reactions?
   1. Ototoxicity
   2. Nephrotoxicity
   3. Neuromuscular blockage
   4. Cardiotoxicity

9. A nurse is caring for a severely ill client with a gram-negative bacterial infection who has been prescribed aminoglycosides. Which of the following tasks should the nurse perform as part of the preadministration assessment for the client? **Select all that apply.**
   1. Swab-infected site for client's culture and sensitivity.
   2. Monitor vital signs every 4 hours.
   3. Document findings in client's chart.
   4. Obtain specimen for urinalysis.
   5. Ensure that blood is drawn for hepatic/renal function tests.

10. A nurse is caring for a client who is being administered aminoglycosides. Which of the following vital sign assessments is the *best* indicator of the adverse reaction of neuromuscular blockade?
    1. Temperature
    2. Pulse
    3. Respiration rate
    4. Blood pressure

Antibacterial Drugs That Interfere With DNA/RNA Synthesis

- Explain the uses, general drug actions, contraindications, precautions, interactions, and adverse reactions of antibacterial drugs that interfere with DNA/RNA synthesis.
- Distinguish preadministration and ongoing assessment activities the nurse should perform on the client taking an antibacterial drug that interferes with DNA/RNA synthesis.
- List nursing diagnoses particular to a client receiving an antibacterial drug that interferes with DNA/RNA synthesis.
- Examine ways to promote an optimal response to therapy, how to manage adverse reactions, and important points to keep in mind when educating clients about the use of antibacterial drugs that interfere with DNA/RNA synthesis.

SECTION I: ASSESSING YOUR UNDERSTANDING

Activity A FILL IN THE BLANKS

1. _____ are the primary class of bactericidal drugs affecting the bacterial cell by interfering with the synthesis of DNA.

2. When given _____, the client should be monitored frequently because the medications can be irritating to the tissue.

3. _____ is a miscellaneous drug used to treat anaerobic bacterial infections.

4. When taking any antibacterial, overgrowth of other bacteria or elimination of normal flora can result in _____.

5. When taking fluoroquinolones, _____ _____, especially in those older than 60 years, is a serious adverse reaction.

Activity B DOSAGE CALCULATION

1. A client is prescribed 500 mg of rifaximin every 12 hours. The drug is available in the form of 500-mg tablets. How many tablets should the nurse administer per dose?

   _____

   _____

2. A client with a bacterial infection is prescribed ciprofloxacin to be administered intravenously. The prescribed dosage for ciprofloxacin is 500 mg/kg. The client weighs 65 kg. The ciprofloxacin is available in a concentrated form of 100 mg/mL. How much of the drug solution should have been prepared for the nurse to administer?

   _____

   _____

3. A client with bronchitis is prescribed 400 mg of moxifloxacin every 12 hours. The drug is available in the form of 400-mg tablets. The nurse instructs the client to take how many tablets every 12 hours?

_____

_____

4. A client with pneumonia is prescribed 300 mg of levofloxacin IV daily. The drug is available in a concentrated solution form of 25 mg/mL. How many mL of the solution will be mixed into the IV secondary set for infusion?

_____

_____

Activity C MATCHING

1. Match the drugs that interact adversely with fluoroquinolones in Column A with their common uses in Column B.

Column A

____ **1.** Theophylline

____ **2.** Cimetidine

____ **3.** Oral anticoagulants

____ **4.** Nonsteroidal anti-inflammatory drugs (NSAIDs)

Column B

a. Blood thinners

b. Relief of pain and inflammation

c. Management of respiratory problems

d. Management of GI upset

2. Match the adverse reactions given in Column A with their definitions in Column B.

Column A

____ **1.** Candidiasis

____ **2.** Tendonitis

____ **3.** Pseudomembra-nous colitis

____ **4.** Photosensitivity

Column B

a. Organism frequently the cause of fungal infections

b. Exaggerated skin rash when exposed to sun

c. Inflammation of the connective tissues attaching muscles and bones

d. Infection caused by the bacteria _Clostridium difficile_

Activity D SHORT ANSWERS

A nurse's role in managing clients who are administered IV fluoroquinolones involves monitoring and managing interventions that aid in their recovery. A client in acute pain due to tissue injury is prescribed intravenous fluoroquinolones.

1. What assessment should the nurse perform when caring for the client who is administered IV fluoroquinolones?

_____

_____

2. A nurse has analyzed assessment data and selected the following nursing diagnoses for this client:

■ **Acute pain** related to tissue injury during drug therapy
■ **Anxiety** related to fever and hospitalization
■ **Deficient knowledge** related to drug routine complexity

How will the nurse evaluate the effectiveness of the treatment plan?

_____

_____

_____

Activity E CHART THE FINDING

Continue to chart the following temperature findings for a client with a bacterial infection:

1. *The bacteria are not sensitive to the antibacterial drug ordered.*

2. *The bacteria are sensitive to the antibacterial drug ordered.*

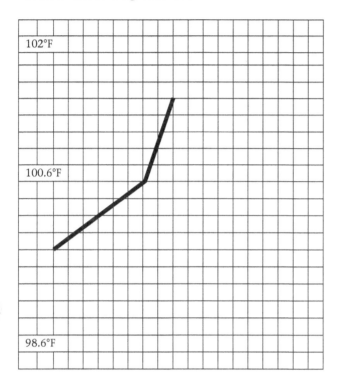

SECTION II: APPLYING YOUR KNOWLEDGE

Activity F CASE STUDY

 Betty Peterson is a 54-year-old woman. She is hospitalized for kidney stone pain. The primary health care provider orders ciprofloxacin (Cipro) 400 mg every 12 hours IV for 2 days and then Cipro 500 mg by mouth every 12 hours for 12 more days.

1. What preadministration assessments should be completed prior to starting Mrs. Peterson on Cipro?

_____

_____

2. Cipro is available in a solution of 10 mg/mL. How many mL of solution in the syringe pump will the clinical pharmacist have prepared for the nurse to administer one 400-mg dose?

_____

_____

Now Map It Out! Use the templates provided in the appendix to add information and make client connections on a concept map.

You have two new clients to map in Chapter 9 from the textbook and here in the study guide. Using the concept mapping template for Betty Peterson, map out this new situation above. Draw out the possible medical problem and teaching needs of the client. Then make another concept map with Mr. Park in the long-term care facility.

SECTION III: PRACTICING FOR NCLEX

Activity G NCLEX-STYLE QUESTIONS

Answer the following questions.

1. A nurse is assigned to care for a client who has developed a serious bacterial infection. The client has been prescribed ciprofloxacin to be administered orally. Which of the following body systems will most likely experience an adverse reaction from the administration of ciprofloxacin?

    1. Respiratory
    2. Genitourinary
    3. Gastrointestinal
    4. Cardiovascular

2. A nurse has been caring for a client who was treated for bacterial infection. The client is now scheduled to receive treatment on an outpatient basis. Which of the following instructions should the nurse offer to the client and client's family under continuing care?

    1. Complete full course of treatment.
    2. Always take the drug with food.
    3. Avoid drinking any alcoholic beverages.
    4. Monitor for adverse symptoms for 3 days.

3. A nurse is caring for a 35-year-old client with pneumonia. The primary health care provider has prescribed ciprofloxacin in a single 800-mg dose to be given intravenously to the client. The available dosage of this drug is 2 g/5 mL. How much of the drug should the nurse give in the injection?
   1. 2 mL
   2. 1 mL
   3. 15 mL
   4. 4 mL

4. The nurse is preparing client teaching materials regarding sun exposure while taking anti-infective drugs. Photosensitivity is most severe with which of the following drugs?
   1. Ciprofloxacin
   2. Ofloxacin
   3. Levofloxacin
   4. Gemifloxacin

5. For clients who may not be proficient in the English language, drug names can be confusing. A pill that is formulated to release the drug over time may be referred to by different names. Which of the following would you tell the client is the name of this type of medication? **Select all that apply.**
   1. Controlled release
   2. Extended release
   3. Immediate release
   4. Sustained release

6. A client with a urinary tract infection is administered ofloxacin. At a follow-up clinic visit, the nurse is required to conduct an ongoing assessment of the client. What are the assessment tasks the nurse has to perform that would indicate the client continues to have a UTI? **Select all that apply.**
   1. Monitor for decrease in pulse and respiratory rate.
   2. Monitor vital signs of the client.
   3. Observe for increase in temperature in the client.
   4. Ask client about urinary frequency.
   5. Document initial signs of any infection in the client.

7. Pseudomembranous colitis is a serious infection. Which of the following organisms is primarily responsible for this condition?
   1. *Helicobacter pylori*
   2. Group A beta-hemolytic (β-hemolytic) streptococci
   3. *Staphylococcus aureus*
   4. *Clostridium difficile*

8. A nurse is assigned to care for a client who has to be administered an anti-infective drug intramuscularly. Which of the following nursing interventions should the nurse perform when caring for this client receiving an intramuscular anti-infective drug? **Select all that apply.**
   1. Check the infusion site every 2 hours.
   2. Rotate the injection sites.
   3. Inspect previous injection sites.
   4. Assess for vein irritation.
   5. Administer no more than 3 mL per dose.

9. A nurse is required to care for a client who is to be administered a fluoroquinolone. The nurse knows that under which of the following conditions should fluoroquinolone be administered cautiously?
   1. Client with a history of seizures
   2. Client with renal failure
   3. Client with neuromuscular disorders
   4. Client who is elderly

10. When caring for a client who is receiving an antibacterial drug, a nurse is required to monitor for symptoms of a bacterial superinfection of the bowel. Which of the following symptoms should a nurse monitor for in the client? **Select all that apply.**
   1. Diarrhea/bloody diarrhea
   2. Vomiting
   3. Abdominal cramping
   4. Lesions
   5. Rectal bleeding

11. A nurse is caring for a client who is receiving fluoroquinolones through the intravenous route. Which of the following nursing interventions should the nurse perform to reduce the occurrence of phlebitis or thrombophlebitis?

  1. Check the rate of infusion every 2 hours.
  2. Inspect the vein used for infusion frequently.
  3. Alternate the vein used for infusion.
  4. Raise the arm above the heart during infusions.

12. A nurse is caring for a client with a sexually transmitted infection. The client is to be administered a fluoroquinolone. Which of the following should the nurse ensure to confirm that fluoroquinolone is not contraindicated in the client?

  1. Client is not younger than 18 years.
  2. Client does not have preexisting hearing loss.
  3. Client does not have myasthenia gravis.
  4. Client does not have Parkinson disease.

13. A nurse is caring for a client who is being administered fluoroquinolones. Which of the following instructions should the nurse offer to assist the client to protect herself against photosensitive reactions? **Select all that apply.**

  1. Wear brimmed hats.
  2. Wear long-sleeve clothing.
  3. Venture out preferably on hazy days.
  4. Wear sunscreen.
  5. Wear very light makeup.

CHAPTER

10

Antitubercular Drugs

Learning Objectives

- Discuss the drugs used in the treatment of mycobacteria for tuberculosis (TB).
- Explain the uses, general drug actions, contraindications, precautions, interactions, and general adverse reactions associated with the administration of the antitubercular drugs.
- Distinguish important preadministration and ongoing assessment activities the nurse should perform on the client taking an antitubercular drug.
- List nursing diagnoses particular to a client taking an antitubercular drug.
- Describe directly observed therapy (DOT).
- Examine ways to promote an optimal response to therapy, how to manage adverse reactions, and important points to keep in mind when educating clients about the use of the antitubercular drugs.

SECTION I: ASSESSING YOUR UNDERSTANDING

Activity A FILL IN THE BLANKS

1. Neurotoxicity and hepatitis may be seen with the administration of _____.

2. People with human _____ virus are at risk for tuberculosis (TB) because of their compromised immune systems.

3. _____ tuberculosis is the term used to distinguish TB affecting other body organs from infection with the *Mycobacterium tuberculosis* bacillus and the infection that remains in the lungs.

4. When isoniazid (INH) is taken with foods containing _____, an exaggerated sympathetic nerve-type response can occur.

5. The initial phase of standard protocol TB treatment is for the administration of rifampin, isoniazid, pyrazinamide, and ethambutol for a minimum of _____ months.

Activity B DOSAGE CALCULATION

1. A client has been prescribed 150 mg of isoniazid per day. Each tablet of isoniazid contains 100 mg of the drug. How many tablets will need to be administered to the client in each dose?

_____

_____

2. A physician prescribes 600 mg of rifampin per day for a client. Rifampin is available as 300-mg tablets. How many tablets will need to be administered to the client per day?

_____

_____

3. The dose for pyrazinamide is 25 mg/kg/day. If the client weighs 80 kg, how many tablets will be dispensed as part of the DOT, if the tablets are 500 mg each?

_____

_____

Activity C MATCHING

1. Match the drugs in Column A with the effects of their interaction with isoniazid in Column B.

Column A	Column B
____ **1.** Antacid	**a.** Increases serum level of second drug
____ **2.** Anticoagulant	**b.** Greater hepatitis risk
____ **3.** Phenytoin	**c.** Increases risk for bleeding
____ **4.** Alcohol	**d.** Reduces absorption of isoniazid

Activity D SHORT ANSWERS

A nurse's role in managing clients who are diagnosed with TB and administered antitubercular drugs involves instructing the clients about adverse reactions and precautions to be taken during recovery. Answer the following questions regarding the nurse's role in the management of such situations.

1. The nurse is caring for a 24-year-old client with TB. What assessments should the nurse perform as part of the preadministration interview when providing care for this client?

   _____

   _____

2. The client is discharged from an acute care facility and will now be followed on an outpatient basis. What instructions should the nurse offer the client and client's family to decrease the chances of nonadherence?

   _____

   _____

3. A nurse has analyzed assessment data and selected the following nursing diagnoses for this client:

   ■ **Risk of injury** related to extremity numbness due to neurotoxicity
   ■ **Malnutrition less than body requirements** related to gastric upset and general poor health status
   ■ **Altered Health Maintenance** related to indifference, lack of knowledge, long-term treatment regimen, and other factors

How will the nurse evaluate the effectiveness of the treatment plan?

_____

_____

Activity E WORD FIND PUZZLE

Find the six words about prophylactic use of INH in latent TB hidden in the puzzle.

Q	U	I	E	S	C	E	N	T
C	B	X	A	T	V	R	D	Z
H	Y	D	C	D	I	O	A	P
R	O	P	K	B	Y	Z	J	X
O	T	U	J	R	C	H	Y	R
N	P	O	S	I	T	I	V	E
I	D	V	Z	E	D	V	G	C
C	R	I	X	O	H	A	B	T
Z	J	K	A	N	Y	O	N	E
D	A	B	C	Y	P	J	L	K
K	V	O	R	D	I	X	A	D

Word Hints

_____ members and other close associates of the client diagnosed with active TB

_____, a term meaning it causes no symptoms

Those whose tuberculin skin test has become _____ in the last 2 years

_____ positive, or clients with AIDS with a significant skin test reaction

_____ younger than 35 with a positive skin test

Those with a _____ illness at risk for developing the disease

SECTION II: APPLYING YOUR KNOWLEDGE

Activity F CASE STUDY

Kosal Chey, 55 years of age, lives in a large apartment complex. After conversation with his neighbor, Betty Peterson, he presented to the neighborhood free clinic 2 days ago with a 2-week history of coughing, sputum production, and night sweats. The nurse administered a TST skin test to Mr. Chey. He returns today for the nurse to read the test, which is positive. The primary health care provider decides to treat Mr. Chey for active TB.

1. What other assessments were made that determined Mr. Chey should be treated for active TB rather than latent TB?

   _____

   _____

2. What ongoing assessment should the nurse make while Mr. Chey is taking the antitubercular drugs?

   _____

   _____

Now Map It Out! Use the templates provided in the appendix to add information and make client connections on a concept map.

You have read about Betty Peterson's concerns and learned about the disease process and treatment of TB in Chapter 10 of the textbook. Using the information in the case study above, map out this relationship and determine if this situation regarding Betty Peterson warrants a follow-up by the clinic providers?

SECTION III: PRACTICING FOR NCLEX

Activity G NCLEX-STYLE QUESTIONS

Answer the following questions.

1. A nurse is caring for a client who has been taking rifampin. Which of the following adverse reactions should the nurse monitor for in the client?
   1. Myalgia
   2. Jaundice
   3. Reddish-orange color of bodily fluids
   4. Dermatitis and pruritus

2. A nurse is caring for a client recently diagnosed with active TB; the drug ethambutol is to be administered. As the nurse reviews the client history, which of the following conditions would contraindicate the use of ethambutol in this client? **Select all that apply.**
   1. Client is younger than 13 years.
   2. Client has cataract.
   3. Client has a hypersensitivity to the drug.
   4. Client has diabetes mellitus.
   5. Client has a history of gout.

3. A nurse has been caring for a client with active TB in an acute care facility. To promote adherence, an alternative dosing regimen of twice weekly is recommended. How can this modification of schedule help the client adhere to long-term therapy?
   1. Decreases gastric upset and promotes nutrition
   2. Promotes fluid balance in the client's body
   3. Prevents the occurrence of neuropathy
   4. Prevents the occurrence of liver dysfunction

4. Which of the following drugs should be monitored for interactions when the client is taking rifampin? **Select all that apply.**
   1. Oral anticoagulants
   2. Digoxin
   3. Oral contraceptives
   4. Colchicine
   5. Allopurinol

5. A client with TB is administered pyrazinamide as prescribed. The nurse caring for the client suspects that the client is developing signs of hepatotoxicity as an adverse reaction of pyrazinamide. Which of the following manifestations of a hepatotoxic reaction should the nurse look for in the client?
   1. Jaundiced skin
   2. Epigastric distress
   3. Yellow-orange tears
   4. Hematologic changes

6. A new nurse is assigned to the TB clinic and is learning about drugs new to her. The nurse knows that under which of the following conditions is the use of rifampin contraindicated?
   1. Clients who have tested positive for HIV
   2. Clients with hepatic or renal impairment
   3. Clients with diabetes mellitus
   4. Clients with diabetic retinopathy

7. Which of the following individuals are especially susceptible to TB? **Select all that apply.**
   1. Those living in crowded conditions
   2. People with HIV
   3. Children younger than 6 years
   4. Adults older than 30 years
   5. Clients with severe COPD

8. How is TB transmitted from person to person?
   1. Contact with infected blood
   2. Fecal-oral transmission
   3. Inhalation of infected droplets
   4. Contact with sweat

9. TB can affect which of the following organs? **Select all that apply.**
   1. Lungs
   2. Liver
   3. Kidneys
   4. Spleen
   5. Uterus

10. Which of the following are true of antitubercular drugs? **Select all that apply.**
    1. Treat active cases of TB.
    2. Prophylaxis to prevent the activation of TB.
    3. Render the client noninfectious to others.
    4. Treat dormant cases of TB.

11. Active TB may be difficult to diagnose in clients infected with HIV because of their immune system deficiency. Which of the following can be used to determine if a client with HIV and a negative skin test has active TB? **Select all that apply.**
    1. X-ray studies
    2. Blood tests
    3. Sputum analyses
    4. Urinalysis
    5. Physical examinations

12. A client in the initial phase of TB treatment develops a decrease in visual acuity and changes in color perception. Which drug may be causing this reaction?
    1. Ethambutol
    2. Isoniazid
    3. Pyrazinamide
    4. Rifampin

CHAPTER 11

Antiviral Drugs

Learning Objectives

- Explain the uses, general drug actions, adverse reactions, contraindications, precautions, and interactions of antiviral drugs.
- Distinguish important preadministration and ongoing assessment activities the nurse should perform on the client receiving an antiviral/antiretroviral drug.
- List nursing diagnoses particular to a client taking an antiviral drug.
- List possible goals for a client taking an antiviral/antiretroviral drug.
- Examine ways to promote an optimal response to therapy and manage adverse reactions, and special considerations to keep in mind when educating the client and the family about the antiviral/antiretroviral drugs.

SECTION I: ASSESSING YOUR UNDERSTANDING

Activity A FILL IN THE BLANKS

1. To reproduce, the virus needs the cellular material of another _____ _____.

2. More than _____ viruses have been identified as capable of producing disease.

3. _____, also called Norvir, is contraindicated if the client is taking bupropion (Wellbutrin), zolpidem (Ambien), or an antiarrhythmic drug.

4. _____ are not effective against viral infections.

5. _____ drugs are used in the treatment of human immunodeficiency virus (HIV) and acquired immune deficiency syndrome (AIDS).

Activity B DOSAGE CALCULATION

1. A primary health care provider has prescribed 120 mg/kg of Foscavir per day to be given intravenously. The strength of the drug in the available solution is 24 mg/mL. How many mL of the solution should the nurse administer to the client who weighs 65 kg?

2. The primary health care provider has prescribed intravenous acyclovir to a client. The standard dosage of the drug is 5 mg/kg to be given once a day. The client weighs 50 kg. The drug available in solution is 50 mg/mL. How many mL of drug solution will the nurse expect to be prepared for one dose?

3. The primary health care provider has prescribed 500 mg of famciclovir every 8 hours for a client with shingles. The drug is available in 250-mg tablets. How many tablets should the nurse instruct the client to take per dose?

4. The primary health care provider has prescribed 5 mg/kg of cidofovir for a client. The injectable drug is available 50 mg/mL. The drug is infused in a secondary IV infusion. How many mL of the drug will be added to the IVPB if the client weighs 40 kg?

_____

_____

5. The primary health care provider is prescribing didanosine to a client with HIV. The dose is 400 mg if the client weighs over 60 kg and 250 mg if the client weighs less than 60 kg. What will be the dose for a client who weighs 125 lb?

_____

_____

Activity C MATCHING

1. Match the drugs that interact adversely with antivirals in Column A with their common uses in Column B.

Column A

____ **1.** Probenecid

____ **2.** Cimetidine

____ **3.** Ibuprofen

____ **4.** Imipenem/ cilastatin

Column B

a. Gout treatment

b. Pain relief

c. Anti-infective agent

d. Relief of gastric upset, heartburn

2. Match the drugs that interact adversely with antiretrovirals in Column A with their common uses in Column B.

Column A

____ **1.** Antifungals

____ **2.** Clarithromycin

____ **3.** Sildenafil

____ **4.** Opioid analgesics

Column B

a. Treat bacterial infection

b. Relieve pain

c. Eliminate or manage fungal infections

d. Treat erectile dysfunction

Activity D SHORT ANSWERS

A nurse's role in managing clients who are being administered antiviral drugs includes observing and monitoring their progress and performing any necessary assessments. Answer the following questions, which involve the nurse's role in management of such situations.

1. A client is diagnosed with herpes simplex virus (HSV) and the primary health care provider has prescribed antiviral drugs. What should the nurse assess for before administering the antiviral drug?

_____

_____

2. A client has hepatitis B and the primary health care provider has prescribed an antiviral drug. What ongoing assessments should the nurse perform while administering the antiviral drug to the client?

_____

_____

Activity E **VIRAL SUDOKU PUZZLE**

FLU	HZV			HCV				
HPV			CMV	RSV	FLU			
	RSV	HSV					HPV	
HSV				HPV				HZV
HIV			HSV		HZV			CMV
HCV				HBV				HPV
	HPV					HBV	HSV	
			HIV	CMV	RSV			FLU
				HSV			HCV	RSV

SECTION II: APPLYING YOUR KNOWLEDGE

Activity F **CASE STUDY**

 Johnnie Atain is a neighbor living in Betty Peterson's apartment complex. He is a 35-year-old man who has been HIV positive for 5 years. He is currently taking a combination of medications as part of HAART. Johnnie presents to the free neighborhood clinic complaining of pain in his mouth, loss of appetite, and white patches on his tongue and throat.

1. While triaging Mr. Atain, what information should the nurse obtain?

_____

_____

_____

2. Mr. Atain tells the nurse he is depressed having to take many medications for the HIV and wants to try some natural alternatives. He has been told to take St. John's wort because it will help lift his mood in addition to having antiviral effects. How should the nurse respond to his questions about the herbal preparation St. John's wort?

_____

_____

_____

Now Map It Out! Use the templates provided in the appendix to add information and make client connections on a concept map.

You have read in the textbook how herbal therapy can be contraindicated when certain drugs are taken (as in the case of Mr. Atain taking St. John's wort with antiretroviral medications). It was Betty Peterson who encouraged Johnnie Atain to try the herbal supplement, St. John's wort, because she feels better taking it herself. Look at your map for Betty Peterson. Do you see any medical conditions or issues on her map that would make her decide to use the herbal supplement St. John's wort as a treatment? Using the information provided here, map out this relationship and determine if and when there is an herbal/drug interaction in Betty's future.

SECTION III: PRACTICING FOR NCLEX

Activity G NCLEX-STYLE QUESTIONS

Answer the following questions.

1. A nurse is to administer ribavirin to a client with RSV. Which of the following points should the nurse keep in mind while administering the drug? Select all that apply.
   1. Discard and replace the solution every 24 hours.
   2. The drug can worsen respiratory status.
   3. The drug increases risk of nephrotoxicity.
   4. The drug should be administered with a small-particle aerosol generator.
   5. The drug induces anorexia and weight loss.

2. A client on an antiretroviral drug is also taking clarithromycin. Which of the following are the effects of the antiretroviral therapy when it is combined with clarithromycin?
   1. Increased serum level of the antiretroviral
   2. Increased serum level of both drugs
   3. Risk of toxicity
   4. Decreased effectiveness of the antiretroviral

3. A client with HSV-1 has been prescribed antiviral therapy. Before beginning the treatment, which of the following assessments is most appropriate considering the client's infection?
   1. Save a sample of client's urine.
   2. Record client's temperature.
   3. Inspect areas with lesions.
   4. Check client's blood pressure.

4. In which of the following cases should a nurse monitor for phlebitis in a client?
   1. When client is given drugs orally
   2. If drugs are given intramuscularly
   3. When client is given drugs intravenously
   4. If the drug is given transdermally

5. In which of the following client populations should the nurse exercise caution and monitor for exacerbation of problems while caring for clients who are taking indinavir?
   1. Renal impairment
   2. Cardiac disorders
   3. Sulfonamide allergy
   4. History of bladder stone formation

6. A clinical pharmacist is required to prepare and administer didanosine powder to a client with HIV. Which of the following points should be kept in mind while mixing and administering the drug?
   1. Administer drug with meals.
   2. Mix with no more than 2 ounces of water.
   3. Avoid generating and inhaling dust.
   4. Refrigerate solution.

7. The primary health care provider has prescribed 800 mg of acyclovir per dose. The drug is available in 200-mg capsules. How many capsules should the nurse administer to the client per dose?
   1. 1
   2. 2
   3. 4
   4. 8

8. Which of the following represents a route of entry for viruses into the body? Select all that apply.
   1. Insect bite
   2. Contact on intact skin
   3. Needle stick
   4. Inhalation
   5. Ingestion

9. Which of the following are caused by a virus? Select all that apply.
   1. Common cold
   2. Impetigo
   3. Wart
   4. Influenza
   5. Hepatitis C

10. Highly active antiretroviral therapy (HAART) is used to treat which of the following infections?
    1. HIV
    2. HSV
    3. Cytomegalovirus (CMV)
    4. Rotavirus

11. How are retroviruses different from viruses? Select all that apply.

    1. Human immunodeficiency virus is an example of a retrovirus.

    2. Retroviruses contain an enzyme called reverse transcriptase.

    3. RNA is the primary component of the retrovirus instead of DNA.

    4. DNA is the primary component of the retrovirus instead of RNA.

    5. CMV is an example of a retrovirus.

CHAPTER 12

Antifungal and Antiparasitic Drugs

Learning Objectives

- Differentiate between superficial and systemic fungal infections.
- Compare and contrast helminthic infections, protozoal infections, and amebiasis.
- Explain the uses, general drug actions, adverse reactions, contraindications, precautions, and interactions of antifungal and antiparasitic drugs.
- Distinguish important preadministration and ongoing assessment activities the nurse should perform on the client receiving an antifungal and antiparasitic drug.
- List nursing diagnoses particular to a client taking an antifungal and antiparasitic drug.
- List possible goals for a client taking an antifungal and antiparasitic drug.
- Examine ways to promote an optimal response to therapy, how to manage adverse reactions, and important points to keep in mind when educating the client and family about antifungal and antiparasitic drugs.

SECTION I ASSESSING YOUR UNDERSTANDING

Activity A FILL IN THE BLANKS

1. _____ fungal infections are serious infections that occur when fungi gain entrance into the interior of the body.

2. _____ mycotic infections occur on the surface of, or just below, the skin or nails.

3. _____ is an aminoglycoside with amebicidal activity and is used to treat intestinal amebiasis.

4. _____ damage is the most serious adverse reaction to the use of amphotericin B.

5. Since many people travel worldwide, many travelers are treated _____ to prevent parasitic infection.

Activity B DOSAGE CALCULATION

1. A child has been prescribed 3 mg/lb/day of griseofulvin, to be administered in two equal doses every day. The available drug is in the form of a 125 mg/5 mL suspension. If the child weighs 83.5 lb, how many mL should the parent administer for each dose?

_____

_____

2. A client with a nail infection has been prescribed 200 mg of itraconazole daily. The drug is available in the form of 100-mg capsules at the pharmacy. The client lives in a remote area and wants to be sure they have the entire amount of drug needed for two separate 7-day courses of treatment. What is the total number of capsules required for this client?

_____

_____

3. A group of volunteer student nurses is going overseas. The malaria prophylaxis treatment is chloroquine 500 mg weekly on the same day for 8 weeks. The available chloroquine tablet is 250 mg. How many tablets should be given to each student nurse for the entire course of treatment?

_____

_____

Activity C SEQUENCING AND MATCHING

1. *Write the correct sequence for the life cycle of malaria in the boxes provided.*

1. In the liver, the parasite invades red blood cells

2. Mosquito picks up the parasite from the infected host

3. Infected mosquito injects the parasite into the host, and it migrates to the liver

4. RBCs rupture, spreading the parasite throughout the body

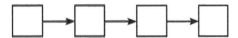

2. *Match the antifungal drugs in Column A with their uses in Column B.*

Column A

____ **1.** Terbinafine

____ **2.** Ketoconazole

____ **3.** Griseofulvin

____ **4.** Miconazole

____ **5.** Micafungin

Column B

a. Treat ringworm infections

b. Treat nail bed fungal infections

c. Fungal prevention in stem cell transplantation

d. Treat systemic fungal infections

e. Treat vaginal infections

3. *Match the antiparasitic drugs in Column A with their effect on infections in Column B.*

Column A

____ **1.** Albendazole

____ **2.** Chloroquine

____ **3.** Nitazoxanide

____ **4.** Hydroxychloroquine

Column B

a. Besides malaria, used to treat autoimmune disorders

b. Used to kill tapeworms

c. Prevention of malaria

d. Treat *Giardia* diarrhea

Activity D SHORT ANSWERS

A nurse's role in managing a client who is prescribed an antifungal drug involves preadministration assessment. Answer the following question, which involves the nurse's role in management of clients on antifungal therapy.

1. A client with a vaginal yeast infection is prescribed an antifungal drug. What preadministration assessments should the nurse conduct before an antifungal drug is prescribed?

_____

_____

A nurse's role in managing clients who are administered anthelmintic drugs involves teaching the client or family members how to prevent spread of the infection. Answer the following question, which involves the nurse's role in the management of such situations.

2. A client with a pinworm infection has been recommended an anthelmintic drug. What should the client be taught to prevent the spread of pinworm to other family members?

_____

_____

Activity E CROSSWORD PUZZLE

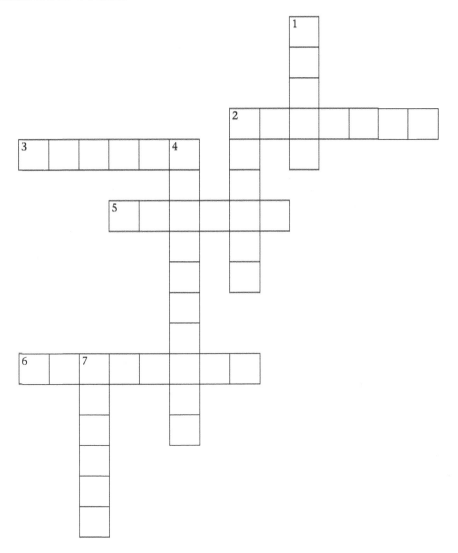

Across

2. An herbal microbial oil
3. Suffix meaning retards growth of fungi
5. A single-celled, colorless plant
6. An organism that lives in or on another organism

Down

1. Suffix meaning deadly to fungi
2. Yeast infection of the mouth
4. Term for quinidine toxicity
7. The fever and chills associated with administering amphotericin B by IV infusion

SECTION II APPLYING YOUR KNOWLEDGE

Activity F CASE STUDY

 Johnnie Atain is a neighbor living in Betty Peterson's apartment complex. He is a 35-year-old man who has been HIV positive for 5 years. He is currently taking a combination of medications as part of HAART therapy. Johnnie presents to the free neighborhood clinic complaining of pain in his mouth, loss of appetite, and white patches on his tongue and throat.

1. Which of Johnnie's medications or medical conditions put him at risk for a fungal infection?

_____

_____

_____

2. The primary health care provider diagnoses Johnnie with oral candidiasis and prescribes nystatin 500,000 units QID for 7 days. Nystatin suspension is available as 100,000 units/mL. How many mL will be in each dose and how should Johnnie be taught to use the suspension?

_____

_____

_____

Now Map It Out! Use the templates provided in the appendix to add information and make client connections on a concept map.

Mr. Atain tells the nurse he is lucky to have a nice neighbor like Betty. She too had a kidney infection (with kidney stones) and was given a prescription for Cipro. Lucky for him, her pain was gone after about a week, so she stopped the pills and had some extras on hand. Betty gave these to Johnnie and he has taken three of them to get a "jump start" on this possible mouth infection. How has this increased Johnnie's risk for a fungal infection, and what risk does this cause Betty for not taking her entire course of medication? Find the issue on Betty Peterson's concept map.

SECTION III PRACTICING FOR NCLEX

Activity G NCLEX-STYLE QUESTIONS

Answer the following questions.

1. A client with a fungal infection is seen at the health care clinic. The primary health care provider prescribes topical administration of an antifungal drug. What kinds of reactions should the nurse teach the client to monitor for?
   1. Dehydration
   2. Nausea
   3. Stinging
   4. Diarrhea

2. The nurse is documenting the history of a client who is to be started on itraconazole therapy. In which of the conditions is itraconazole contraindicated?
   1. Bone marrow suppression
   2. Severe liver disease
   3. History of heart failure
   4. History of asthma

3. What care should the nurse take when administering an IV solution of amphotericin B?
   1. Ensure that the IV solution is protected from light.
   2. Freeze the unused IV solution.
   3. Ensure that the IV solution is used within 48 hour.
   4. Store the drug in a heated environment.

4. A client has been prescribed intravenous administration of amphotericin B to cure a fungal infection. What adverse reactions should a nurse monitor for in the client? **Select all that apply.**
   1. Vomiting
   2. Hypertension
   3. Chills and shaking
   4. Fever

5. A client presents with a toenail fungal infection. She is planning a wedding and wishes to wear open-toed shoes. It has been explained to her that the reaction to the treatment is slow. As a result, the client is anxious and upset. What is the best intervention the nurse can do to help reduce the anxiety of the client undergoing antifungal treatment?

    1. Check the client's blood pressure.
    2. Encourage the client to verbalize feelings.
    3. Provide the client with a warm blanket.
    4. Keep the client away from light.

6. A client was admitted to an acute care facility for severe diarrhea due to a *Giardia* infection. As part of the discharge teaching, the nurse needs to instruct the client how to prevent spread of the infection. Which is the most important instruction that the nurse should include in the client's teaching plan?

    1. There should be no sexual contact while lesions are present.
    2. Precautions to avoid sunlight should be taken when going outdoors.
    3. Physical activities should be avoided.
    4. Towels should be kept separate from those of other family members.

7. A client undergoing treatment with ketoconazole is soon to be discharged. What reactions for the ketoconazole drug should the nurse instruct the client to expect?

    1. Unusual fatigue, yellow skin, and darkened urine
    2. Fever, sore throat, or skin rash
    3. Headache, dizziness, and drowsiness
    4. Nausea, vomiting, or diarrhea

8. A nurse is planning an overseas mission where they will be required to care for acutely ill clients with malaria. Which of the following interventions are nurses expected to perform?

    1. Record vital signs of the client every 12 hour.
    2. Observe the client every 4 hour for malaria symptoms.
    3. Collect urine samples of the client and send for testing.
    4. Carefully measure and record the fluid intake and output.

9. For which of the following client populations is the antimalarial drug quinine contraindicated?

    1. Clients with myasthenia gravis
    2. Clients with thyroid disease
    3. Clients with blood dyscrasias
    4. Clients with diabetes

10. While in a pediatric acute care facility, it is discovered that a client may have a pinworm infection. Which of the following interventions should the nurse perform?

    1. Save stool samples during the first day of treatment only.
    2. Follow hospital procedure for transporting stool to the laboratory.
    3. Visually inspect stools only if client reports anything unusual.
    4. Use any container to save a sample of the stool.

11. A woman has been prescribed pyrantel for roundworms after getting the infection from her child. Which of the following should the nurse tell the client when educating her about taking an anthelmintic drug?

    1. Use birth control pills instead of the barrier method for contraception.
    2. Discontinue dosage as soon as symptoms disappear.
    3. Use chlorine bleach to disinfect toilet facilities or shower stall after bathing.
    4. Take the drug with milk and not water, unless the client is lactose intolerant.

12. Which of the following adverse reactions is associated with paromomycin?
    1. Vertigo, hypotension
    2. Nephrotoxicity and ototoxicity
    3. Thrombocytopenia
    4. Peripheral neuropathy

13. Which of the following pieces of information should a nurse give to a client who has been prescribed metronidazole?
    1. Take the drug with meals or immediately afterward.
    2. Avoid alcohol for the first week of treatment.
    3. Take cimetidine for gastric upset or other stomach problems.
    4. Wear protective clothing to guard against photosensitivity.

Drugs Used to Manage Pain

CHAPTER 13

Nonopioid Analgesics: Salicylates and Nonsalicylates

Learning Objectives

- Discuss in general terms how pain is defined and the challenges of understanding the client's pain experience.
- Distinguish the types, uses, general drug actions, common adverse reactions, contraindications, precautions, and interactions of the salicylates and acetaminophen.
- Explain important preadministration and ongoing assessment activities the nurse should perform for the client taking salicylates or acetaminophen.
- List nursing diagnoses particular to a client taking salicylates or acetaminophen.
- Discuss the ways to promote an optimal response to therapy, how to manage common adverse reactions, and important points to keep in mind when educating clients about the use of salicylates or acetaminophen.

SECTION I ASSESSING YOUR UNDERSTANDING

Activity A FILL IN THE BLANKS

1. The analgesic action of the salicylates is due to the inhibition of _____, which are fatty acid derivatives found in almost every tissue of the body and bodily fluid.

2. Aspirin prolongs bleeding time by inhibiting the aggregation (clumping) of _____.

3. _____ is a reduction in all cellular components of the blood.

4. The use of aspirin may be involved in the development of _____ syndrome in children who have chickenpox or influenza.

5. _____, a ringing sound in the ear, is one of the symptoms of salicylism.

Activity B DOSAGE CALCULATION

1. A client has been prescribed 650 mg of aspirin every 4 hours. The available tablets are 325 mg. How many tablets will the nurse administer to the client per dose?

_____

_____

2. The primary care provider prescribes 500 mg of Dolobid orally, every 8 hours, for a client. The available tablets are 250 mg. How many tablets will the nurse administer to the client in each dose?

_____

_____

3. Bufferin, 2000 mg daily, has been recommended for a client. The available tablet contains 650 mg of salicylate. Will a TID administration exceed the recommended dose?

_____

_____

4. A client has been prescribed 600 mg of acetaminophen every day, to be taken in equally divided doses every 6 hours. The client has the drug in the form of a 300-mg tablet. What will the dose be every 6 hours and how many tablets should the client take for each dose?

_____

_____

5. A client can take 650 mg of buffered aspirin every 4 hours. The available tablets are 325 mg. How many tablets will the nurse administer to the client each time if the tablets are to be administered every 8 hours?

_____

_____

6. A client is prescribed 650 mg of Ecotrin every 4 hours. The nurse has 325-mg tablets. How many tablets should the nurse administer every 4 hours?

_____

_____

Activity C MATCHING

1. Match the drugs that interact adversely with salicylates in Column A with the likely effect they may have when taken with salicylates from Column B.

Column A

____ **1.** Anticoagulant

____ **2.** Activated charcoal

____ **3.** Antacid

____ **4.** Carbonic anhy- drase inhibitor

Column B

a. Decreased effects of the salicylates

b. Increased risk for bleeding

c. Increased risk for salicylism

d. Decreased absorption of the salicylates

2. Match the nursing diagnoses in Column A with their related factors from the textbook in Column B.

Column A

____ **1.** Impaired comfort

____ **2.** Chronic or acute pain

____ **3.** Impaired phys- ical mobility

____ **4.** Risk for poisoning

Column B

a. Peripheral nerve damage and/or tissue inflammation due to the aspirin therapy

b. Increased use of salicylate or acetaminophen

c. Fever of the disease process (e.g., infection or surgery)

d. Muscle and joint stiffness

Activity D SHORT ANSWERS

A nurse's role in managing discomfort of clients involves assisting them with relieving their pain. The nurse also helps administer drugs and provide physical comfort. Briefly answer the following questions, which involve the nurse's role in the management of such situations.

1. What is the difference between acute and chronic pain?

_____

_____

_____

2. A client had been prescribed salicylates. How can the nurse monitor and manage this client's discomfort?

_____

_____

_____

Activity E CROSSWORD PUZZLE

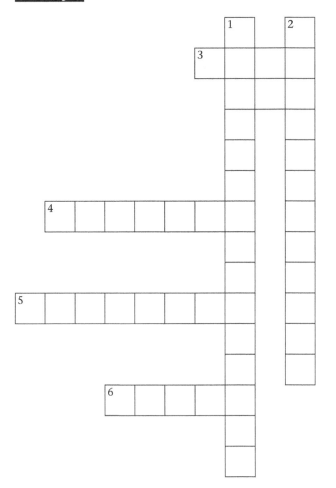

Across

3. The unpleasant sensory and emotional perception associated with actual or potential tissue damage
4. Pain with a duration of more than 6 months
5. An early sign of salicylism
6. Pain with a duration of less than 3–6 months

Down

1. The primary adverse reaction of salicylates (two words)
2. The condition of rheumatoid arthritis that is reduced by salicylates

SECTION II APPLYING YOUR KNOWLEDGE

Activity F CASE STUDY

 Janna Wong is a 16-year-old gymnast. Her mother calls the clinic upset about one of Janna's friends. Mrs. Wong tells the nurse the young girl overdosed on acetaminophen and is very ill in the children's hospital. She wants to know how to keep the same thing from happening to her daughter. Many cases of acetaminophen overdose are caused by people taking more than the recommended daily limit without realizing it (no more than 3250 mg per day). This happens because people are not aware of the number of over-the-counter products that contain acetaminophen, such as cold and flu remedies. Additionally, when combined with alcohol (which is in many cold relievers), this can increase the risk of drug toxicity. Discuss how Mrs. Wong and her daughter Janna can be active learners in understanding the safe use of acetaminophen.

1. What should the nurse tell Mrs. Wong about the safe use of acetaminophen?

_____

_____

_____

2. Try this activity; discuss what you find with your classmates and how you could explain the activity to others.

   a. Write out what you typically take as cold or flu remedies when you are ill.

   _____

   _____

   b. Look at the drug labels in your home or at the store. Add up the amount of acetaminophen you typically take in a 24-hour period for a cold or flu. How close are you to the daily limit?

   _____

   _____

Now Map It Out! Use the templates provided in the appendix to add information and make client connections on a concept map.

When talking about her friends, Janna shares with you that she keeps healthy by purchasing and taking DayQuil and NyQuil when she feels head congestion. She says the liquid keeps her in top shape for competition on the school gymnastic team. As you map out Janna's problems, can you find any situation that would lead to a potential overdose of acetaminophen in her situation, too?

SECTION III PRACTICING FOR NCLEX

Activity G NCLEX-STYLE QUESTIONS

Answer the following questions.

1. A client has been prescribed salicylates as an analgesic agent. Which of the following adverse reactions caused by salicylates should the nurse monitor for?
   1. Skin eruptions
   2. GI bleeding
   3. Jaundice
   4. Neurologic disorders

2. For which of the following clients are salicylates contraindicated? **Select all that apply.**
   1. Clients with hypersensitivity to the drug
   2. Clients with a history of heart failure
   3. Clients with influenza or viral illness
   4. Clients with bleeding disorders
   5. Clients with hepatic disorders

3. Which of the following symptoms can be observed in a client with salicylate levels between 150 and 250 mcg/mL?
   1. Nausea
   2. Respiratory alkalosis
   3. Hemorrhage
   4. Asterixis

4. Which of the following is an effect of combining loop diuretics with acetaminophen?
   1. Increased possibility of toxicity
   2. Decreased effect of acetaminophen
   3. Increased risk for bleeding
   4. Decreased effectiveness of the diuretic

5. Which of the following informational facts should a nurse provide to a client who has been prescribed salicylates regarding their purchase and storage?
   1. Do not use over-the-counter drugs containing aspirin.
   2. Include paprika, licorice, prunes, and raisins in the diet.
   3. Store the drug in a cool, ventilated area.
   4. Purchase salicylates in small amounts.
   5. Notify the physician before surgery or a dental procedure.

6. Which of the following adverse reactions should a nurse monitor for in a client who has been administered a salicylate?
   1. GI bleeding
   2. Hypoglycemia
   3. Pancytopenia
   4. Hemolytic anemia

7. In which of the following instances can aspirin be used to treat clients?
   1. Clients with hemophilia
   2. Clients with rheumatoid arthritis
   3. Clients with severe postoperative pain
   4. Clients taking anticoagulants

8. A client has been prescribed acetaminophen. Which of the following are signs of acetaminophen toxicity that the nurse should monitor for in the client?
   1. Malaise
   2. Increased anxiety
   3. Hyperglycemia
   4. Bradycardia

9. When time is used to describe the duration of pain, which of the following terms are used? **Select all that apply.**
   1. Acute
   2. Traumatic
   3. Chronic
   4. Postoperative
   5. Neuropathic

10. Which of the following are classified as acute pain? **Select all that apply.**
    1. Postoperative pain
    2. Procedural pain
    3. Osteoarthritis pain
    4. Fibromyalgia pain
    5. Diabetic neuropathic pain

11. Chronic pain is classified as pain that lasts for more than how long?
    1. 1 week
    2. 1 month
    3. 6 weeks
    4. 6 months

12. Which of the following are examples of chronic pain? **Select all that apply.**
    1. Fibromyalgia pain
    2. Postoperative pain
    3. Traumatic pain
    4. Rheumatoid arthritis pain
    5. Osteoarthritis pain

Nonopioid Analgesics: Nonsteroidal Anti-Inflammatory Drugs (NSAIDs) and Migraine Headache Medications

Learning Objectives

- Discuss the importance of good pain assessment.
- Compare and contrast standardized methods to assess pain in different client populations.
- Explain the uses, general drug actions, common adverse reactions, contraindications, precautions, and interactions of the nonsteroidal anti-inflammatory drugs (NSAIDs).
- Describe the types, general drug actions, common adverse reactions, contraindications, precautions, and interactions of drugs used to treat migraine headaches.
- Distinguish important preadministration and ongoing assessment activities the nurse should perform on the client taking an NSAID.
- List nursing diagnoses particular to a client taking an NSAID.
- Examine the ways to promote an optimal response to therapy, how to manage common adverse reactions, and important points to keep in mind when educating clients about the use of NSAIDs.

SECTION I ASSESSING YOUR UNDERSTANDING

Activity A FILL IN THE BLANKS

1. Two basic measures necessary for pain assessment in any client population are _____ and _____.

2. NSAIDs inhibit prostaglandin synthesis by blocking the action of the enzyme _____.

3. _____ is a COX-2 drug associated with an increased risk of serious cardiovascular thrombosis, myocardial infarction (MI), and stroke.

4. Most _____ for pain relief are available over the counter without a prescription.

5. _____ syndrome may occur in children if aspirin or NSAIDs are taken.

6. NSAIDs are prescribed for the pain and _____ associated with arthritis.

Activity B DOSAGE CALCULATION

1. A client has been prescribed 150 mg of diclofenac orally per day. Diclofenac is available as 50-mg tablets. How many tablets will the nurse administer to the client per day?

_____

_____

2. A client has been prescribed 100 mg of indomethacin orally per day. The drug is available in 50-mg tablets. How many tablets will the nurse administer to the client per day?

_____

_____

3. A client has been prescribed Vimovo 325 mg orally in two doses a day. The drug is available in 325-mg tablets. How many tablets will the nurse administer to the client each time?

_____

_____

4. A client has been prescribed a daily dose of 200 mg of flurbiprofen orally, to be divided into two equal doses. The drug is available in 100-mg tablets. How many tablets will the nurse administer to the client in each dose?

_____

_____

5. A client has been prescribed a daily dose of 400 mg of meclofenamate orally in four divided doses. The drug is available as 100-mg tablets. How many tablets will the nurse administer to the client per dose?

_____

_____

Activity C MATCHING

1. Match the NANDA nursing diagnosis in Column A with the discomforts faced by clients in Column B.

Column A

____ **1.** Impaired Physical Mobility

____ **2.** Impaired Skin Integrity

____ **3.** Acute or Chronic Pain

Column B

a. 5HT agonist use

b. Peripheral tissue damage

c. Muscle and joint stiffness

2. Match the drugs that interact with NSAIDs in Column A with their interacting effects in Column B.

Column A

____ **1.** Anticoagulants

____ **2.** Hydantoins

____ **3.** Acetaminophen

____ **4.** Diuretics

Column B

a. Increased risk of renal impairment

b. Increased excretion of extracellular fluid

c. Increased effectiveness of the anticonvulsant

d. Increased risk of bleeding

Activity D SHORT ANSWERS

A nurse's role in managing clients who are being administered NSAIDs involves monitoring the clients and implementing interventions that aid in their recovery. Answer the following questions, which involve the nurse's role in the management of such situations.

1. What conditions are treated with NSAIDs?

_____

_____

_____

2. Why is good pain assessment important?

_____

_____

_____

3. A nurse is caring for a client taking an NSAID for moderate pain. NSAIDs can have adverse reactions on the sensory organs. What sensory reactions should the nurse monitor for in this client?

_____

_____

Activity E **CROSSWORD PUZZLE**

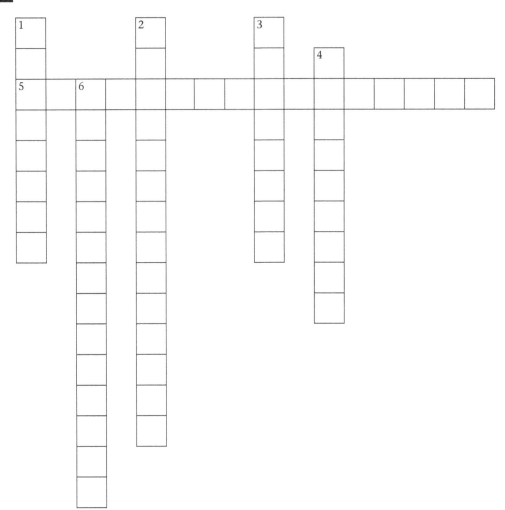

Across

5. GI adverse reactions are common because NSAIDS block this enzyme

Down

1. A basic component of a good pain assessment
2. Inhibition of these allows NSAIDs to reduce inflammation
3. Type of headache believed to be caused by vascular spasms
4. A subjective basic component of a good pain assessment
6. Type of serious problem such as thrombosis, MI, and stroke

SECTION II APPLYING YOUR KNOWLEDGE

Activity F CASE STUDY

 Mr. Park, aged 77 years, presents to the clinic today complaining of knee and hip pain. He has hypertension. His medications include an antihypertensive and aspirin. He has tried acetaminophen in the past to treat his joint pain, but with little relief. The primary health care provider diagnoses him with osteoarthritis. In the textbook, the drug Celebrex was considered, yet due to cost it was changed and a prescription for ibuprofen 800 mg q8hr PRN pain was written. The primary health care provider has asked the nurse to bring Mr. Park the prescription.

1. What should the nurse tell Mr. Park about taking the ibuprofen with his other medications?

_____

_____

2. What important aspects of ibuprofen administration should the nurse educate Mr. Park about?

_____

_____

Now Map It Out! Use the templates provided in the appendix to add information and make client connections on a concept map.

Here is where you begin to see the effects of polypharmacy, when multiple drugs interact with one another. Using the concept map template for Mr. Park, draw out the possible medical problems and drugs being used by this client. What are the results of how some of these drugs interact? What new problems may we now see?

SECTION III PRACTICING FOR NCLEX

Activity G NCLEX-STYLE QUESTIONS

Answer the following questions.

1. A client with rheumatoid arthritis has been administered an NSAID. Which GI system adverse reactions should the nurse monitor for in the client? **Select all that apply.**
   1. Epigastric pain
   2. Appendicitis
   3. Abdominal distress
   4. Indigestion
   5. Intestinal ulceration

2. A nurse documents the history of a client who is to be started on NSAID therapy. In which of the following conditions is ibuprofen recommended for use?
   1. Clients with sulfonamide allergy
   2. Clients with peptic ulceration
   3. Clients with cardiac disease
   4. Clients with a history of stroke

3. A nurse is assigned to care for a client prescribed an NSAID. Which of the following conditions should the nurse assess for before administering the NSAID to the client?
   1. Visual disturbances
   2. Skin reactions
   3. Dizziness
   4. Bleeding disorders

4. A nurse is caring for a client undergoing NSAID treatment. Which of the following should the nurse suggest to the client to promote an optimal response to therapy?
   1. Avoid exercise.
   2. Restrict to a liquid diet.
   3. Take medication with food.
   4. Restrict mobility.

5. A client has been prescribed indomethacin for rheumatoid disorders. Which of the following conditions should the nurse monitor for during the ongoing administration of the NSAID to the client?
   1. Skin eruptions
   2. Diarrhea
   3. Rash
   4. GI bleeding

6. A 68-year-old client is prescribed an NSAID for arthritis. Why should treatment for the older adult begin with a reduced dosage that is increased slowly?
   1. Increased risk of inflammation
   2. Increased risk of erythema
   3. Increased RBC count
   4. Increased risk of serious ulcer diseases

7. A client being treated for arthritis is to be discharged. Which of the following instructions should the nurse include in the client's teaching plan? **Select all that apply.**
   1. Avoid physical activities during drug therapy.
   2. Do not use the drugs on a regular basis unless the primary health care provider is notified.
   3. Keep towels separate from those of other family members.
   4. Avoid use of aspirin.
   5. Take the drug with a full glass of water or with food.

8. Blocking of which of the following enzymes is responsible for the pain-relieving effects of NSAIDs?
   1. Cyclooxygenase-1
   2. Cyclooxygenase-2
   3. Cyclooxygenase-3
   4. Cyclooxygenase-4

9. The most common side effects caused by NSAIDs involve which of the following?
   1. Stomach
   2. Lungs
   3. Liver
   4. Peripheral nerves

10. A hypersensitivity to which of the following medications is a contraindication for all NSAIDs?
    1. Acetaminophen
    2. Hydrochlorothiazide
    3. Aspirin
    4. Lisinopril

11. Which of the following NSAIDs appear to work by specifically inhibiting cyclooxygenase-2, without inhibiting cyclooxygenase-1?
    1. Celecoxib
    2. Ibuprofen
    3. Naproxen
    4. Meloxicam

12. Blocking of which of the following enzymes is responsible for the gastrointestinal side effects caused by NSAIDs?
    1. Cyclooxygenase-2
    2. Cyclooxygenase-3
    3. Cyclooxygenase-1
    4. Cyclooxygenase-4

CHAPTER 15

Opioid Analgesics and Antagonists

Learning Objectives

- Explain how pain intensity is used to determine treatment using opioids and nonopioid analgesics.
- Discuss the uses, general drug actions, general adverse reactions, contraindications, precautions, and interactions of the opioid analgesics and antagonists.
- Distinguish important preadministration and ongoing assessment activities the nurse should perform on the client taking an opioid analgesic or antagonist.
- List nursing diagnoses particular to a client taking an opioid analgesic or antagonist.
- Examine ways to promote optimal response to therapy, how to manage adverse reactions, and important points to keep in mind when educating clients about the use of opioid analgesics and antagonists.

SECTION I ASSESSING YOUR UNDERSTANDING

Activity A FILL IN THE BLANKS

1. The most widely used opioid, _____ sulfate, is an effective drug for moderately severe to severe pain.

2. A drug that is a(n) _____ has a greater affinity for a cell receptor than an opioid drug, and by binding to the cell it prevents a response to the opioid.

3. Most opioid analgesics are derived from _____ or a synthetic substance like it.

4. _____ is an illegal narcotic substance in the United States and is not used in medicine.

5. Older adults, _____ clients, or debilitated clients may have a reduced initial opioid dose until their response to the drug is known.

Activity B DOSAGE CALCULATION

1. A primary health care provider prescribes 30 mg of codeine orally four times a day for a client. The available tablets are 60 mg. How many tablets will the nurse instruct the client to take in each dose?

   _____

   _____

2. A primary health care provider prescribes 60 mg of methadone per day. Each tablet contains 30 mg of the drug. How many tablets will the nurse need to administer to the client in each dose?

   _____

   _____

3. A primary health care provider prescribes 100 mg of tramadol daily to a client. Tramadol is available in the form of Ultram tablets, each tablet containing 50 mg of tramadol. How many Ultram tablets will the nurse teach the client to take daily?

_____

_____

4. A client is prescribed fentanyl 50 mcg IV 30 minute before a GI procedure. The available vial has a dosage strength of 0.05 mg/1 mL. How much fluid will the nurse need to draw up to administer to the client?

_____

_____

5. A primary health care provider prescribes 250 mg of morphine sulfate daily to a client. Each 5 mL of Roxanol oral solution contains 100 mg of morphine sulfate. How much Roxanol oral solution will the nurse need to administer to the client daily?

_____

_____

Activity C OUT IN THE COMMUNITY

Question 1. Many people are fearful of pain management because of the way narcotic street drugs are associated with addiction. As nurses we are fearful of overmedicating clients, too. To be good client educators, we need to understand these fears. In this activity, you ask what people think about opiates.

Class question: If a person was terminally ill, what is the greatest fear when considering strong drugs like morphine sulfate for pain management?

Activity

1. Ask the question above to four different people; say the words exactly as stated above. Write down what they tell you.

2. Count the number of times the people call the strong drugs *narcotics*. Do they use the term *opioid*?

Report the following in your class discussion:

3. Compare the responses with other students. Do you see certain fears named repeatedly?

4. How many times did the word *narcotic* get mentioned? Relate this to your readings.

Activity D SHORT ANSWERS

A nurse's role in managing clients who are prescribed opioid analgesics involves helping the clients deal with acute/chronic pain. The nurse also assists clients in coping with their drug regimens. Answer the following questions, which involve the nurse's role in managing such situations.

1. A postsurgical client is prescribed morphine sulfate through a PCA infusion pump. What educational points should the nurse instruct the client regarding use of the PCA infusion pump?

_____

_____

2. A nurse has analyzed the assessment data and selected the following nursing diagnoses for this client:

   ■ **Altered breathing pattern** related to pain and effects on breathing center by opioids
   ■ **Injury risk** related to dizziness or lightheadedness from opioid administration
   ■ **Constipation** related to the decreased GI motility caused by opioids
   ■ **Malnutrition** related to anorexia caused by opioids
   ■ How will the nurse evaluate the effectiveness of the treatment plan?

_____

_____

3. How is pain intensity used to determine treatment using opioids and nonopioid analgesics?

_____

_____

Activity E CROSSWORD PUZZLE

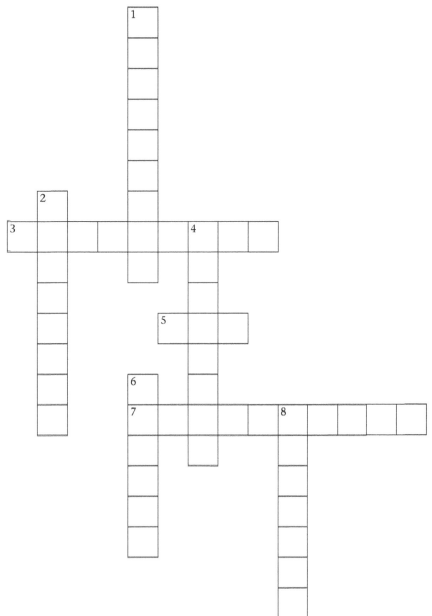

Across

3. The body's physical adaptation to a drug
5. A self-administered pump that allows clients to control the administration of their drug following a painful procedure
7. Tool that directs the use of both opioid and nonopioid treatment of mild to severe pain (two words)

Down

1. Effects of opioid drugs that include respiratory depression, decreased gastrointestinal motility, and miosis
2. The drug other opioids are compared to when attempting to determine dosing or conversion between drug types
4. A term referring to the properties of a drug to produce numbness or a stupor-like state
6. A term used for drugs that change the pain sensation by attaching to receptor sites in the brain producing an analgesic, sedative, and euphoric effect
8. A drug that binds with a receptor and stimulates the receptor to produce a therapeutic response

SECTION II APPLYING YOUR KNOWLEDGE

Activity F CASE STUDY

 Alfredo Garcia, aged 55 years, is being seen in the clinic in preparation for an endoscopy. He was told opiates are used during the procedure, and he is concerned about addiction potential.

1. How should the nurse address Mr. Garcia's concerns?

   _____

   _____

2. After the procedure, what information should be included regarding the opiate he was given?

   _____

   _____

Now Map It Out! Use the templates provided in the appendix to add information and make client connections on a concept map.

During the procedure, a fast-acting sedative and fentanyl are used for conscious sedation. Draw this out on Mr. Garcia's concept map and view his other health issues. Do you see any places where there may be the potential for an interaction? What nursing interventions are important to carry out after the procedure to reduce potential problems based upon his premapped out conditions?

SECTION III PRACTICING FOR NCLEX

Activity G NCLEX-STYLE QUESTIONS

Answer the following questions.

1. A client is prescribed an opioid analgesic for the treatment of pain. Which preadministration assessment is the most critical to conduct before the administration of an opioid analgesic?
   1. Obtain client's blood pressure.
   2. Assess the intensity and location of pain.
   3. Monitor client's pulse rate.
   4. Assess client's respiratory rate.

2. A nurse is caring for a client who would like to try medical marijuana for pain relief. Which of the following should the nurse confirm to ensure that the use of medical marijuana does not impact treatment in the client?
   1. Client is not taking anticoagulants.
   2. Client is not taking acetaminophen.
   3. Client does not have acute ulcerative colitis.
   4. Client does not have a history of seizure disorders.

3. A terminally ill client is prescribed an opioid analgesic for pain relief. The nurse notices that the client has developed severe anorexia due to the opioid treatment. What is the priority task for a client with imbalanced nutrition due to prolonged administration of an opioid?
   1. Ensure an increase in client's fluid intake.
   2. Assess client's food intake after each meal.
   3. Complement client's meal with protein supplements.
   4. Record client's bowel movements daily.

4. Opioid-naïve clients are most at risk for which of the following when administered a drug such as meperidine?
   1. Hypertension
   2. Respiratory depression
   3. Diarrhea
   4. Physical dependence

5. When a surgical client experiences a decrease in respirations, for which of the following reasons is naloxone used cautiously?
   1. Return of intense pain
   2. Vomiting
   3. Dizziness
   4. Headache

6. A client is being administered opioid analgesics in an ambulatory procedure clinic. Which of the following observations made by the nurse would require immediate attention by the primary health care provider? **Select all that apply.**
   1. Decrease in respiratory rate
   2. Change in pulse quality
   3. Decrease in blood pressure
   4. Increase in body weight
   5. Increase in body temperature

7. A nurse is assigned to care for a client who has been prescribed opioid therapy. Which of the following statements in the client's health history will require cautious use of opioid analgesics by the nurse? **Select all that apply.**
   1. Undiagnosed abdominal pain
   2. Age is 13 years
   3. Hepatic or renal impairment
   4. Client is hypoxic
   5. A fungal infection

8. A client on opioid therapy is also prescribed barbiturates (sedative), under close supervision. Which of the following risks is likely to occur in this client?
   1. Bacterial infections
   2. Hypertension
   3. Respiratory depression
   4. Hypothyroidism

9. A client who was being treated for severe diarrhea with opioid analgesics has recovered and is to be discharged. Which of the following instructions should the nurse include in the client's teaching plan?
   1. Avoid traveling
   2. Avoid alcohol
   3. Avoid exercising
   4. Avoid starchy food

10. Which of the following is considered the gold standard in pain management?
   1. Morphine sulfate
   2. Codeine
   3. Oxymorphone
   4. Hydrocodone

11. Which of the body systems does not adapt and compensate for the secondary effects of opioids?
   1. GI system
   2. Respiratory system
   3. Cardiovascular system
   4. Nervous system

12. Lactating females may use opioid analgesics, but they should wait how long after taking an opioid analgesic to breastfeed the infant?
   1. 2–4 hours
   2. 4–6 hours
   3. 6–8 hours
   4. 8–10 hours

13. The benefit of PCA postoperative medication includes which of the following? **Select all that apply.**
   1. Drug is delivered before pain happens.
   2. Client must wait for the nurse to administer.
   3. Ambulation occurs sooner.
   4. Less drug is used.

CHAPTER 16

Anesthetic Drugs

Learning Objectives

- State the uses of local anesthesia, methods of administration, and nursing responsibilities when administering a local anesthetic.
- Describe the purpose of a preanesthetic drug and the nursing responsibilities associated with the administration of a preanesthetic drug.
- Identify several drugs used for local, regional, conscious sedation, and general anesthesia.
- List and briefly describe the four stages of general anesthesia.
- Discuss important nursing responsibilities associated with caring for a client receiving a preanesthetic drug and during the postanesthesia care (recovery room) period.

SECTION I: ASSESSING YOUR UNDERSTANDING

Activity A FILL IN THE BLANKS

1. A _____ block is a type of regional anesthesia produced by injection of a numbing drug into or near a nerve trunk.

2. _____ anesthesia is the provision of a pain-free state for the entire body.

3. _____ is a loss of feeling or sensation.

4. A nurse _____ is a registered nurse with a master's degree and special training who is qualified to administer anesthetics.

5. An _____ is a physician with special training in administering anesthesia.

6. A preanesthetic drug that decreases secretions of the upper respiratory tract is called a _____ blocking drug.

Activity B SEQUENCING

1. Write the correct sequence of body reactions as general anesthesia is given and the client progresses through the four stages of anesthesia.

1. The client is ready for the surgical procedure to begin.

2. Respiratory arrest, and vital signs cease.

3. Muscles become rigid and sounds are exaggerated.

4. The client loses consciousness.

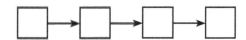

Activity C MATCHING

1. Match the various types of local anesthesia in Column A with their application in Column B.

Column A	Column B
___ 1. Spinal anesthesia	a. Injection of anesthetic around nerves
___ 2. General anesthesia	b. Application of the anesthetic to the surface of the skin
___ 3. Regional anesthesia	c. Injection of a local anesthetic drug into the subarachnoid space
___ 4. Topical anesthesia	d. Inhalation of gas for anesthesia

2. Match the drugs used for general anesthesia in Column A with their specific actions in Column B.

Column A

____ **1.** Lidocaine

____ **2.** Midazolam

____ **3.** Propofol

____ **4.** Ketamine

Column B

a. Used for surgical procedures that do not require the relaxation of skeletal muscles

b. Used for continuous sedation of intubated or respiratory-controlled clients in intensive care units

c. Used for conscious sedation before minor procedures

d. Used for local anesthesia of tissues for suturing

Activity D **SHORT ANSWERS**

A nurse is required to care for clients who are to be administered anesthesia. A number of nursing interventions are associated with the administration of anesthesia. Answer the following questions, which involve the nurse's role in managing such situations.

1. A nurse observes an abnormal laboratory test finding that was included in the client's chart shortly before surgery. What should be the nurse's immediate reaction?

_____

_____

2. What unique postoperative nursing intervention is carried out for a client with regional anesthesia?

_____

_____

3. What factors should a nurse be aware of that influence the choice of general or regional anesthesia?

_____

_____

Activity E **CROSSWORD PUZZLE**

Across

3. This type of anesthesia requires multiple drugs and stages to achieve a state where surgical procedures can be performed without pain, movement, or memory

5. The person whose responsibility it is to assist, maintain, and recover a client who has been given an anesthetic

6. This type of anesthesia includes topical, local infiltration, and regional pain relief

Down

1. A drug pertaining to status before administration of an anesthetic agent; it must be given on time

2. The term for the loss of feeling or sensation

4. Clients need this after general anesthesia

SECTION II: APPLYING YOUR KNOWLEDGE

Activity F CASE STUDY

Mr. Park, age 77 years, is admitted to the hospital to undergo surgery to his hip. He has no other chronic medical conditions besides his arthritis and is in good health. His only medication is Lortab 5/500 mg, and he is allergic to penicillin.

1. As the preoperative nurse, what are your responsibilities to Mr. Park?

_____

_____

_____

2. As part of preanesthesia, the physician has ordered Mr. Park to receive midazolam 5 mg, 45 minutes prior to surgery. Midazolam is available in a 1-mg/mL vial. How much would the nurse need to prepare to administer to the client? What should the nurse assess before administration of the medication?

_____

_____

_____

Now Map It Out! Use the templates provided in the appendix to add information and make client connections on a concept map.

Find the data indicating the cause of a surgical procedure. Include the preoperative sedative on Mr. Park's concept map. From your chapter readings and review of your concept map, can you tell why he is being given midazolam and not glycopyrrolate? Do you anticipate any potential problems from using this drug preoperatively in Mr. Park's case?

SECTION III: PRACTICING FOR NCLEX

Activity G NCLEX-STYLE QUESTIONS

Answer the following questions.

1. Which of the following stages of general anesthesia begins with a loss of consciousness?
   1. I
   2. II
   3. III
   4. IV

2. Which of the following effects of topical anesthesia should a nurse be aware of when caring for a client?
   1. Decreased anxiety and apprehension
   2. Desensitized skin or mucous membranes
   3. Loss of feeling in the lower extremities
   4. Cardiovascular stimulation

3. Which of the following should the nurse perform as postoperative interventions after the administration of anesthesia?
   1. Review client's laboratory test records.
   2. Administer a hypnotic agent to the client.
   3. Position the client to prevent aspiration of vomitus.
   4. Monitor client's blood pressure every 12 hours.

4. A client who is in the operating room is experiencing an increase in his respiratory secretions. The nurse knows that which of the following has occurred during the preanesthesia period?
   1. Client's anesthesia records were not reviewed.
   2. The drug was not administered on time.
   3. Client's respiratory status was not assessed.
   4. Client's IV lines were not well assessed.

5. A nurse is caring for a client who is to receive local anesthesia for the suturing of a wound. Which of the following interventions should the nurse perform when caring for this client? **Select all that apply.**
   1. Observe if there is any oozing.
   2. Apply dressing to the surgical areas.
   3. Observe the client for any signs of bleeding.
   4. Assess the client's pulse every 5–15 minutes.
   5. Exercise caution in administering opioids.

6. A nurse is assigned to care for a client who is to receive anesthesia. Which of the following should the nurse confirm to ensure that the use of preanesthetic drugs is not contraindicated in this client?
   1. Client is not older than 60 years.
   2. Client does not need anesthesia on their extremities.
   3. Client is not younger than 13 years.
   4. Client does not have a low body weight.

7. A pregnant client is admitted to an acute care facility for a C-section delivery. The primary health care provider decides to administer a transsacral block as anesthesia. What type of anesthetic is the transsacral block?
   1. Topical anesthesia
   2. Conduction block
   3. General anesthesia
   4. Spinal block

8. A nurse is assigned to care for a client who is to be administered local anesthesia. Which of the following should the nurse confirm to ensure that the use of epinephrine along with the local anesthesia is not contraindicated in the client?
   1. Client does not have anemia.
   2. Client does not have low blood pressure.
   3. Client is not older than 60 years.
   4. Client does not need anesthesia for their extremities.

9. Which of the following is an example of regional anesthesia?
   1. Spinal anesthesia
   2. Topical anesthesia
   3. Local infiltration anesthesia
   4. General anesthesia

10. Which type of anesthesia may be applied by the nurse with a cotton swab or sprayed on the area to be desensitized?
    1. Local infiltration anesthesia
    2. General anesthesia
    3. Topical anesthesia
    4. Conduction block anesthesia

11. Which type of anesthesia is commonly used for the suturing of small wounds?
    1. Local infiltration anesthesia
    2. General anesthesia
    3. Conduction block anesthesia
    4. Spinal anesthesia

12. A nurse may be asked to administer which of the following drugs prior to a colonoscopy in order to help the client relax?
    1. Midazolam
    2. Meperidine
    3. Lidocaine
    4. Fentanyl

Drugs That Affect the Central Nervous System

Central Nervous System Stimulants

- List the three classes of CNS stimulants.
- Explain the uses, general drug actions, general adverse reactions, contraindications, precautions, and interactions of CNS stimulants.
- Distinguish important preadministration and ongoing assessment activities the nurse should perform on the client taking a CNS stimulant.
- List nursing diagnoses particular to a client taking a CNS stimulant.
- Examine ways to promote an optimal response to drug therapy, how to manage common adverse drug reactions, and important points to keep in mind when educating clients about the use of CNS stimulants.

SECTION I: ASSESSING YOUR UNDERSTANDING

Activity A FILL IN THE BLANKS

1. Analeptics increase the depth of respirations by stimulating special receptors located in the _____ arteries and upper aorta.

2. Modafinil analeptic is used to treat _____.

3. Amphetamines are _____ drugs that stimulate the CNS.

4. The drug doxapram increases the respiratory rate by stimulating the _____.

5. When a CNS stimulant is administered with anesthetics, there is an increased risk of cardiac _____.

Activity B DOSAGE CALCULATION

1. A nurse working the night shift has been prescribed 200 mg of modafinil 1 hour before the shift starts. The available tablets are 100 mg each. How many tablets will the nurse take before going to work?

   _____

   _____

2. A client has been prescribed 0.5 mg/kg of doxapram to be administered intravenously for respiratory depression. The drug is available in 20-mg/mL vials. If the client weighs 80 kg, how many mL of the drug solution should be administered to the client?

   _____

   _____

3. A client has been prescribed 50 mg of atomoxetine once a day. The tablets are available in 25 mg each. How many tablets will the nurse teach the parent to administer to the client daily?

   _____

   _____

4. An adult client with ADHD has been prescribed a starting dose of 30 mg of lisdexamfetamine once daily. The available tablets are 20 mg each. How many tablets will the nurse instruct the client to take daily?

_____

_____

5. A client has been prescribed 35 mg of phendimetrazine three times daily, to be taken over a period of 6 days. The available tablets are 35 mg each. How many tablets will the nurse instruct the client to take each dose?

_____

_____

Activity C MATCHING

1. Match the drug in Column A with the likely interaction effect when combined with a CNS stimulant in Column B.

Column A

____ **1.** Anesthetics

____ **2.** Theophylline

____ **3.** Modafinil

Column B

a. Decreased effect of the oral contraceptive

b. Increased risk of cardiac arrhythmias

c. Increased risk of hyperactive behaviors

Activity D SHORT ANSWERS

A nurse's role in managing clients who are administered CNS stimulants involves understanding the effects of the drug and performing appropriate interventions depending on the type of drug administered. Answer the following questions, which involve the nurse's role in managing such situations.

1. A nurse caring for a postsurgical client receives an order for CNS stimulant treatment for respiratory depression. What are the nursing assessments and interventions while caring for a client with an ineffective breathing pattern who is being administered CNS stimulants?

_____

_____

_____

2. A nurse is teaching the family of a client with ADHD who is starting CNS stimulant treatment. What strategies should the nurse instruct the family to use for beginning therapy, dosing, and tracking results?

_____

_____

_____

Activity E WORD FIND PUZZLE

A	H	P	C	B	M	X	K
N	O	D	K	A	Z	P	N
A	M	X	A	P	N	E	A
L	B	H	D	K	P	O	R
E	U	P	H	O	R	I	C
P	A	Z	D	B	C	V	O
T	V	C	P	E	A	M	L
I	K	W	T	S	D	H	E
C	P	B	O	I	X	Z	P
O	D	M	C	T	V	B	S
H	A	P	K	Y	O	E	Y

Word Hints

1. A drug that stimulates the respiratory center of the brain

2. An intense feeling of excitement and happiness

3. Abbreviation for a disorder characterized by inattention, hyperactivity, and impulsivity

4. Chronic disorder that results in recurrent attacks of drowsiness and sleep during daytime

5. Stimulants are used to promote daytime wakefulness in obstructive sleep

_____

6. BMI over 30 kg/m²

7. Hyper _____

SECTION II: APPLYING YOUR KNOWLEDGE

Activity F CASE STUDY

 Alfredo Garcia was seen at the clinic regarding hypertension. As part of his care, the primary health care provider suggests weight reduction. Mr. Garcia expresses frustration over attempting to lose weight and always gaining it and more back. Mr. Garcia weighs 215 lb and is 5'6" tall. Access the Internet to find a BMI calculator.

1. Determine Mr. Garcia's BMI. Based on the guidelines in the Client Teaching for Improved Client Outcomes: Using Anorexiants for Weight Loss, is he a candidate to use a stimulant for weight reduction?

   _____

   _____

   _____

2. The nurse should review Mr. Garcia's MAR for which specific medications that may interact adversely with anorexiants?

   _____

   _____

   _____

Now Map It Out! Use the templates provided in the appendix to add information and make client connections on a concept map.

You have two new clients to map in Chapter 17 from the textbook and here in the study guide. Using the Drug Summary Tables, look at some of the drugs that may be recommended for both Mr. Garcia and his weight issues as well as Janna Wong's possible ADHD. Make a note of drug interactions and the drugs you already know these two clients are currently taking.

SECTION III: PRACTICING FOR NCLEX

Activity G NCLEX-STYLE QUESTIONS

Answer the following questions.

1. A nurse is caring for a client who is receiving CNS stimulants. Which of the following adverse reactions should the nurse monitor for in this client?
   1. Bradycardia
   2. Hyperactivity
   3. High blood pressure
   4. Elevated temperature

2. In which of the following clients are the use of CNS stimulants contraindicated?
   1. Liver disorders
   2. Acute ulcerative colitis
   3. Ventilation disorder
   4. Bone marrow suppression

3. Which of the following interventions should the nurse perform as part of the ongoing assessment after administering an analeptic?
   1. Send blood sample for a platelet count test.
   2. Check pulse rate and blood pressure every hour.
   3. Monitor consciousness levels every 5–15 minutes.
   4. Monitor respiratory rate for 5 minutes after administration.

4. Which is the best explanation for using a stimulant for hyperactive behavior?
   1. Hyperactive behavior stops when the pulse speeds up.
   2. The euphoric feeling makes hyperactivity lessen.
   3. Distracting neurotransmission is lessened.
   4. Norepinephrine is blocked and never put in the synapse.

5. CNS stimulants have been prescribed for a child with ADHD. Which of the following points should the nurse include in the teaching plan? **Select all that apply.**
   1. Monitor the child's eating patterns.
   2. Teach the parents the importance of preparing nutritious meals.
   3. Provide a light breakfast so that the child stays alert.
   4. Advise parents to give OTC sleeping pills in case of insomnia.
   5. Check the child's height and weight measurements to monitor growth.

6. A client is prescribed an anorexiant as part of obesity treatment. Which is the most important assessment the nurse should perform as part of the preadministration process?
   1. Record blood pressure
   2. Observe urinary output
   3. Measure weight
   4. Measure blood glucose

7. Which of the following structures make up the parts of the central nervous system (CNS)? **Select all that apply.**
   1. Brain
   2. Spinal cord
   3. Sensory nerve endings
   4. Autonomic nervous system

8. The analeptics are CNS stimulants that do which of the following? **Select all that apply.**
   1. Dilate coronary and peripheral blood vessels
   2. Improve flow in the limbic system of the brain
   3. Slow down the digestive system
   4. Stimulate the respiratory center of the brain
   5. Decrease function of the endocrine system

9. Anorexiants are primarily used for which purposes?
   1. Treat ADHD
   2. Suppress the appetite
   3. Suppress the cardiovascular system
   4. Stimulate the respiratory system

10. Which of the following medications is used to treat narcolepsy and does not cause cardiac and other systemic stimulatory effects like other CNS stimulants?
   1. Provigil
   2. Caffeine
   3. Dopram
   4. Focalin

11. Most anorexiants are classified in which pregnancy category?
   1. Category A
   2. Category B
   3. Category C
   4. Category X

12. Pediatric clients given atomoxetine (Strattera) should be monitored closely for which of the following?
   1. Suicidal ideation
   2. Hypertension
   3. Dyspnea
   4. Hyperglycemia

Antidementia Drugs

- Compare and contrast the clinical manifestations of Alzheimer disease (AD).
- Explain the uses, general drug actions, general adverse reactions, contraindications, precautions, and interactions associated with the administration of antidementia drugs.
- Distinguish important preadministration and ongoing assessment activities the nurse should perform with the client taking an antidementia drug.
- List nursing diagnoses particular to a client taking an antidementia drug.
- Examine ways to promote an optimal response to therapy, how to manage common adverse reactions, and important points to keep in mind when educating clients about the use of antidementia drugs.

SECTION I ASSESSING YOUR UNDERSTANDING

Activity A FILL IN THE BLANKS

1. Dementia is a major issue in _____ disease.

2. Acetylcholine is a transmitter in the _____ neuropathway.

3. Antidementia drugs slow the progression of but do not cure _____.

4. In Alzheimer disease, specific pathologic changes occur in the cortex of the _____.

5. Antidementia drugs are not used to treat acute confusion, also known as _____.

Activity B DOSAGE CALCULATION

1. A client with dementia in a memory care unit is prescribed 15 mg of donepezil per day. Donepezil is available in the form of 10-mg tablets. How many tablets will the nurse have to administer to the client in each dose?

   _____

   _____

2. The caregiver of a client with dementia is going on vacation. She is setting up a medication box and wants to be sure there is enough medicine at home while she is gone. Memantine is supplied in 10-mg tablets and the daily dose of memantine is 20 mg. How many tablets does she need to load into the medication box for a 10-day period?

   _____

   _____

3. A client with dementia comes to respite care with a container of rivastigmine for administration. The caregiver is exhausted and says there is a total of 18 mg of rivastigmine for the client and it is to be administered over the next 3 days. The drug is to be given twice a day. The rivastigmine is supplied in 1.5-mg capsules. As the nurse attempts to reconcile the medication, determine the dose prescribed for the client.

   _____

   _____

4. Rivastigmine comes in a transdermal patch which is changed every 3 days. Patch 1 delivers 4.6 mg/24 hours or 9 mg total. Patch 2 delivers 9.5 mg/24 hours or 18 mg total. If the primary health care provider decides to order a transdermal patch in place of oral medications for the client in the aforementioned question, which patch should be chosen?

_____

_____

Activity C MATCHING

1. Match the antidementia drugs given in Column A with the corresponding adverse reactions given in Column B.

Column A

___ **1.** Donepezil

___ **2.** Memantine

___ **3.** Rivastigmine

___ **4.** Galantamine

Column B

a. Vomiting

b. Dyspepsia

c. Confusion

d. Muscle cramps

2. Match the drugs that interact adversely with an antidementia drug in Column A with their common uses in Column B.

Column A

___ **1.** Anticholinergics

___ **2.** Nonsteroidal anti-inflammatory drugs

___ **3.** Theophylline

Column B

a. Breathing problem

b. Decrease of bodily secretions

c. Pain relief

Activity D SHORT ANSWERS

A nurse's role in managing clients who are being administered antidementia drugs involves assessing and implementing interventions that aid in their support and monitoring the clients for the occurrences of adverse reactions of the drug administration. Answer the following questions, which involve the nurse's role in the management of such situations.

1. A client is administered an antidementia drug for treating mild to moderate dementia of Alzheimer disease. What preadministration assessments should the nurse perform in clients who are prescribed antidementia drugs?

_____

_____

2. The combination of disease factors and type of drug administered can make meals less appealing to the client. What are some interventions a nurse should perform to maximize appetite and support the client at mealtimes?

_____

_____

Activity E CROSSWORD PUZZLE

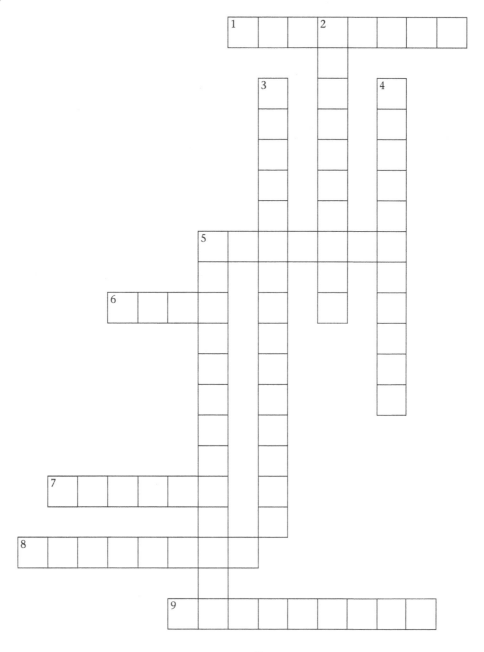

Across

1. An acute, temporary state of mental confusion
5. The type of protein plaques that tangle in nerve tissue
6. Abbreviation for screening test for cognition
7. Herb used for promoting memory
8. Progressive decrease in cognitive function
9. Generic name for the drug Namenda

Down

2. Cholinesterase, a class of drugs that delays the breakdown of acetylcholine
3. The branch of the autonomic nervous system concerned with conserving body energy
4. Medication delivery system that involves the skin
5. The neurotransmitter that transmits impulses across the parasympathetic branch of the autonomic nervous system

SECTION II APPLYING YOUR KNOWLEDGE

Activity F CASE STUDY

 Mrs. Moore is an 85-year-old Caucasian female. She seems forgetful and confused at times. Her son calls the clinic concerned about his mother. He is fearful that if she is diagnosed with Alzheimer disease he could catch it too. Using the guidelines presented in the textbook, answer the following questions.

1. Explain the stages for Alzheimer disease.

   _____

   _____

2. The physician writes Mrs. Moore a prescription for donepezil (Aricept) 5 mg daily. What adverse effects should the nurse review with her son?

   _____

   _____

Now Map It Out! Use the templates provided in the appendix to add information and make client connections on a concept map.

Using information regarding prescriptions for Mrs. Moore's symptoms of dementia, map out the symptoms, medication prescribed, adverse reactions, and subsequent findings when she presented for an x-ray examination. Can you cross-link any of the mapping data for this case study?

SECTION III PRACTICING FOR NCLEX

Activity G NCLEX-STYLE QUESTIONS

Answer the following questions.

1. A client is prescribed antidementia drugs for the treatment of dementia. Which of the following adverse reactions should the nurse monitor for in the client?
   1. Diarrhea
   2. High blood pressure
   3. Seizure disorders
   4. Renal dysfunction

2. Clients with Alzheimer disease are prescribed cholinesterase inhibitors so as to slow the progression of dementia. What causes the dementia?
   1. Low levels of acetylcholine
   2. Diabetes mellitus
   3. Too much iron in the diet
   4. Bladder obstruction

3. Other than the mental changes, which body system is most disrupted by adverse reactions of antidementia drugs or the disease process of dementia?
   1. Cardiovascular system
   2. Musculoskeletal system
   3. Genitourinary system
   4. Gastrointestinal system

4. A nurse is caring for a client with dementia of Alzheimer disease. Which of the following is an effect of the interaction of nonsteroidal anti-inflammatory drugs with cholinesterase inhibitors?
   1. Asthma
   2. Sick sinus syndrome
   3. Increased risk of GI bleeding
   4. Increased risk of theophylline toxicity

5. A client with a history of ulcer disease is administered a cholinesterase inhibitor for treating Alzheimer disease. Which of the following conditions should the nurse monitor for when caring for the client?
   1. Bleeding
   2. Respiratory distress
   3. Jaundice
   4. Goiter

6. A nurse is caring for a client receiving antidementia drugs. The drug is known to cause the adverse reactions of dizziness and syncope that can place the client at risk for injury. Which of the following interventions should the nurse implement in order to reduce the risk of injury? **Select all that apply.**
   1. Use physical restraints.
   2. Monitor client every 12 hours.
   3. Keep bed in low position.
   4. Use soft bedding.
   5. Use night lights.

7. Ginkgo, one of the oldest herbs in the world, is thought to improve memory and brain function and to enhance circulation to the brain, heart, limbs, and eyes. In which of the following clients is the use of ginkgo contraindicated?
   1. Clients receiving MAOI antidepressants
   2. Clients receiving sedatives and hypnotics
   3. Clients receiving opioid analgesics
   4. Clients receiving anticholinergic drugs

8. A nurse is caring for a client receiving antidementia drugs for the treatment of Alzheimer disease. Why is it important for the nurse to pay proper attention to the dosing of medication?
   1. Helps to decrease the adverse GI reactions
   2. Helps the client to recover faster
   3. Helps the client to maintain normal temperature
   4. Helps to decrease variations in the pulse rate

9. NMDA receptor antagonists are utilized for the treatment of which of the following medical conditions?
   1. Myasthenia gravis
   2. Alzheimer disease
   3. Glaucoma
   4. Urinary retention

10. Which of the following is a cholinesterase inhibitor available in a transdermal patch for drug administration?
    1. Memantine (Namenda)
    2. Rivastigmine (Exelon)
    3. Donepezil (Aricept)
    4. Galantamine (Razadyne)

11. People fearful of having memory problems may take which of the following herbal products, which has been used to improve mental performance?
    1. Ginkgo
    2. Garlic
    3. Kava
    4. Willow bark

12. New staging is proposed for Alzheimer disease, in which mild cognitive impairment (MCI) defines stage 2. Which of the following is involved in MCI?
    1. Changes in thinking are noted by strangers.
    2. Other causes of memory loss are ruled out.
    3. Functional ability declines significantly.
    4. Anxiety is not a factor in the illness progression.

CHAPTER 19

Antianxiety Drugs

- Explain the uses, general drug actions, general adverse reactions, contraindications, precautions, and interactions associated with the administration of antianxiety drugs.
- Distinguish important preadministration and ongoing assessment activities the nurse should perform on the client taking an antianxiety drug.
- List nursing diagnoses particular to a client taking an antianxiety drug.
- Examine ways to promote an optimal response to therapy, how to manage common adverse reactions, and important points to keep in mind when educating clients about the use of antianxiety drugs.

SECTION I: ASSESSING YOUR UNDERSTANDING

Activity A FILL IN THE BLANKS

1. Drugs used to treat anxiety are called _____.

2. Anxiety is a _____ feeling, yet as anxiety increases it can interfere with day-to-day functioning.

3. Psychiatric anxiety disorders (that need long-term treatment) use _____ for treatment instead of antianxiety drugs.

4. _____ administration is indicated primarily in acute states when it is difficult to have the client take the medication by mouth.

5. _____ symptoms occur if benzodiazepines are taken for more than 3 months and discontinued abruptly.

Activity B DOSAGE CALCULATION

1. A client is prescribed 0.25 mg of alprazolam orally three times a day. The drug is available in 0.5-mg tablets. How many tablets should the nurse administer to the client for each dose?

   _____

   _____

2. A client is prescribed 30 mg of oxazepam orally four times a day around the clock. At what interval should the nurse administer the drug, which is available in 15-mg tablets?

   _____

   _____

3. A client is prescribed 15 mg of Buspar daily. The tablet is available in 5-mg doses. How many tablets are needed to meet the daily dose?

   _____

   _____

4. A primary health care provider prescribes 25 mg of chlordiazepoxide orally four times a day for a client. The drug is available in 10-mg tablets. How many tablets will the nurse administer to the client in each dose?

   _____

   _____

5. A primary health care provider prescribes 5 mg of clonazepam every 12 hours for the first 3 days. How many milligrams of the drug would the nurse administer to the client over 3 days?

_____

_____

Activity C MATCHING

1. Match the drug in Column A with the likely interaction effect when combined with an antianxiety drug in Column B.

Column A

____ **1.** Alcohol

____ **2.** Digoxin

____ **3.** Antipsychotic

____ **4.** Analgesic

Column B

a. Increased risk for central nervous system (CNS) depression

b. Increased risk for convulsions

c. Increased risk for digitalis toxicity

d. Increased risk for sedation and respiratory depression

2. Match the drugs in Column A with their actions in Column B.

Column A

____ **1.** Buspirone

____ **2.** Hydroxyzine

____ **3.** Chlordiazepoxide

Column B

a. Acts on the hypothalamus

b. Acts by enhancing the actions of a natural brain chemical GABA (gamma [γ]-aminobutyric acid)

c. Acts on the brain's serotonin receptors

Activity D SHORT ANSWERS

A nurse's role in managing clients who are being administered antianxiety drugs involves monitoring the clients and implementing interventions that aid in their recovery. Answer the following questions, which involve the nurse's role in managing such situations.

1. A client with anxiety has been prescribed alprazolam. What should the nurse assess for in this client before administering the first dose of alprazolam?

_____

_____

2. A client receiving alprazolam complains of constipation. What interventions should the nurse perform to ensure the client's well-being?

_____

_____

Activity E CROSSWORD PUZZLE

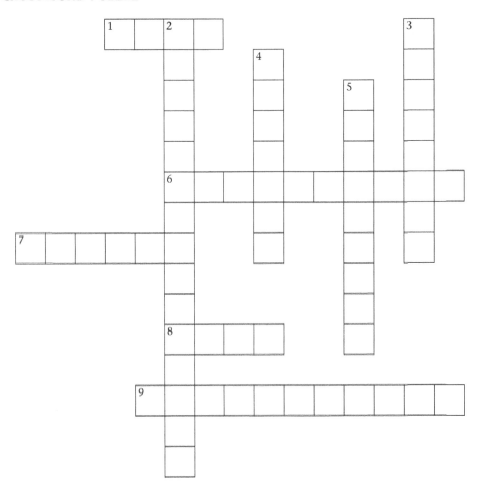

Across

1. Abbreviation of the neurotransmitter inhibitor that is involved in the regulation of sleep and anxiety.
6. A psychological compulsion or craving to use a substance to obtain a pleasurable experience.
7. An unsteady gait; muscular incoordination.
8. Abbreviation for a mental health condition triggered by a terrifying event.
9. Another term for antianxiety drugs.

Down

2. The primary class of antianxiety drugs.
3. A dependence where negative body withdrawal symptoms result from abrupt discontinuation.
4. A feeling of apprehension, worry, or uneasiness.
5. Response to a drug requiring increasingly larger dosages to obtain the desired effect.

SECTION II: APPLYING YOUR KNOWLEDGE

Activity F CASE STUDY

 Mrs. Moore is an 85-year-old woman. Due to worsening dementia, she is often agitated. The physician has written an order for Mrs. Moore to receive lorazepam (Ativan) 0.5 mg TID PRN.

1. What are some things to consider as the nurse caring for Mrs. Moore with regard to the lorazepam?

_____

_____

_____

2. What should the nurse's ongoing assessment consist of for Mrs. Moore?

_____

_____

_____

Now Map It Out! Use the templates provided in the appendix to add information and make client connections on a concept map.

Using information regarding prescriptions for Mrs. Moore's symptoms of dementia and agitation, map out the symptoms, medication prescribed, and adverse reactions. Are there any drug–drug interactions that you should be concerned about?

SECTION III: PRACTICING FOR NCLEX

Activity G NCLEX-STYLE QUESTIONS

Answer the following questions.

1. A nurse is caring for a client who is receiving antianxiety drugs. Which of the following is an adverse reaction the nurse should monitor the client for?
   1. Seizures
   2. Diarrhea
   3. Abdominal cramps
   4. Bradycardia

2. A client prescribed digoxin for cardiac problems is prescribed diazepam for an anxiety event. Which of the following drug interactions should the nurse monitor for in the client?
   1. Increased risk for central nervous system depression
   2. Increased risk for respiratory depression
   3. Increased risk for sedation
   4. Increased risk for digitalis toxicity

3. The primary health care provider has diagnosed a client with anxiety due to withdrawal from alcohol. Which of the following should the nurse relate to alcohol withdrawal?
   1. Diarrhea
   2. Acute panic
   3. Dry mouth
   4. Lightheadedness

4. A nurse is caring for a client with anxiety. The client is to be administered lorazepam. Which of the following is a contraindication for lorazepam administration?
   1. Younger than 25 years
   2. Lactation
   3. Anxiety
   4. Parkinson disease

5. A client being treated for anxiety is to be discharged. Which of the following instructions should the nurse include in the client's teaching plan?
   1. Avoid sunlight
   2. Avoid alcohol
   3. Avoid yogurt
   4. Avoid sour cream

6. A nurse is assigned to care for an older, agitated client who will be administered IM doxepin. Which of the following safety measures should the nurse take while administering the IM doxepin?
   1. Administer the drug intramuscularly on the gluteus muscle.
   2. Monitor for hearing or kidney problems.
   3. Administer the drug intramuscularly on the arms.
   4. Monitor for secondary bacterial or fungal infections.

7. A client on alprazolam therapy has discontinued treatment for a week. Which of the following is a withdrawal symptom the nurse should monitor the client for?
   1. Diarrhea
   2. Dizziness
   3. Metallic taste
   4. Dry mouth

8. Antianxiety drugs are also referred to as which of the following?
   1. Anxiolytics
   2. Opioids
   3. NSAIDs
   4. Anesthetics

9. Which of the following is the best way to approach a client with ineffective coping?
   1. "You are not still feeling anxious, are you?"
   2. "You need to take all your meds to feel better."
   3. "Tell me about your day?"
   4. "Are you starting to drink again?"

10. Which of the following exerts its anxiolytic effect by acting on the brain's serotonin receptors?
    1. Buspirone (Buspar)
    2. Lorazepam (Ativan)
    3. Doxepin (Sinequan)
    4. Hydroxyzine (Vistaril)

11. Which of the following exerts its anxiolytic effect by acting on the hypothalamus and brainstem reticular formation?
    1. Buspirone (Buspar)
    2. Doxepin (Sinequan)
    3. Hydroxyzine (Vistaril)
    4. Diazepam (Valium)

12. How early can benzodiazepine withdrawal occur in a client?
    1. 7 days
    2. 12 hours
    3. 1 day
    4. 2 months

Sedatives and Hypnotics

Learning Objectives

- Differentiate between a sedative and a hypnotic.
- Explain the uses, general drug actions, adverse reactions, contraindications, precautions, and interactions of sedatives and hypnotics.
- Distinguish important preadministration and ongoing assessment activities the nurse should perform with the client taking a sedative or hypnotic.
- List nursing diagnoses particular to a client taking a sedative or hypnotic.
- Examine ways to promote an optimal response to therapy, how to manage common adverse reactions, and important points to keep in mind when educating clients about the use of sedatives or hypnotics.

SECTION I: ASSESSING YOUR UNDERSTANDING

Activity A FILL IN THE BLANKS

1. Sleep deprivation may interfere with the _____ process of a client.

2. Sedatives and hypnotics are primarily used to treat _____.

3. A _____ is a drug that induces drowsiness or sleep.

4. Drinking beverages containing caffeine contributes to _____.

5. _____ is a hormone produced by the pineal gland in the brain.

6. A _____ is a drug that produces a relaxing, calming effect.

Activity B DOSAGE CALCULATION

1. A client is prescribed 0.5 mg of triazolam (Halcion) twice a day. Triazolam is available in 1-mg tablets. How many tablets in total will the client take each day?

   _____

   _____

2. A client is prescribed 15 mg of temazepam per day. The available tablet of temazepam contains 5 mg of the drug. How many tablets will the nurse have to administer to the client in each dose?

   _____

   _____

3. A client is prescribed 10 mg of zaleplon at bedtime. The available zaleplon tablet contains 5 mg of the drug. How many tablets of zaleplon will the nurse have to administer to the client?

   _____

   _____

4. A client is prescribed 2 mg of estazolam orally at bedtime. Estazolam is available in the form of 1-mg tablets. How many tablets will the nurse have to administer to the client?

_____

_____

5. A client is prescribed 10 mg of zolpidem orally at bedtime. Zolpidem is available in 10-mg tablets. How many tablets of the drug will the nurse have to administer to the client?

_____

_____

Activity C MATCHING

1. Match the types of drugs in Column A with their common uses in Column B.

Column A

____ 1. Antidepressants

____ 2. Opioid analgesics

____ 3. Antihistamines

____ 4. Phenothiazines

____ 5. Cimetidine

Column B

a. Pain relief

b. Management of gastric upset

c. Management of depression

d. Relief of allergy symptoms

e. Management of agitation and psychotic symptoms

2. Match the key terms in Column A with their definitions in Column B.

Column A

____ 1. Ataxia

____ 2. Hypnotics

____ 3. Sedatives

Column B

a. Produce a relaxing, calming effect

b. Unsteady gait

c. Induce drowsiness or sleep

Activity D SHORT ANSWERS

A nurse's role in managing clients who are being administered sedative and hypnotic drugs involves monitoring clients and implementing interventions that aid in their recovery. Answer the following questions, which involve the nurse's role in managing such situations.

1. A client is prescribed a sedative. What assessments should the nurse perform before administering the drug?

_____

_____

2. List nursing diagnoses specific to a client taking a sedative or hypnotic.

_____

_____

Activity E WORD FIND PUZZLE

Find the word INSOMNIA and the seven words causing it hidden in the puzzle.

Z	I	D	A	R	L	Q	O
B	N	E	W	J	O	B	C
T	S	Y	Q	V	D	A	H
R	O	T	L	Z	W	H	E
Q	M	L	R	J	O	T	A
A	N	X	I	E	T	Y	D
L	I	O	D	T	S	Z	A
P	A	I	N	L	D	S	C
W	O	Z	R	A	T	L	H
C	H	A	N	G	E	S	E

SECTION II: APPLYING YOUR KNOWLEDGE

Activity F **CASE STUDY**

 Lillian Chase is a 36-year-old woman. She presents to the clinic with a chief complaint of insomnia. The primary health care provider writes Lillian a prescription for temazepam (Restoril) 15 mg at bedtime as needed for sleep.

1. Is temazepam (Restoril) a sedative or a hypnotic?

   _____

   _____

   _____

2. What is the difference between a sedative and a hypnotic?

   _____

   _____

   _____

Now Map It Out! Use the templates provided in the appendix to add information and make client connections on a concept map.

Two clients, Mr. Phillip and Ms. Chase, have been prescribed sleeping aids. After you read the case study in Chapter 21 (the next chapter) of the textbook, map out symptoms and look at each of the concept maps. Are there any contraindications at this time for these medications? How should prescribing practices be different for these two clients?

SECTION III: PRACTICING FOR NCLEX

Activity G **NCLEX-STYLE QUESTIONS**

Answer the following questions.

1. A nurse is caring for a client who has been administered hypnotics for insomnia. Which of the following is a criterion for evaluating the effectiveness of the treatment?
   1. Decreased level of consciousness
   2. Normal respiration rate
   3. Improved sleep pattern
   4. Decrease in restlessness

2. A client in an acute care facility has convulsions and is prescribed a sedative. Which of the following should the nurse record before administration of the drug?
   1. Platelet count
   2. Blood pressure
   3. Hematocrit
   4. Blood sugar

3. A nurse is caring for a client who is to undergo surgery. The client is prescribed preoperative sedation. For which adverse reactions should the nurse monitor this client?
   1. Nausea
   2. Headache
   3. Restlessness
   4. Anxiety

4. Which of the following client conditions should alert the nurse to use sedatives and hypnotics cautiously?
   1. Hearing impairment
   2. Hyperglycemia
   3. Glucose intolerance
   4. Renal impairment

5. A nurse is caring for a client who has been prescribed a nonbenzodiazepine as a temporary sleep aid. How soon does the body build a tolerance to these drugs?
   1. 3 days
   2. 2 weeks
   3. 1 month
   4. 2 years

6. How many people in the United States are affected by sleep/wake disturbances?
   1. 700,000
   2. 4.5 million
   3. 40 million
   4. 3 billion

7. Bedtime snacks high in fat should not be served to clients taking which of the following drugs? **Select all that apply.**
   1. Triazolam
   2. Eszopiclone
   3. Zaleplon
   4. Ramelteon

8. A client is seen at the clinic with insomnia related to chronic headache. The client is prescribed a sedative. Which of the following are benefits of sedatives? **Select all that apply.**
   1. Relaxing effect
   2. Nausea
   3. Calming effect
   4. Dizziness
   5. Drowsiness

9. Sedatives and hypnotics are used to primarily treat which of the following?
   1. Insomnia
   2. Anxiety
   3. Hypertension
   4. Depression

10. Grapefruit juice should not be served to clients taking which of the following drugs? **Select all that apply.**
    1. Triazolam
    2. Temazepam
    3. Zaleplon
    4. Ramelteon

11. In which client would you most likely prescribe a sedative to produce sleep instead of a hypnotic?
    1. 14-year-old girl
    2. 35-year-old man
    3. 45-year-old obese woman
    4. 72-year-old man

12. Benzodiazepines are classified in which pregnancy category?
    1. Category A
    2. Category X
    3. Category B
    4. Category C

Antidepressant Drugs

- Define depression and identify symptoms of a major depressive disorder (MDD).
- Compare and contrast the different types of antidepressant drugs.
- Explain the uses, general drug actions, general adverse reactions, contraindications, precautions, and interactions of the antidepressant drugs.
- Distinguish important preadministration and ongoing assessment activities that the nurse should perform on the client taking an antidepressant drug.
- List nursing diagnoses particular to a client taking an antidepressant drug.
- Examine ways to promote an optimal response to therapy, how to manage common adverse reactions, and important points to keep in mind when educating clients about the use of antidepressant drugs.

SECTION I: ASSESSING YOUR UNDERSTANDING

Activity A FILL IN THE BLANKS

1. _____ is used with antidepressants in treating major depressive disorders.

2. _____ of a depressive mood is when a person is at the greatest risk for self-harm.

3. Clinical depression is characterized by a dysphoric mood lasting at least _____ _____.

4. Older men with prostatic enlargement are at increased risk for urinary retention when they take _____ antidepressants.

5. The therapeutic effects of the antidepressants may take _____ to _____ weeks to be seen.

Activity B DOSAGE CALCULATION

1. A primary health care provider prescribes 150 mg of amitriptyline per day for a client. The available tablets are 50 mg. How many tablets should the nurse administer to the client daily?

   _____

   _____

2. A client is prescribed 50 mg of amoxapine three times a day. The drug is available in 25-mg tablets. How many tablets should the nurse administer to the client for each dose?

   _____

   _____

3. A client is prescribed 60 mg of duloxetine (Cymbalta) daily. The available capsules contain 30 mg of duloxetine. How many capsules are needed each day to meet the prescribed drug dosage?

   _____

   _____

4. A client is prescribed 20 mg of citalopram (Celexa) a day. The drug is available in 20-mg tablets. How many tablets should the client take each evening?

_____

_____

5. A primary health care provider has prescribed paroxetine 20 mg/day for a client. The client is given all medications via a gastro tube. The available oral solution is paroxetine 10 mg/5 mL. How many mL should the nurse administer to the client daily?

_____

_____

6. A client has been prescribed 60 mg of fluoxetine (Prozac) per day to be administered once in the morning. The drug is available in 20-mg tablets. How many tablets should the nurse administer to the client daily?

_____

_____

Activity C OUT IN THE COMMUNITY

Older adults are sometimes overlooked for depression assessment. Depression is infrequently discussed because of an association with the stigma of mental illness. To be good clinical practitioners, we need to practice asking about depressive mood. In this activity, you will find a depression assessment tool and practice asking the associated questions.

Class question: *Do we overlook geriatric clients for depressive symptoms?*

Activity

1. Go to your computer and search for "geriatric depression assessment scale." How many do you find?

2. You want to find a simple tool. Looking at a couple of the tools found, note how many questions you are required to ask the client. Write that down now.

3. Download an easy-to-use tool, take it to the clinic, and try interviewing a client. Was it hard to use?

Report the following in your class discussion:

1. How many tools did you find on the Internet to assess for depression?

2. Did the client have trouble answering the questions? Was it easy to assess for depression?

Activity D SHORT ANSWERS

A nurse's role in administering antidepressant drugs involves assisting clients in managing the common adverse reactions of the drugs. The nurse also educates clients about the use of these drugs. Answer the following questions, which involve the nurse's role in managing such situations.

1. How is clinical depression treated?

_____

_____

_____

2. What are the different types of antidepressants? Which are most commonly used?

_____

_____

_____

3. How do antidepressants affect neurotransmission?

_____

_____

_____

Activity E SUDOKU PUZZLE

Complete the puzzle with abbreviations for antidepressants and neurotransmitters.

			CNS		SNRI			
	SSRI			MAOI		SNRI	TCA	CNS
	SNRI		SERO	SSRI		MAOI		DNRI
SERO	DNRI	EPI	SNRI	DOPA		TCA		MAOI
SNRI				CNS				DOPA
CNS		MAOI		TCA		DNRI	SNRI	SSRI
TCA		DNRI		EPI	DOPA		MAOI	
MAOI	CNS	SNRI		SERO			DOPA	
			MAOI		CNS			

SECTION II: APPLYING YOUR KNOWLEDGE

Activity F CASE STUDY

 Jane Smith is the daughter of Betty Peterson; she is 27 years of age. She presents to the primary health care provider's office for follow-up after giving birth to her first child 6 weeks ago. The triage nurse notices that Mrs. Smith has a monotonous speech pattern and is slow to answer questions.

1. The nurse suspects Mrs. Smith might be depressed. What are other symptoms of depression that the nurse should attempt to identify?

_____

_____

2. The primary health care provider diagnoses Mrs. Smith with depression and gives her a prescription for escitalopram (Lexapro) 10 mg daily. What information should be included in the nurse's teaching plan for educating Mrs. Smith about her medication?

_____

_____

Now Map It Out! Use the templates provided in the appendix to add information and make client connections on a concept map.

Mrs. Smith is concerned about taking a drug for depression after witnessing her mother, Betty, and the adverse reactions she experienced on antidepressants. When asked Betty Peterson states she has been taking an antidepressant almost since Jane was born. The drug prescribed for her is amitriptyline. Add this new data to Betty's concept map. Does it help explain any reactions you have read about in Betty's care?

SECTION III: PRACTICING FOR NCLEX

Activity G NCLEX-STYLE QUESTIONS

Answer the following questions.

1. A nurse is caring for a client who is prescribed a tricyclic antidepressant drug for depression. Which of the following is a common adverse reaction to the drug?
   1. Photosensitivity
   2. Hypertensive episodes
   3. Severe convulsions
   4. Nervous system depression

2. A client undergoing antidepressant therapy calls a local health care facility. They heard on TV that if an antidepressant is taken one should not be eating grapefruit. Which of the following drugs should the nurse screen the client for that grapefruit is contraindicated?
   1. Duloxetine
   2. Sertraline
   3. Venlafaxine
   4. Bupropion

3. A nurse is caring for a client undergoing antidepressant therapy. The client is also prescribed warfarin for circulatory disorders. For which of the following risks should the nurse monitor the client?
   1. Increased risk for bleeding
   2. Increased risk for hypotension
   3. Increased anticholinergic symptoms
   4. Increased risk for nervous system depression

4. A nurse is caring for a client with major depressive disorder and bulimia nervosa. The client is prescribed fluoxetine, a selective serotonin reuptake inhibitor (SSRI). Which of the following is a typical adverse reaction of this type of drug for which the nurse should monitor the client?
   1. Vertigo
   2. Blurred vision
   3. Somnolence
   4. Tremor

5. A client under treatment with monoamine oxidase inhibitor (MAOI) antidepressants shows symptoms including a headache followed by a sore neck, nausea, vomiting, sweating, fever, chest pain, dilated pupils, and bradycardia indicative of hypertensive crisis. Which of the following factors needs immediate attention?
   1. Blood pressure
   2. Blood sugar
   3. Temperature
   4. Respiration rate

6. A nurse is preparing a client to see the primary health care provider regarding depressed mood in the community mental health clinic. Which of the following activities should the nurse perform as part of the preadministration assessment? **Select all that apply.**
   1. Obtain a complete medical history.
   2. Obtain blood pressure measurements.
   3. Obtain a complete blood count.
   4. Obtain blood sugar levels.
   5. Obtain pulse and respiratory rate.

7. A nurse is caring for a client receiving MAOI antidepressants. The nurse instructs the client to avoid foods containing tyramine. Which of the following is the result of tyramine interacting with an MAOI antidepressant?
   1. Blurred vision
   2. Hypertensive crisis
   3. Orthostatic hypotension
   4. Photosensitivity

8. A nurse is caring for a client undergoing antidepressant therapy. The nurse observes the client showing signs of orthostatic hypotension. What intervention should the nurse perform in this case?
   1. Instruct the client to change positions slowly.
   2. Instruct the client to drink plenty of fluids.
   3. Monitor the client for hyperglycemia.
   4. Monitor the client's vital signs frequently.

9. A nurse is caring for a client who has been prescribed fluoxetine. When is the best time to administer an SSRI?
   1. At bedtime
   2. With dinner
   3. In the morning
   4. With lunch

10. Anticholinergic effects such as dry mouth, sedation, and urinary retention are common adverse events occurring with the use of which of the following classes of antidepressants?
    1. Tricyclic antidepressants
    2. SSRIs
    3. MAOIs
    4. Serotonin norepinephrine reuptake inhibitors

11. Which of the following drugs exerts its effect by inhibiting the activity of monoamine oxidase, leading to increases in epinephrine, norepinephrine, dopamine, and serotonin?
    1. Sertraline (Zoloft)
    2. Amitriptyline
    3. Bupropion (Wellbutrin)
    4. Phenelzine (Nardil)

12. Which of the following antidepressants should not be used with the smoking cessation products?
    1. Bupropion (Wellbutrin)
    2. Sertraline (Zoloft)
    3. Phenelzine (Nardil)
    4. Amitriptyline

Antipsychotic Drugs

Learning Objectives

- Explain the uses, general drug actions, general adverse reactions, contraindications, precautions, and interactions associated with the administration of antipsychotic drugs.
- Distinguish important preadministration and ongoing assessment activities the nurse should perform on the client taking an antipsychotic drug.
- List nursing diagnoses for a client taking an antipsychotic drug.
- Examine ways to promote an optimal response to therapy, how to manage common adverse reactions, and important points to keep in mind when educating clients about the use of antipsychotic drugs.

SECTION I: ASSESSING YOUR UNDERSTANDING

Activity A FILL IN THE BLANKS

1. The term _____ refers to a spectrum of disorders that affect mood and behavior.

2. Antipsychotic drugs are thought to act by inhibiting or blocking the release of the neurotransmitter _____ in the brain.

3. Atypical or second-generation antipsychotics act upon _____ receptors as well as the dopamine receptors in the brain.

4. _____ affect is the absence of an emotional response to any situation or condition.

5. The term _____ syndrome refers to a group of adverse reactions occurring in the extrapyramidal portion of the nervous system as a result of antipsychotic drugs.

Activity B DOSAGE CALCULATION

1. A primary health care provider prescribes 4 mg of risperidone daily for a client with psychiatric disorders. Risperidone is available in 4-mg tablets. How many tablets will the nurse administer to the client?

_____

_____

2. An inpatient client refuses to take their risperidone. The nurse calls the primary health care provider, who prescribes a dose of risperidone 8 mg to be given now. The injectable drug suspension comes in a dose of 12.5 mg/2 mL. How many mL should the nurse administer to the client?

_____

_____

3. A primary health care provider prescribes a total of 80 mg of ziprasidone (Geodon) per day in two divided doses for a client having manic episodes of bipolar disorder as well as psychosis. The available ziprasidone capsule is 40 mg. How many capsules will the nurse administer to the client in each dose?

_____

_____

4. A primary health care provider prescribes 15 mg of aripiprazole (Abilify) daily for a manic client whose mouth has been wired shut after repair of the jaw following a fight. Aripiprazole is available as an oral solution of 1 mg/mL. How many mL should the nurse administer the client in a single dose?

_____

_____

5. A primary health care provider prescribes 5 mg of thiothixene (Navane) two times a day for a client with psychosis. Navane is available in 5-mg capsules. How many capsules will the nurse administer to the client in each dose?

_____

_____

Activity C MATCHING

1. Match the drugs in Column A with the likely interaction effect when combined with an antipsychotic in Column B.

Column A

____ **1.** Anticholinergic drugs

____ **2.** Immunologic drugs

____ **3.** Antacids

____ **4.** Loop diuretics

Column B

a. Decreased effectiveness of lithium

b. Increased risk for TD and psychotic symptoms

c. Increased risk for lithium toxicity

d. Increased severity of bone marrow suppression

2. Match the conditions in Column A with their manifestations in Column B.

Column A

____ **1.** Hallucinations

____ **2.** Delusions

____ **3.** Flattened affect

____ **4.** Anhedonia

Column B

a. False beliefs that cannot be changed with reason

b. Finding no pleasure in activities that are normally pleasurable

c. False perceptions having no basis in reality

d. Absence of an emotional response to any situation or condition

Activity D SHORT ANSWERS

A nurse's role in managing clients being administered antipsychotic drugs involves monitoring and performing interventions for serious manifestations of acute psychosis. Answer the following questions, which involve the nurse's role in managing such situations.

1. What should a nurse assess for in the client before administering the first dose of an antipsychotic drug?

_____

_____

_____

2. A client receiving an antipsychotic is showing signs of escalating aggressiveness. What nursing interventions should be performed for the client who is given a parenteral injection of an antipsychotic drug?

_____

_____

_____

Activity E **CROSSWORD PUZZLE**

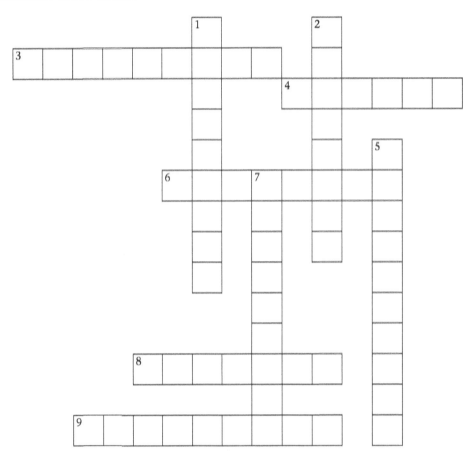

Across

3. Term meaning extreme restlessness and increased motor activity
4. The inability to finish a sentence when communicating
6. The neurotransmitter that plays a major part in schizophrenia
8. Type of dyskinesia with rhythmic, involuntary movements
9. Term meaning lack of joy or pleasurable feelings

Down

1. Term meaning the spectrum of disorders that affect mood and behavior
2. A false belief that cannot be changed with reason
5. When client repeatedly gets admitted to mental health unit
7. Term meaning inability to determine and initiate goals and activities

SECTION II: APPLYING YOUR KNOWLEDGE

Activity F CASE STUDY

 Joe Chase (brother of Lillian) is a 38-year-old man with a diagnosis of schizoaffective disorder. He is admitted to a mental health inpatient facility after he stopped taking his medications and suffered a manic episode. His prior medications consisted of quetiapine (Seroquel) 300 mg at bedtime and lithium 300 mg TID. The primary health care provider decides to restart Mr. Chase's quetiapine (Seroquel), but instead of restarting the lithium, the primary health care provider starts Mr. Chase on olanzapine (Zyprexa) 10 mg daily.

1. What should you as the nurse discuss with Mr. Chase regarding his new medication olanzapine (Zyprexa)?

_____

_____

2. What laboratory work would need to be obtained, and how frequently, now that Mr. Chase is taking both quetiapine and olanzapine?

_____

_____

Now Map It Out! Use the templates provided in the appendix to add information and make client connections on a concept map.

In the textbook, Mrs. Moore's daughter is questioning whether starting quetiapine (Seroquel) would also be appropriate for her mother. Which generation antipsychotic is this drug? What are some of the adverse reactions seen with quetiapine use? Look at your concept map for Mrs. Moore. Are there any medical conditions that would contraindicate this drug use? Now add this prescription to her map. What monitoring becomes more evident when you add this drug?

SECTION III: PRACTICING FOR NCLEX

Activity G NCLEX-STYLE QUESTIONS

Answer the following questions.

1. A client who was administered an antipsychotic has developed photosensitivity. What should the nurse include in client teaching?
    1. Ask the client to minimize alcohol use.
    2. Ask the client to avoid natural sunlight.
    3. Suggest the client use tanning beds.
    4. Suggest the client drink at least five glasses of water per day.

2. A nurse has administered clozapine to a client. Which of the following adverse reactions should the nurse monitor for in the client?
    1. Rashes
    2. Polyuria
    3. Dystonia
    4. Neutropenia

3. A client is displaying violent behavior, and antipsychotic drugs have to be given parenterally. Which of the following interventions should the nurse perform while administering the drug?
    1. Administer the drug intravenously to the client.
    2. Ensure the injection site has minimal muscle mass.
    3. Ensure the client remains upright after the injection.
    4. Ensure that assistance is available for securing the client.

4. A nurse is required to give antipsychotic drugs to a client orally. Which of the following interventions should the nurse perform during the drug administration?
    1. Give drugs individually, not together.
    2. Confirm whether the drug has been swallowed by asking the client.
    3. Mix the drug in liquids such as fruit juices, tomato juice, or milk.
    4. Compel the client to swallow the drug if they refuse to do so.

5. A client with schizophrenia has been prescribed clozapine. Which of the following points should the nurse include in the teaching program?

   1. Purchase a month's supply of the drug.
   2. Schedule WBC count tests every 2 weeks.
   3. Continue WBC testing for 1 week after end of therapy.
   4. Monitoring for bone marrow suppression will be done weekly.

6. As the nurse is interviewing, the newly admitted mental health client, who begins to cry. Which of the following interventions should the nurse perform?

   1. Reach out and touch the client.
   2. Sit empathetically and listen.
   3. Tell the client you will return later.
   4. Hand the client a tissue.

7. A client with schizophrenia has been prescribed asenapine. If symptoms of hypotension and sedation are observed after administration of the drug, which of the following interventions should the nurse perform to minimize the risk of injury to the client?

   1. Administer the drug with food.
   2. Administer the drug with a calcium supplement.
   3. Administer the drug every 8 hours.
   4. Administer the drug at bedtime.

8. A client who has undergone antipsychotic drug therapy is being discharged from an inpatient facility. Which of the following points should the nurse include in the teaching plan? **Select all that apply.**

   1. Report any unusual changes or physical effects.
   2. Inform the client about the risks of EPS and TD.
   3. Decrease dosage if the symptoms increase.
   4. Take the drug on an empty stomach.
   5. Avoid exposure to the sun.

9. Which of the following is a symptom of psychosis that is defined as finding no pleasure in activities that are normally pleasurable?

   1. Anhedonia
   2. Delusions
   3. Hallucinations
   4. Flattened affect

10. Typical antipsychotic medications are thought to exert their effects in which of the following ways?

   1. Stimulating the release of dopamine in the brain
   2. Inhibiting the release of dopamine in the brain
   3. Inhibiting the release of acetylcholine in the brain
   4. Stimulating GABA receptors in the brain

11. Which of the following antipsychotics is used as an antiemetic and can be administered rectally to a client?

   1. Chlorpromazine
   2. Aripiprazole
   3. Clozapine
   4. Haloperidol

12. What is the name of the tool used to monitor clients for involuntary movements?

   1. MOVE
   2. FACES
   3. AIMS
   4. MDS

Drugs That Affect the Peripheral Nervous System

CHAPTER 23

Adrenergic Drugs

Learning Objectives

- Discuss the activity of the autonomic nervous system, specifically the sympathetic branch.
- Compare and contrast the types of shock, physiologic responses of shock, and the use of adrenergic drugs in the treatment of shock.
- Explain the uses, general drug actions, contraindications, precautions, interactions, and adverse reactions associated with the administration of adrenergic vasopressor drugs.
- Distinguish important preadministration and ongoing assessment activities the nurse should perform on the client taking an adrenergic drug.
- List nursing diagnoses particular to a client taking an adrenergic drug.
- Examine ways to promote an optimal response to therapy, how to manage common adverse reactions, and important points to keep in mind when educating clients about the use of adrenergic drugs.

SECTION I: ASSESSING YOUR UNDERSTANDING

Activity A FILL IN THE BLANKS

1. Adrenergic drugs are useful in improving hemodynamic status by improving _____ contractility and increasing heart rate.

2. The autonomic nervous system is divided into the _____ and the parasympathetic nervous branches.

3. Supine _____ is a potentially dangerous adverse reaction that can occur when a client is taking midodrine.

4. Adrenergic drugs are classified as pregnancy category _____ and are used with extreme caution during pregnancy.

5. _____ are drugs that raise the blood pressure because of their ability to constrict blood vessels.

Activity B SEQUENCING

1. Write the correct sequence of self-injection using an autoinjector such as the EpiPen for an allergic reaction in the boxes provided.

1. Check for clear solution and take off the activation cap.

2. If alone, contact emergency medical services.

3. Retain the container until seen by medical personnel.

4. Firmly jab the outer thigh, hold in place for 10 seconds.

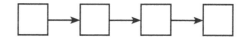

Activity C MATCHING

1. Match the drug names in Column A with their corresponding contraindications in Column B.

Column A	Column B
____ 1. Isoproterenol	a. Narrow-angle glaucoma
____ 2. Dopamine	b. Tachyarrhythmias
____ 3. Midodrine	c. Ventricular fibrillation
____ 4. Epinephrine	d. Severe hypertension

2. Match the drugs in Column A with the likely interaction effect when combined with an adrenergic drug in Column B.

Column A

_____ **1.** Antidepressants

_____ **2.** Oxytocin

_____ **3.** Bretylium

_____ **4.** Dilantin

Column B

a. Increased risk of hypertension

b. Increased risk of bradycardia

c. Increased sympathomimetic effect

d. Increased risk of arrhythmias

Activity D **SHORT ANSWERS**

A nurse's role in managing clients who are being administered adrenergic drugs involves monitoring and interventions. Answer the following questions, which involve the nurse's role in managing such situations.

1. A client is admitted to the emergency department in hypovolemic shock. The primary care provider has ordered an adrenergic drug. What should the nurse assess for in the client before administering the first dose?

_____

_____

2. The nurse is monitoring a client receiving metaraminol. What are the appropriate nursing interventions involved during the ongoing administration of metaraminol?

_____

_____

Activity E **CHART THE FINDING**

Continue to chart the following blood pressure findings for a client following a car accident:

1. **The client is hemorrhaging internally and in hypovolemic shock.**

2. **The client in shock is successfully treated with an adrenergic drug.**

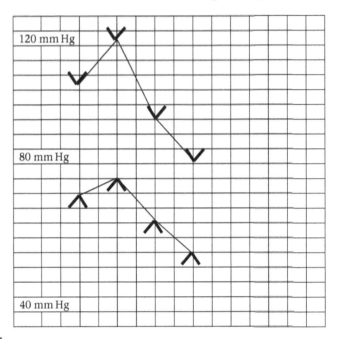

SECTION II: APPLYING YOUR KNOWLEDGE

Activity F **CASE STUDY**

Lillian Chase, a 36-year-old woman, was involved in a motor vehicle accident. She was in shock and preliminary examination showed significant head trauma, a spinal cord injury, a knee injury, and several lacerations and contusions. Her blood pressure is 85/60 mm Hg.

1. Based on these findings, which type of shock was Ms. Chase likely suffering from?

_____

_____

2. Besides hypotension, what other symptoms of shock might the ED nurse have observed in Ms. Chase?

_____

_____

Now Map It Out! Use the templates provided in the appendix to add information and make client connections on a concept map.

Lillian is administered an adrenergic agent for her hypotension and admitted to the acute care facility for observation. During shift change, the following day the care assistant comes to you with a blood pressure reading of 180/120 mm Hg. Map out the above data from Lillian's accident and observe the data you already have on your map. Any reason to see an abrupt change in her blood pressure?

SECTION III: PRACTICING FOR NCLEX

Activity G NCLEX-STYLE QUESTIONS

Answer the following questions.

1. A nurse is required to administer metaraminol for a client who is taking digoxin. The client is at an increased risk for which of the following adverse reactions?
   1. Epigastric distress
   2. Pheochromocytoma
   3. Cardiac arrhythmias
   4. Decrease in blood pressure

2. For which of the following clients is isoproterenol contraindicated?
   1. Clients with narrow-angle glaucoma
   2. Clients with tachycardia
   3. Clients with hypotension
   4. Clients with pheochromocytoma

3. A 65-year-old client has been prescribed isoproterenol. Which of the following should the nurse report immediately to the primary health care provider?
   1. Feeling of nausea
   2. Changes in pulse rate
   3. Severe headache
   4. Urinary urgency

4. A client has been prescribed midodrine. Which of the following is an adverse effect of midodrine that the nurse should monitor for?
   1. Supine hypertension
   2. Tachycardia
   3. Orthostatic hypotension
   4. Respiratory distress

5. A nurse is caring for a client who has been administered metaraminol. Which of the following changes should the nurse report immediately to the primary health care provider?
   1. Consistent fall in blood pressure
   2. Rise in blood glucose levels
   3. Decrease in gastric motility
   4. Increase in the heart rate

6. A client is experiencing insomnia during epinephrine therapy. Which of the following interventions should the nurse perform while caring for the client? **Select all that apply.**
   1. Identify circumstances that disturb sleep.
   2. Draw curtains over windows.
   3. Provide bedtime back rub to the client.
   4. Give frequent sips of tea and coffee.
   5. Administer drugs only during daytime.

7. A nurse observes leakage of norepinephrine from the IV line. Which of the following interventions should the nurse perform to minimize tissue injury?
   1. Discontinue old IV line immediately.
   2. Do not add another IV line unless instructed.
   3. Move the head of the bed to an elevated position.
   4. Mix alkaline solutions with norepinephrine infusions.

8. The adrenergic branch of the autonomic nervous system is also known by which of the following names?
   1. Parasympathetic nervous system
   2. Sympathetic nervous system
   3. Central nervous system
   4. Somatic nervous system

9. Which of the following is stimulated during the body's fight, flight, or freeze response to a stressful condition?
   1. Sympathetic nervous system
   2. Parasympathetic nervous system
   3. Central nervous system
   4. Somatic nervous system

10. Which of the following is the primary neurotransmitter of the sympathetic nervous system?
    1. Norepinephrine
    2. Dopamine
    3. Serotonin
    4. Acetylcholine

11. Which of following adrenergic receptors is responsible for the vasoconstriction of peripheral blood vessels?
    1. Alpha$_1$ receptors
    2. Alpha$_2$ receptors
    3. Beta$_1$ receptors
    4. Beta$_2$ receptors

12. Which of following adrenergic receptors is responsible for decreased tone, motility, and secretions of the GI tract?
    1. Alpha$_2$ receptors
    2. Beta$_1$ receptors
    3. Alpha$_1$ receptors
    4. Beta$_2$ receptors

CHAPTER 24

Adrenergic Blocking Drugs

Learning Objectives

■ List the four types of adrenergic blocking drugs.
■ Discuss the uses, general drug actions, general adverse reactions, contraindications, precautions, and interactions of the adrenergic blocking drugs.
■ Discuss important preadministration and ongoing assessment activities the nurse should perform on the client taking an adrenergic blocking drug.
■ List nursing diagnoses particular to a client taking an adrenergic blocking drug.
■ Explain ways to promote an optimal response to therapy, how to manage common adverse reactions, nursing actions that may be taken to minimize orthostatic or postural hypotension, and important points to keep in mind when educating clients about the use of adrenergic blocking drugs.

SECTION I: ASSESSING YOUR UNDERSTANDING

Activity A FILL IN THE BLANKS

1. _____ is the substance that transmits nerve impulses across the sympathetic branch of the autonomic nervous system.

2. _____ drugs block the transmission of norepinephrine in the sympathetic system.

3. Antiadrenergic drugs _____ transmission of the nerves that produce the fight, flight, or freeze response.

4. Beta-adrenergic (β-adrenergic) blocking drugs are often called beta _____ by clients.

5. _____ is a narrowing or blockage of the drainage channels between the anterior and posterior chambers of the eye.

6. As a result of using a beta-adrenergic blocker, the heart rate becomes _____.

Activity B DOSAGE CALCULATION

1. A client has been prescribed 10 mg of bisoprolol daily. The drug is dispensed from the pharmacy in the form of a 5-mg tablet. How many tablets should the client take each day?

_____

_____

2. A client with hypertension has been prescribed 15 mg of pindolol twice daily. The drug is dispensed from the local pharmacy as 15-mg tablets. The client is taking a flight and would like enough medication for a 10-day trip. What is the total number of tablets required for this client?

_____

_____

3. A client has been prescribed 10 mg of alfuzosin daily. The available drug is in the form of a 10-mg tablet. How many tablets should the client take each day?

_____

_____

4. A client with benign prostatic hyperplasia (BPH) has not felt relief after 2 weeks of drug therapy. The primary health care provider increases the dose from 5 to 7.5 mg of doxazosin daily. The client still has 5-mg tablets at home and wishes to use them all before getting a new prescription. How many tablets should the client take each day?

_____

_____

5. A client has been prescribed 10 mg of prazosin every 24 hours. The drug is dispensed in the form of a 5-mg tablet. How many tablets should the client take each day?

_____

_____

Activity C MATCHING

1. Match the drug in Column A with the likely interaction effect when combined with a beta-adrenergic blocker in Column B.

Column A

___ 1. Clonidine

___ 2. Lidocaine

___ 3. Antidepressants (MAOIs, SSRIs)

___ 4. Loop diuretics

Column B

a. Increased effect of the beta blocker, bradycardia

b. Increased risk of paradoxical hypertensive effect

c. Increased risk of hypotension

d. Increased serum level of the beta blocker

2. Match the drugs that interact adversely with antiadrenergics in Column A with their common uses in Column B.

Column A

___ 1. Adrenergics

___ 2. Levodopa

___ 3. Lithium

___ 4. Anesthetic agents

Column B

a. Surgery

b. Treatment of mania

c. Management of cardiovascular problems

d. Management of Parkinson disease

Activity D SHORT ANSWERS

A nurse's role in managing a client who is prescribed adrenergic blocking drugs involves assisting the client through preadministration assessment and monitoring. Answer the following questions, which involve the nurse's role in the management of clients on adrenergic blocking drug therapy.

1. A client is prescribed an adrenergic blocking drug. The nurse will teach the client or family how to perform a blood pressure measurement at home. What skills should the nurse monitor in a teach-back session?

_____

_____

_____

Activity E CROSSWORD PUZZLE

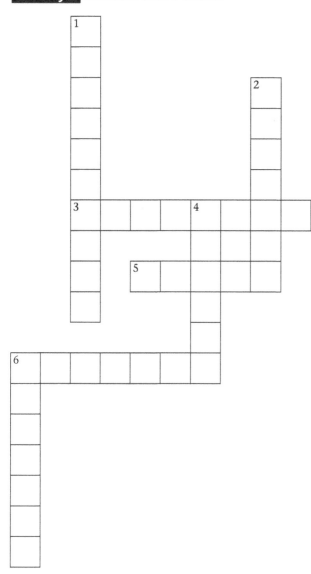

Describe the effect that a sympatholytic drug would have on each body system.

Across

3. Prostate muscle contractions
5. The heart rate
6. Bladder muscles

Down

1. Pupil of the eye
2. Blood vessels
4. Process of bronchodilation
6. Blood pressure

SECTION II: APPLYING YOUR KNOWLEDGE

Activity F CASE STUDY

Alfredo Garcia's mother, Maria, is a Spanish-speaking woman, aged 83 years. She presents to the ED via ambulance with nausea and substernal chest pain. After being assessed by the ED primary health care provider, it is determined that Mrs. Garcia is having an acute MI. The primary health care provider orders metoprolol (Lopressor) three bolus doses of 5 mg IV.

1. Prior to administering the three bolus doses of metoprolol (Lopressor) to Mrs. Garcia, what should the nurse's preadministration include?

   _____

   _____

2. Mrs. Garcia's anxiety is escalating because she does not speak English and her son, Alfredo, has not arrived in the ED yet. What should the nurse do?

   _____

   _____

Now Map It Out! Use the templates provided in the appendix to add information and make client connections on a concept map.

Both Alfredo and his mother have been seen and prescribed the same medication. Review your concept map for Mr. Garcia and the data on his mother from her event in the ED. Do you see any similarities?

SECTION III: PRACTICING FOR NCLEX

Activity G NCLEX-STYLE QUESTIONS

Answer the following questions.

1. A client with pheochromocytoma is admitted to a health care facility. The primary health care provider prescribes phentolamine, an alpha-adrenergic blocking drug, to the client. Which of the following reactions should the nurse monitor for in the client?
   1. Diarrhea
   2. Orthostatic hypotension
   3. Tachycardia
   4. Bronchospasm

2. The clinic nurse is documenting the history of a client who is to begin alpha-adrenergic blocking drug therapy. In which of these conditions are alpha-adrenergic blocking drugs contraindicated?
   1. Renal disease
   2. Pheochromocytoma
   3. Coronary artery disease
   4. Emphysema

3. A nurse is caring for an older client. The primary health care provider has prescribed a beta-adrenergic blocking drug to the client. What should the nurse monitor for in the older client when administering a beta-adrenergic blocking drug?
   1. Vascular insufficiency
   2. Occipital headache
   3. Dizziness
   4. CNS depression

4. A nurse is caring for a client who has been administered prazosin. For which of the following adverse reactions should the nurse monitor the client who is administered peripherally acting antiadrenergic drugs?
   1. Dry mouth
   2. Drowsiness
   3. Malaise
   4. Lightheadedness

5. A nurse is caring for a client who has been prescribed the sympatholytic drug propranolol by the primary health care provider. What nursing interventions should the nurse perform when the client is administered the sympatholytic drug?
   1. Measure the apical pulse rate.
   2. Measure the body temperature.
   3. Measure the weight.
   4. Measure the respiration rate.

6. A nurse at an eye care center is assigned to prepare a teaching plan for a client undergoing adrenergic blocking drug therapy for glaucoma. Which of the following should the nurse include in the teaching plan of the client?
   1. Inform the client to monitor his own pulse and blood pressure.
   2. Inform the client to take drugs as directed with food or on an empty stomach.
   3. Tell the client to contact the primary health care provider if change in vision occurs.
   4. Ask the client to keep ambulating often.

7. A client in an acute psychiatric unit has been routinely taking an antiadrenergic drug. The client has also been given haloperidol for the treatment of psychosis. Which of the following interactions should the nurse monitor for in the client?
   1. Increased risk of lithium toxicity
   2. Increased risk of psychotic behavior
   3. Increased risk of hypertension
   4. Increased effect of anesthetic

8. The use of an alpha-adrenergic blocker will result in which of the following client outcomes?
   1. Vasoconstriction
   2. Vasodilation
   3. Tachypnea
   4. Bradycardia

9. Which of the following medications is an alpha-adrenergic (α-adrenergic) blocker?
    1. Phentolamine
    2. Metoprolol
    3. Losartan
    4. Lisinopril

10. In which organ are the majority of the beta-adrenergic receptors found?
    1. Heart
    2. Kidney
    3. Brain
    4. Liver

11. BPH is treated with which category of antiadrenergic drug?
    1. Alpha blockers
    2. Topical beta blockers
    3. Centrally acting
    4. Peripherally acting

12. Which of the following is an example of an alpha/beta-adrenergic blocking drug?
    1. Metoprolol (Lopressor)
    2. Losartan (Cozaar)
    3. Lisinopril (Prinivil)
    4. Carvedilol (Coreg)

Cholinergic Drugs

- Discuss important aspects of the parasympathetic nervous system.
- Explain the uses, drug actions, general adverse reactions, contraindications, precautions, and interactions of cholinergic drugs.
- Distinguish important preadministration and ongoing assessment activities the nurse should perform on the client taking a cholinergic drug.
- List nursing diagnoses particular to a client taking a cholinergic drug.
- Examine ways to promote an optimal response to therapy, how to manage common adverse reactions, and important points to keep in mind when educating the client about the use of cholinergic drugs.

SECTION I: ASSESSING YOUR UNDERSTANDING

Activity A FILL IN THE BLANKS

1. _____ receptors stimulate the smooth muscle.

2. Cholinergic drugs mimic the activity of the _____ nervous system.

3. _____ is the substance that transmits nerve impulses across the parasympathetic branch of the autonomic nervous system.

4. Drugs that inhibit the enzyme acetylcholinesterase are called _____.

5. _____ receptors stimulate the skeletal muscles in the parasympathetic nerve branch of the autonomic nervous system.

Activity B DOSAGE CALCULATION

1. A primary health care provider prescribes 120 mg of Mestinon four times a day for the treatment of myasthenia gravis. Mestinon is available as 60-mg tablets. How many tablets should the care provider anticipate administering each day?

2. A client has been prescribed 10 mg of bethanechol three times a day for the treatment of urinary retention. Bethanechol is available as 5-mg tablets. How many tablets should the long-term care nurse administer to the client in a single dose?

3. A primary health care provider has prescribed 240 mg of Mestinon per dose for myasthenia gravis. If the daily dose of Mestinon is 720 mg, how many doses per day is the client given?

Activity C MATCHING

1. Match the cholinergic drugs in Column A with their uses in Column B.

Column A

____ **1.** Edrophonium

____ **2.** Bethanechol

____ **3.** Pyridostigmine

Column B

a. Treatment of myasthenia gravis

b. Diagnosis of myasthenia gravis

c. Acute nonobstructive urinary retention

Activity D SHORT ANSWERS

A nurse's role in managing clients with myasthenia gravis involves monitoring them and implementing interventions that aid in their recovery. Answer the following questions, which involve the nurse's role in the management of such situations.

1. A client with myasthenia gravis has been recommended pyridostigmine to help reduce symptoms of the disease. What should a nurse assess for in the client before administering the first dose?

_____

_____

2. A client is undergoing treatment for myasthenia gravis. What should the nurse explain to the client about the disorder and the drug to be administered for myasthenia gravis?

_____

_____

Activity E WORD FIND

Find five words describing the parasympathetic system.

P	B	S	A	F	P	G	J	C	D	K
A	L	Q	C	U	E	M	H	K	O	F
R	H	J	E	D	L	Z	I	Y	P	X
A	C	O	T	B	Q	U	D	S	O	C
S	N	G	Y	K	O	J	Y	A	V	I
Y	Z	I	L	X	R	P	E	O	S	W
M	U	S	C	A	R	I	N	I	C	Z
P	D	F	H	O	S	O	W	U	V	Q
A	K	Y	O	P	T	L	X	M	B	R
T	I	O	L	S	C	I	O	G	J	L
H	G	B	I	A	Q	Z	N	F	E	Y
E	S	U	N	J	E	D	P	I	R	H
T	X	I	E	H	M	B	F	Y	C	G
I	Q	D	M	K	F	U	J	X	O	L
C	H	O	L	I	N	E	R	G	I	C

SECTION II: APPLYING YOUR KNOWLEDGE

Activity F CASE STUDY

 Mr. Park, a 77-year-old man who has recently had a surgical procedure, is having difficulty urinating after surgery. The primary health care provider has requested that the nurse check for urinary retention before prescribing medication.

1. Prior to administering a medication for urinary retention, what should the nurse's preadministration assessment include?

_____

_____

2. If Mr. Park is given a cholinergic drug for urinary retention, when will it work?

_____

_____

Now Map It Out! Use the templates provided in the appendix to add information and make client connections on a concept map.

Here is another situation where the effects of polypharmacy may occur. In both the study guide and the textbook, we learn Mr. Park is prescribed preoperative medications, and we are faced with possibly adding a cholinergic agent in this chapter. Review your concept map for Mr. Park. Are there any possible drug interactions that would occur if a cholinergic drug was taken? What new problems may we now see?

SECTION III: PRACTICING FOR NCLEX

Activity G NCLEX-STYLE QUESTIONS

Answer the following questions.

1. A nurse is caring for a client who uses a cholinergic drug for glaucoma. Which of the following adverse effects should the nurse monitor for during the topical administration of cholinergic drugs?
   1. Temporary reduction of visual acuity
   2. Increased ocular tension
   3. Decreased sweat production
   4. Anaphylactic shock

2. A client has been prescribed a cholinergic drug. What should the nurse instruct the client about the medication?
   1. Tell the client not to take the drug for a day once every 7 days.
   2. Instruct the client in English, and encourage him to learn the language.
   3. Emphasize the importance of uninterrupted therapy.
   4. Instruct the client that record-keeping is unnecessary.

3. A client with myasthenia gravis has been prescribed pyridostigmine. The client informs the nurse that he has respiratory problems and is taking corticosteroids. Which of the following interactions between the two drugs should the nurse anticipate in the client?
   1. Increased neuromuscular blocking effect
   2. Decreased effect of the cholinergic
   3. Increased absorption of the cholinergic
   4. Decreased serum level of corticosteroids

4. What happens to selected body systems when the parasympathetic neuropathway is stimulated? **Select all that apply.**
   1. Blood vessels constrict.
   2. Blood is diverted to the GI system.
   3. Dry mouth occurs.
   4. Heart rate slows.
   5. Pupils of the eye constrict.

5. A client is undergoing cholinergic drug therapy. Which of the following drugs does the nurse administer cautiously with this client?
   1. Salicylates
   2. Analgesics
   3. Aminoglycoside antibiotics
   4. Antidiabetics

6. A nurse is caring for a client with myasthenia gravis. The client has been administered pyridostigmine. What symptoms would indicate drug overdose? **Select all that apply.**
   1. Drooping of the eyelids
   2. Rapid fatigability of the muscles
   3. Salivation
   4. Clenching of the jaw
   5. Muscle rigidity and spasm

7. A client in the acute care facility is being treated for urinary retention. What is the role of the nurse when caring for the client being administered cholinergic therapy?
   1. Instruct the client to void before the drug is administered.
   2. Encourage the client to take the drug with milk to enhance absorption.
   3. Place the call light and items that client might need within easy reach.
   4. Encourage the client to have five to seven glasses of water after drug administration.

8. Which of the following interventions should the nurse perform if the client develops diarrhea after administering the urecholine drug orally? **Select all that apply.**
   1. Ensure that bedpan or bathroom is readily available.
   2. Check for blood stains in the stool.
   3. Encourage the client to ambulate to assist the passing of flatus.
   4. Encourage the client to increase his fibrous food intake.
   5. Keep a record of the number, consistency, and frequency of stools.

9. The stimulation of which of the following receptors in the parasympathetic nervous system stimulates smooth muscle?
   1. Muscarinic receptors
   2. Nicotinic receptors
   3. Alpha-adrenergic (α-adrenergic) receptors
   4. Beta-adrenergic (β-adrenergic) receptors

10. The stimulation of which of the following receptors in the parasympathetic nervous system stimulates skeletal muscle?
    1. Muscarinic receptors
    2. Nicotinic receptors
    3. Alpha-adrenergic receptors
    4. Beta-adrenergic receptors

11. Which of the following is the enzyme responsible for deactivating acetylcholine, the primary neurotransmitter in the parasympathetic nervous system?
    1. Acetylcholinesterase
    2. DNA gyrase
    3. Protease
    4. Lipase

12. Which of the following is an example of a direct-acting cholinergic that acts like the neurotransmitter acetylcholine?
    1. Bethanechol
    2. Pyridostigmine
    3. Pilocarpine
    4. Edrophonium

26

Cholinergic Blocking Drugs

Learning Objectives

- Explain the uses, general drug actions, general adverse reactions, contraindications, precautions, and interactions of the cholinergic blocking drugs (also called anticholinergic drugs and cholinergic blockers).
- Distinguish important preadministration and ongoing assessment activities the nurse should perform on the client taking a cholinergic blocking drug.
- List nursing diagnoses particular to the client taking a cholinergic blocking drug.
- Examine ways to promote an optimal response to therapy, how to manage common adverse reactions, and important points to keep in mind when educating clients taking cholinergic blocking drugs.

SECTION I: ASSESSING YOUR UNDERSTANDING

Activity A FILL IN THE BLANKS

1. _____ is the primary neurotransmitter in the parasympathetic branch of the autonomic nervous system.

2. Cholinergic blocking drugs inhibit the activity of acetylcholine at the _____ nerve synapse.

3. _____ is a type of visual impairment occurring due to the use of cholinergic blocking drugs, characterized by a difficulty in focusing resulting from paralysis of the ciliary muscle.

4. The nurse should use _____ with caution in clients with asthma.

5. An unexpected or unusual effect of cholinergic blocking drugs is known as drug _____.

Activity B DOSAGE CALCULATION

1. A client with an overactive bladder is prescribed 60 mg of trospium per day divided into three doses. The drug is available in the form of 20-mg tablets. How many tablets should the client take in each dose?

_____

_____

2. The primary health care provider has prescribed 100 mg of flavoxate for a client to be administered four times a day. The available drug is in the form of 100-mg tablets. How many tablets should the client take in each dose?

_____

_____

3. A client in respiratory distress is prescribed 2 puffs of ipratropium for relief, not to exceed 12 inhalations in 24 hours. If the client has used the inhaler every 4 hours around the clock, has the client exceeded the daily dose recommendation?

_____

_____

4. A client is going on a 5-day cruise trip and is worried about becoming seasick. The primary health care provider recommends an OTC product. If the scopolamine tablets are 0.4 mg and the prescribed dose is up to 0.8 mg daily, should the client purchase the 0.4-mg 12 pack or 24 pack?

_____

_____

Activity C MATCHING

1. Match the cholinergic blocking drugs in Column A with their uses in Column B.

Column A	Column B
____ **1.** Atropine	**a.** Treatment of overactive bladder syndrome
____ **2.** Propantheline	
____ **3.** Fesoterodine	**b.** Adjunctive treatment of peptic ulcer
	c. Reduce oral secretions

2. Match the adverse reactions associated with cholinergic blocking drugs in Column A with the measures to lessen their intensity in Column B.

Column A	Column B
____ **1.** Photophobia	**a.** Chew gum or dissolve hard candy in mouth
____ **2.** Dry mouth	
____ **3.** Constipation	**b.** Schedule tasks requiring alertness before the first dose of the drug is taken
____ **4.** Drowsiness	
	c. Wear protective eyewear when outside
	d. Eat foods high in fiber

Activity D SHORT ANSWERS

A nurse's role in caring for clients receiving cholinergic blocking drugs involves monitoring and managing the clients' needs and helping them in their recovery. Answer the following questions, which involve the nurse's role in the management of such situations.

1. A nurse has analyzed assessment data and selected the following nursing diagnoses for this client:

- **Impaired comfort** related to xerostomia
- **Constipation** related to slowing of peristalsis in the GI tract
- **Risk for injury** related to dizziness, drowsiness, mental confusion, impaired vision, or heat prostration

How will the nurse evaluate the effectiveness of the treatment plan?

_____

_____

2. What instructions should the nurse offer an older client's family when monitoring the client receiving cholinergic blocking drugs?

_____

_____

_____

Activity E CROSSWORD PUZZLE

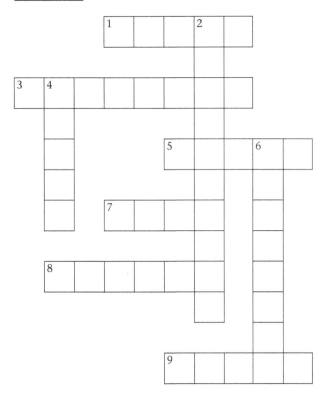

Across

1. A higher rate indicates tissue perfusion problems

3. Increases in hot weather, leading to dehydration

5. If ambulation is an issue, any walkway obstructions

7. Remove these to prevent slipping and injury

8. How people change their fluid intake because they are afraid of urinary urgency

9. Eating more of this will help to reduce constipation

Down

2. These should be worn when outside if photophobic

4. Frequent sips of this will reduce dry mouth

6. This drug is used to dry up secretions before surgery

SECTION II: APPLYING YOUR KNOWLEDGE

Activity F CASE STUDY

Mrs. Moore's daughter is staying at her home. She notes that her 85-year-old mother is getting up to go to the bathroom multiple times at night. She worries that these are symptoms of overactive bladder syndrome. The primary health care provider writes Mrs. Moore a prescription for tolterodine (Detrol LA) 4 mg daily.

1. Discuss the adverse reactions that should be included in the nurse's teaching plan for Mrs. Moore and her daughter.

_____

_____

2. What should the nurse instruct the daughter to observe for in Mrs. Moore because she is an older client taking a cholinergic blocking drug?

_____

_____

Now Map It Out! Use the templates provided in the appendix to add information and make client connections on a concept map.

Here is another situation where the effects of polypharmacy may occur. In the textbook, we learn about drug idiosyncrasy. Mrs. Moore suffers from mental changes. What do you know about the anticholinergic agent described in the above scenario? Review your concept map for Mrs. Moore. Are there any possible drug interactions that would occur if an anticholinergic drug was taken? What new problems may we now see?

SECTION III: PRACTICING FOR NCLEX

Activity G NCLEX-STYLE QUESTIONS

Answer the following questions.

1. In which of the following client conditions should atropine be used cautiously?
   1. Tachyarrhythmias
   2. Myasthenia gravis
   3. Glaucoma
   4. Asthma

2. A client is being administered propantheline for the treatment of a peptic ulcer. After receiving the drug, the client complains of constipation. Which of the following instructions should the nurse provide this client to help relieve constipation?
   1. Consume an antacid after meals for severe constipation.
   2. Increase fluid intake to 2000 mL daily.
   3. Increase the consumption of citrus juices.
   4. Restrict fluid consumption to prevent urinary frequency.

3. A client with bladder overactivity likes to garden. The cholinergic blocking drug prescribed is known to cause heat prostration. What instructions should the nurse offer the client to help lessen the intensity of heat prostration? **Select all that apply.**
   1. Wear loose-fitting clothes.
   2. Sponge the skin with cool water.
   3. Garden early in the morning.
   4. Use fans to cool the body.
   5. Wear sunglasses when outdoors.

4. Glycopyrrolate is administered to a client to reduce bronchial and oral secretions. Which of the following are unintended adverse reactions of the drug and not anticipated actions? **Select all that apply.**
   1. Nausea
   2. Altered taste perception
   3. Tachycardia
   4. Mydriasis
   5. Dry mouth

5. A nurse is caring preoperatively for a 65-year-old client. Which of the following interventions should the nurse perform first when caring for this client as part of the preoperative routine?
   1. Validate atropine administration before giving.
   2. Monitor for changes in the client's pulse rate or rhythm.
   3. Ensure that the client has not received antibiotics recently.
   4. Place the client in the Fowler position.

6. A nurse needs to administer a cholinergic blocking drug preoperatively to a client. Why should the nurse administer the drug to the client at the exact time as prescribed by the primary health care provider?
   1. To avoid abdominal cramping in the client after the drug administration
   2. To ensure effectiveness of the drug after administration of the anesthetic
   3. To allow the drug to produce the greatest effect before administration of the anesthetic
   4. To avoid excessive salivation and make the client feel comfortable

7. A nurse is caring for a client with bladder overactivity. The client has been prescribed oxybutynin by the primary health care provider. Which of the following conditions does the nurse anticipate the client will have to deal with on a daily basis?
   1. Mydriasis
   2. Mouth dryness
   3. Blurred vision
   4. Hesitancy

8. A nurse is caring for a client who has been administered atropine preoperatively to reduce the production of secretions in the respiratory tract. Which of the following drug reactions should the nurse identify as part of the desired response?
   1. Vomiting
   2. Elevated temperature
   3. Low pulse rate
   4. Drowsiness

9. Which of the following is an example of a parasympatholytic drug?

    1. Oxybutynin
    2. Bethanechol
    3. Ambenonium
    4. Pyridostigmine

10. The drug benztropine is used for the treatment of Parkinson disease because it exerts its effect by inhibiting the action of which of the following receptors?

    1. Muscarinic receptors
    2. Nicotinic receptors
    3. Alpha-adrenergic receptors
    4. Beta-adrenergic receptors

11. The cholinergic blocking drug glycopyrrolate is used in conjunction with anesthesia for which of the following reasons?

    1. Increase muscle rigidity
    2. Relaxation
    3. Prolongation of anesthesia
    4. Reduction of oral secretions

12. The nurse should observe clients receiving a cholinergic blocking drug during the hot summer months because these clients are at increased risk of which of the following?

    1. Sunburn
    2. Heart attack
    3. Heat prostration
    4. Dehydration

Drugs That Affect the Neuromuscular System

27

Antiparkinson Drugs

Learning Objectives

- Define the terms *Parkinson disease* and *parkinsonism*.
- Explain the uses, general drug action, adverse drug reactions, contraindications, precautions, and interactions of antiparkinson drugs.
- Distinguish important preadministration and ongoing assessment activities the nurse should perform on the client taking an antiparkinson drugs.
- List nursing diagnoses particular to a client taking an antiparkinson drugs.
- Examine ways to promote an optimal response to therapy, how to manage adverse reactions, and important points to keep in mind when educating clients about the use of antiparkinson drugs.

SECTION I: ASSESSING YOUR UNDERSTANDING

Activity A FILL IN THE BLANKS

1. _____ is a degenerative disorder due to an imbalance of dopamine and acetylcholine.

2. The cardinal signs of Parkinson disease include _____, _____, and slow movement (also known as _____).

3. In Parkinson disease, the gait becomes unsteady and _____.

4. Parkinson-like symptoms may be seen with the use of certain drugs; these movements are also called _____ _____.

5. Restless leg syndrome is a disorder with an _____ urge to move the legs.

Activity B DOSAGE CALCULATION

1. A client with Parkinson disease has been recommended amantadine 400 mg/day in four equally divided doses. The drug is available in 100-mg capsules. To meet the recommended dose, how many tablets should the nurse administer in each dose?

   _____

   _____

2. A client is taking 25 mg Sinemet in each dose. The muscle movements are working well with TID dosing. How many total milligrams is the client taking on a daily basis?

   _____

   _____

3. A client with Parkinson disease is showing increased choreiform movements. Because the client is having swallowing difficulties, IM injection is recommended. The primary health care provider (PHCP) has recommended 0.5 mg of benztropine TID. The drug is available in 1 mg/mL solution. How many mL should the nurse administer to the client in each dose?

   _____

   _____

Activity C MATCHING

1. Match the dopaminergic agents in Column A with their adverse reaction in Column B.

Column A

_____ **1.** Amantadine

_____ **2.** Bromocriptine

_____ **3.** Carbidopa/levodopa

_____ **4.** Rasagiline

Column B

a. Dysphagia

b. Orthostatic hypotension

c. Arthralgia

d. Epigastric distress

2. Match the drugs in Column A with their uses in Column B.

Column A

_____ **1.** Bromocriptine

_____ **2.** Benztropine

_____ **3.** Entacapone

_____ **4.** Apomorphine

Column B

a. Treatment of drug-induced extrapyramidal symptoms

b. Treatment of Parkinson disease "off" episode

c. Treatment of both Parkinson disease and endocrine imbalances

d. Used as adjunct to levodopa/carbidopa in Parkinson disease

Activity D SHORT ANSWERS

A nurse's role in managing Parkinson-like symptoms involves assisting clients with the administration of antiparkinson drugs. The nurse also helps in educating clients and their families about the treatment regimen. Answer the following questions, which involve the nurse's role in the management of such situations.

1. A nurse is assigned to care for a client with Parkinson disease. During preadministration assessment, the nurse has to assess the client's neuromuscular status. What should the nurse observe to assess the neuromuscular status of the client?

_____

_____

2. Lack of balance and the potential for injury are always a concern with Parkinson disease. What are some interventions the nurse can suggest that would help to stabilize or improve balance for the client?

_____

_____

Activity E WORD FIND

Find six words describing Parkinson disease.

Q	O	S	R	V	Y	D	P	G	E	T	G
B	J	A	C	H	A	L	A	S	I	A	D
W	R	K	O	Q	W	E	R	J	X	U	I
Y	U	A	P	I	T	S	K	I	O	R	J
T	K	T	D	N	R	U	I	Y	G	A	T
R	A	H	J	Y	K	W	N	V	I	P	Z
X	W	I	G	D	K	P	S	N	S	W	G
E	N	S	U	T	A	I	O	K	R	J	P
J	Y	I	Q	S	U	T	N	P	O	D	E
G	R	A	B	E	S	Y	I	E	P	S	J
U	P	X	S	Y	I	R	S	T	S	Q	K
A	I	T	D	B	O	E	M	N	Y	I	W
D	R	Y	O	T	D	F	O	A	R	C	A

SECTION II: APPLYING YOUR KNOWLEDGE

Activity F CASE STUDY

Alfredo Garcia comes to the clinic with questions about his brother, who is living in Mexico. He is a newly diagnosed Parkinson disease client and has been prescribed carbidopa/levodopa (Sinemet) 300 mg TID. Answer the following questions about his brother's disease state and medication.

1. Mr. Garcia read on the Internet that the symptoms of Parkinson disease are caused by a depletion of dopamine in the central nervous system, but he wants to know why the medication cannot just be dopamine to supplement the deficiency. What should the nurse answer?

   _____

   _____

2. His mother is quite upset over his brother's new diagnosis. Do an Internet search and see if you can find information about Parkinson disease written in Spanish. Compare the literature to your textbook; is it reliable?

   _____

   _____

Now Map It Out! Use the templates provided in the appendix to add information and make client connections on a concept map.

At this time, Alfredo does not show any signs or symptoms of having the same disease as his brother. Because this is distressing to Mrs. Garcia, she could become even more upset if Alfredo were to be on any medication that also present with extrapyramidal symptoms (those which mimic Parkinson disease symptoms). Using Mr. Garcia's concept map, see if you can identify any drugs that may present with EPS. This will give you a quick review of his current drugs, much like medication reconciliation.

SECTION III: PRACTICING FOR NCLEX

Activity G NCLEX-STYLE QUESTIONS

Answer the following questions.

1. A nurse is caring for a client who has been prescribed carbidopa. After administration of the drug, the nurse observes the occurrence of choreiform and dystonic movements in the client. Which of the following interventions should the nurse perform first when caring for this client?
   1. Monitor vital signs frequently.
   2. Withhold the next dose of the drug.
   3. Offer frequent sips of water.
   4. Observe the client for nausea and fatigue.

2. A nurse is assigned to care for a client with suspected neuroleptic malignant-like syndrome following the abrupt discontinuation of an antiparkinson drug. Which of the following symptoms should the nurse monitor for in the client? **Select all that apply.**
   1. Muscular rigidity
   2. Elevated body temperature
   3. Mental changes
   4. Tachycardia
   5. Orthostatic hypotension

3. A nurse is caring for a client who has been prescribed levodopa for the treatment of Parkinson disease. The client informs the nurse that he is taking antacids for the relief of heartburn. What interaction between the two drugs should the nurse anticipate in the client?
   1. Increased risk of hypertension
   2. Increased risk of dyskinesia
   3. Increased effect of levodopa
   4. Increased risk of cardiac symptoms

4. A nurse is assigned to care for a client who receives catechol-O-methyltransferase (COMT) inhibitors. Which of the following data items from the client's record would the nurse expect to see, indicating that the drug has to be administered cautiously to the client?
   1. Decreased renal function
   2. Tachycardia
   3. History of cardiac arrhythmias
   4. GI tract problems

5. What should be included on the discharge plan when a client is receiving antiparkinson drugs? **Select all that apply.**

   1. Instruct the client to avoid taking vitamin B_6 with levodopa.

   2. Instruct the client to contact the PHCP in case of severe dry mouth.

   3. Instruct the client to avoid consumption of alcohol.

   4. Instruct the client to have small and frequent meals.

   5. Encourage the client to increase intake of vitamin C.

6. A nurse caring for a client undergoing antiparkinson drug therapy observes that the client is vomiting frequently, despite nonpharmacological interventions. Which intervention should the nurse consider next for this client?

   1. Request a change of drug.

   2. Administer the drug before meals.

   3. Administer antacids after meals.

   4. Refrain from giving liquids after meals.

7. Which of the following the nursing interventions indicates the client is showing a good response to therapy with antiparkinson drugs?

   1. Change the antiparkinson drug to another.

   2. Discontinue use of antiparkinson drugs.

   3. Observe the client's behavior at frequent intervals.

   4. Observe a drug holiday as prescribed.

8. A nurse is caring for a client with Parkinson disease. Which of the following conditions would the nurse observe indicating abdominal pain due to constipation in the client?

   1. Change in facial expression

   2. Change in gait

   3. Change in food preferences

   4. Change in sleeping amount

9. Which of the following terms refers to a group of symptoms involving motor movement characterized by tremors, rigidity, and bradykinesia?

   1. Parkinsonism

   2. Myasthenia gravis

   3. Seizure disorder

   4. Anxiety

10. Which of the following drugs is classified as a dopaminergic agent that treats Parkinson-like symptoms by supplementing the amount of dopamine in the brain?

   1. Benztropine (Cogentin)

   2. Ropinirole (Requip)

   3. Carbidopa (Lodosyn)

   4. Tolcapone (Tasmar)

11. Which of the following drugs is classified as a catechol-O-methyltransferase (COMT) inhibitor?

   1. Entacapone (Comtan)

   2. Carbidopa (Lodosyn)

   3. Benztropine (Cogentin)

   4. Ropinirole (Requip)

12. Which of the following drugs is classified as a nonergot dopamine receptor agonist?

   1. Entacapone (Comtan)

   2. Carbidopa (Lodosyn)

   3. Apomorphine (Apokyn)

   4. Benztropine (Cogentin)

13. Which of the following drugs is classified as a cholinergic blocking drug used to treat Parkinson-like symptoms?

   1. Apomorphine (Apokyn)

   2. Entacapone (Comtan)

   3. Carbidopa (Lodosyn)

   4. Benztropine (Cogentin)

28

Antiepileptics

Learning Objectives

- Compare and contrast the different types of drugs used as antiepileptics.
- Explain the general drug actions, uses, adverse reactions, contraindications, precautions, and interactions of antiepileptics.
- Distinguish important preadministration and ongoing assessment activities the nurse should perform with the client receiving an antiepileptic.
- List nursing diagnoses particular to a client taking an antiepileptic.
- Examine ways to promote an optimal response to therapy, how to manage common adverse reactions when administering the antiepileptics, and important points to keep in mind when educating a client about the use of antiepileptics.

SECTION I: ASSESSING YOUR UNDERSTANDING

Activity A FILL IN THE BLANKS

1. Sudden involuntary contraction of the muscles of the body, often accompanied by loss of consciousness, is termed a _____.

2. A _____ may be defined as periodic disturbances of the brain's electrical activity.

3. _____ seizure is a localized seizure in the brain, with no impaired consciousness.

4. Antiepileptics _____ abnormal nerve impulse discharges in the CNS.

5. _____ _____ is an emergency situation characterized by continual seizure activity.

Activity B DOSAGE CALCULATION

1. A client has been prescribed 200 mg of Zonegran twice daily. The available drug is in the form of 100-mg capsules. What is the total number of capsules the client would take for each dose?

   _____

   _____

2. A client has been prescribed 200 mg of Topamax daily. The drug is available in 100-mg capsules. How many capsules are required for this client daily?

   _____

   _____

3. A client is prescribed 250 mg of Depakote to be taken twice daily. Depakote is available in 125-mg tablets. How many tablets should the nurse administer to the client in each dose?

   _____

   _____

4. A client has been prescribed 32 mg of tiagabine daily, this will be split into four doses per day orally. The drug is available in 2-, 4-, 12-, and 16-mg tablets in a pharmacy. Which is the best tablet to be dispensed to the client for both ease and safety?

_____

_____

5. A client has been prescribed 600 mg of oxcarbazepine to be taken twice daily. The drug is available in 300-mg tablets. How many tablets should the nurse administer to the client each time?

_____

_____

Activity C MATCHING

1. Match the antiepileptic drugs in Column A with their uses in Column B.

Column A

____ **1.** Phenytoin

____ **2.** Pregabalin

____ **3.** Levetiracetam

____ **4.** Lorazepam

Column B

a. Neuropathic pain

b. Preanesthetic

c. Long-term seizure control

d. Migraine headache

2. Match the antiepileptic drugs in Column A with their adverse reactions in Column B.

Column A

____ **1.** Carbamazepine

____ **2.** Ethotoin

____ **3.** Clonazepam

____ **4.** Ethosuximide

Column B

a. Urinary frequency, pruritus, urticaria

b. Ataxia, visual disturbances, rash

c. Unsteady gait, aplastic anemia and other blood cell abnormalities

d. Hypotension, nystagmus, slurred speech

Activity D SHORT ANSWERS

A nurse's role in managing a client who is prescribed an antiepileptic drug involves assisting the client with preadministration assessment. The nurse also helps in monitoring clients who are administered antiepileptic drugs. Answer the following questions, which involve the nurse's role in the management of clients on antiepileptic therapy.

1. A client with suspected seizures is admitted to an acute care facility. A visitor comes to the nurse's station and says the client just had a seizure. What bedside assessments should the nurse perform to assess this client?

_____

_____

_____

2. After the preadministration assessment, the client is administered an antiepileptic drug for seizure disorders. What is the nurse's role when caring for the client who is administered an antiepileptic drug?

_____

_____

_____

Activity E CROSSWORD PUZZLE

Activity E CROSSWORD PUZZLE

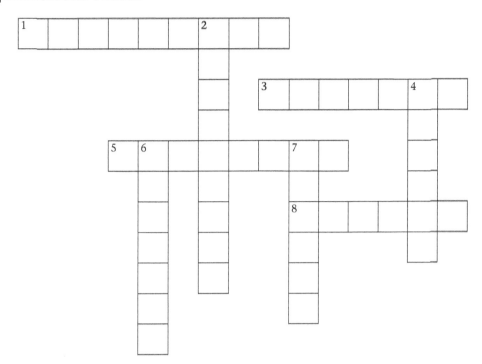

Across

1. Term for the involuntary and constant movement of the eyeball

3. Category of seizures where there is a loss of consciousness during the seizure

5. A chronic, recurring seizure disorder

8. A generalized seizure with loss of muscle tone and in which the person suddenly drops

Down

2. A sudden, forceful muscular contraction

4. Term for an unsteady gait; muscular incoordination

6. Another term for focal seizures with localized seizure activity in the brain, with no impaired consciousness

7. Epilepticus; an emergency situation characterized by continual seizure activity

SECTION II: APPLYING YOUR KNOWLEDGE

Activity F CASE STUDY

Lillian Chase is a woman, aged 36 years. Ms. Chase was hospitalized for neurologic evaluation after actively seizing while in the ED following a motor vehicle accident.

1. What information should the nurse obtain from those who observed the seizure?

_____

_____

2. Ms. Chase is started on phenytoin (Dilantin) 100 mg TID. She comes back to the ED 1 week later with complaints of slurred speech, ataxia, lethargy, dizziness, and nausea. During assessment, the nurse finds that she was taking 300 mg TID. What might the symptoms Ms. Chase is experiencing indicate?

_____

_____

Now Map It Out! Use the templates provided in the appendix to add information and make client connections on a concept map.

Ms. Chase demonstrated a dramatic adverse reaction to the increased dose of phenytoin. Using Lillian's concept map, see if you can identify any drugs that may have contributed an additive or synergistic effect on the phenytoin. This will give you a quick review of her current drugs, again much like medication reconciliation.

SECTION III: PRACTICING FOR NCLEX

Activity G NCLEX-STYLE QUESTIONS

Answer the following questions.

1. A primary health care provider (PHCP) has prescribed carbamazepine to a client with epilepsy at a long-term care facility. Which of the following should the nurse monitor for in the client while administering carbamazepine?
   1. Photosensitivity
   2. Bone marrow depression
   3. Hypotension
   4. Myocardial insufficiency

2. A nurse at a rehabilitative care center is assigned to prepare a teaching plan for a client about to be discharged who will continue hydantoin drug therapy. Which of the following should the nurse include in the teaching plan of the client? **Select all that apply.**
   1. Avoid taking the drugs if you go swimming.
   2. Brush and floss teeth after each meal.
   3. Avoid consumption of discolored capsules.
   4. Notify the PHCP if blurred vision occurs.
   5. Take medication with food.

3. A nurse is caring for a client with tonic–clonic seizures in a long-term care facility. The PHCP has prescribed Dilantin to the client. Which of the hematologic changes in the client should the nurse immediately report to the PHCP?
   1. Sinus bradycardia
   2. Sinoatrial block
   3. Thrombocytopenia
   4. Adams–Stokes syndrome

4. The PHCP has prescribed Lamictal. What instructions should the nurse provide the client receiving Lamictal?
   1. "Eat with food if you are nauseated."
   2. "Report a rash, because it could be an emergency."
   3. "Stop taking if you have no seizures after a week."
   4. "Wear light-colored clothes, for sun protection."

5. A nurse is assigned to care for a client who has been prescribed phenytoin. In which of the following client conditions is the use of phenytoin contraindicated?
   1. History of asthma
   2. Cardiac problems
   3. Hepatic abnormalities
   4. Kidney dysfunction

6. An older client is having a seizure and is to be administered diazepam IV. Which of the following conditions should the nurse monitor for in this specific client?
   1. Gingival hyperplasia
   2. Skin rashes
   3. Throat irritation
   4. Apnea and cardiac arrest

7. A client with seizures has been prescribed the drug phenytoin. Which of the following would indicate drug toxicity?
   1. Client has plasma levels less than 10 mcg/mL.
   2. Phenytoin plasma levels are greater than 20 mcg/mL.
   3. Client has plasma levels greater than 30 mcg/mL.
   4. Phenytoin plasma levels are between 10 and 20 mcg/mL.

8. Simple seizures, motor seizures, and somatosensory seizures are classified as what type of seizure?
   1. Generalized seizures
   2. Tonic–clonic seizures
   3. Focal seizures
   4. Myoclonic seizures

9. Tonic–clonic seizures and myoclonic seizures are classified as what type of seizures?
   1. Generalized seizures
   2. Focal seizures
   3. Somatosensory seizures
   4. Motor seizures

10. Which type of seizure involves a loss of consciousness?
    1. Focal seizures
    2. Somatosensory seizures
    3. Generalized seizures
    4. Motor seizures

11. Which antiepileptic elicits its effects by stabilizing the hyperexcitability postsynaptically in the motor cortex of the brain?
    1. Valproic acid (Depakote)
    2. Phenytoin (Dilantin)
    3. Ethosuximide (Zarontin)
    4. Zonisamide (Zonegran)

12. Which antiepileptic elicits its effects by increasing levels of gamma (γ)-aminobutyric acid (GABA), which stabilizes cell membranes?
    1. Valproic acid (Depakote)
    2. Pregabalin (Lyrica)
    3. Primidone (Mysoline)
    4. Tiagabine (Gabitril)

29

Skeletal Muscle, Bone, and Joint Disorder Drugs

- List the types of drugs used to treat musculoskeletal disorders.
- Explain the uses, general drug actions, adverse reactions, contraindications, precautions, and interactions of the drugs used to treat musculoskeletal disorders.
- Distinguish important preadministration and ongoing assessment activities the nurse should perform on the client taking a drug used to treat musculoskeletal disorders.
- List nursing diagnoses particular to a client taking a drug for the treatment of musculoskeletal disorders.
- Examine ways to promote an optimal response to therapy, how to manage adverse reactions, and important points to keep in mind when educating the client about drugs used to treat musculoskeletal disorders.

SECTION I: ASSESSING YOUR UNDERSTANDING

Activity A FILL IN THE BLANKS

1. The _____ are drugs used to treat musculoskeletal disorders such as osteoporosis and Paget disease.

2. _____ reduces the production of uric acid, thereby decreasing serum uric acid levels and the deposit of urate crystals in joints.

3. Antirheumatic drugs often use the adverse reaction of _____ therapeutically, to decrease the body's autoimmune response.

4. _____ is a condition in which uric acid accumulates in increased amounts in the blood and is often deposited in the joints, causing severe pain.

5. Women taking bisphosphonates orally must remain in the _____ position for at least 30 min after administration.

Activity B DOSAGE CALCULATION

1. A primary health care provider (PHCP) prescribes 6 mg of the drug tizanidine to be given in three equally divided doses daily to a client. Tizanidine is available in 2-mg tablets. How many tablets should the nurse administer in each dose to the client?

_____

_____

2. A PHCP prescribes 100 mg of orphenadrine daily in two equally divided doses to a client. The orphenadrine therapy is to be continued for a period of 7 days. A medication box is purchased to ensure proper administration by the client. The pharmacy dispenses orphenadrine in 50-mg tablets. How many tablets are needed to load the medication box for a 7-day period?

_____

_____

3. A client has been prescribed 1 g of methocarbamol orally for each dose. The drug is available as 500-mg tablets. How many tablets should the client take for each dose?

_____

_____

4. A client alendronate is going out to breakfast on the day she takes her bisphosphonate. If she is meeting friends for breakfast at 8:30 AM, what time does she have to take the alendronate?

_____

_____

5. A client with glucocorticoid-induced osteoporosis is prescribed zoledronic acid to be administered intravenously. The prescribed dosage for zoledronic acid is 5 mg over 15 minutes. The zoledronic acid is available in a concentrated form of 5 mg/100 mL. How much of the drug solution should have been prepared for the nurse to administer?

_____

_____

Activity C MATCHING

1. Match the names of drugs used to treat musculoskeletal disorders given in Column A with the drugs' additional uses (besides musculoskeletal) in Column B.

Column A

____ **1.** Methotrexate

____ **2.** Sulfasalazine

____ **3.** Adalimumab

____ **4.** Probenecid

Column B

a. Crohn disease

b. Adjuvant to antibiotic therapy

c. Cancer chemotherapy

d. Ulcerative colitis

2. Match the musculoskeletal disorders in Column A with their description in Column B.

Column A

____ **1.** Synovitis

____ **2.** Arthritis

____ **3.** Osteoarthritis

____ **4.** Paget disease

Column B

a. Inflammation of a joint involving pain or stiffness

b. Inflammation of the synovial membrane of a joint

c. Chronic bone disorder characterized by abnormal bone remodeling

d. Noninflammatory degenerative joint disease marked by degeneration of the articular cartilage

Activity D SHORT ANSWERS

A nurse's role in managing a client who is prescribed a drug for a musculoskeletal disorder involves assisting the client with a preadministration assessment and monitoring the client with the prescribed drug. Answer the following questions, which involve the nurse's role in the management of clients who are on drug therapy for a musculoskeletal disorder.

1. A client with osteoporosis is prescribed a bisphosphonate drug. What preadministration assessments should the nurse conduct before the administration of a bisphosphonate drug?

_____

_____

2. After the preadministration assessment, the client is administered a drug for the osteoporosis. What ongoing assessment should the nurse perform when caring for a client who is administered a bisphosphonate drug?

_____

_____

Activity E **CROSSWORD PUZZLE**

Find the adverse reactions to musculoskeletal drugs.

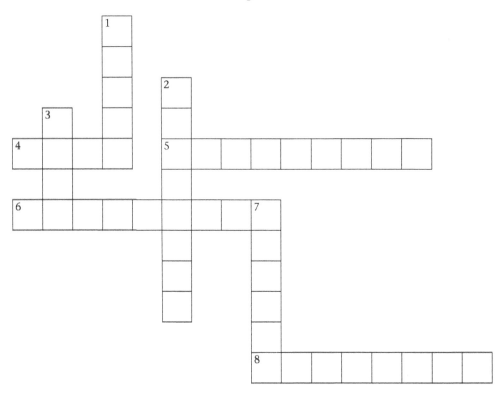

Across

4. Skin _____ could indicate a serious condition, such as Stevens–Johnson syndrome

5. Term meaning fullness or epigastric discomfort

6. At risk for this condition when immunosuppressed

8. Abnormal loss of hair

Down

1. Place where you typically see stomatitis

2. Condition that happens when diazepam is used as a relaxant

3. The increased levels of uric acid from gout cause this severe joint condition

7. GI condition caused by immunosuppressive drugs

SECTION II: APPLYING YOUR KNOWLEDGE

Activity F **CASE STUDY/CONCEPT MAPPING**

Mr. Phillip, an older male, presents to the ED with complaints of a swollen ankle that is painful to the touch.

1. What assessment should the nurse perform prior to the PHCP examining the client?

_____

_____

2. The ED provider diagnoses Mr. Phillip with an acute gout attack. His medical history indicates this is not his first time having a gout attack. The PHCP orders pegloticase 8 mg IV every 2 weeks at the infusion clinic. What specific assessment should the nurse include with each treatment at the clinic?

_____

_____

Now Map It Out! Use the templates provided in the appendix to add information and make client connections on a concept map.

Using introductory information (in Chapter 5 of the textbook), and when you add gout medications to Mr. Phillip's concept map, do you see an interaction? What happens when gout is treated in a person with chronic kidney disease?

SECTION III: PRACTICING FOR NCLEX

Activity G NCLEX-STYLE QUESTIONS

Answer the following questions.

1. A client with osteoporosis is administered bisphosphonate drugs. What adverse reactions should the nurse monitor for in the client?
    1. Dyspepsia
    2. Lethargy
    3. Sleepiness
    4. Constipation

2. An older female client living in a long-term care facility is prescribed alendronate. In which of the following client conditions is the use of alendronate contraindicated?
    1. Hypertension
    2. Hypocalcemia
    3. Insomnia
    4. Diabetes

3. A client with rheumatoid arthritis is administered the disease-modifying antirheumatic drug (DMARD) methotrexate along with sulfa antibiotics. What possible interaction should the nurse monitor for in the client?
    1. Rash
    2. Epigastric distress
    3. Methotrexate toxicity
    4. Theophylline toxicity

4. A client is administered methotrexate for the treatment of rheumatic arthritis. What should the nurse monitor in clients administered with methotrexate? **Select all that apply.**
    1. Hematology
    2. Liver function
    3. Renal function
    4. Pancreatic function
    5. Cardiovascular function

5. A client with rheumatoid arthritis is administered DMARDs. What instructions should the nurse ask the client to follow while taking DMARDs?
    1. Take the drugs with food.
    2. Drink 10 glasses of water a day.
    3. Avoid hazardous tasks in case of drowsiness.
    4. Notify PHCP in the case of diarrhea.

6. A client is administered bisphosphonates for osteoporosis. What ongoing assessments should a nurse perform for clients receiving bisphosphonates for musculoskeletal disorders?
    1. Obtain the client's history of disorders.
    2. Closely monitor the client for adverse reactions.
    3. Appraise the client's physical condition and limitations.
    4. Assess for pain in upper and lower back or hip.

7. A client is administered a drug for a musculoskeletal disorder. What nursing interventions should be used as a general rule for all clients administered a drug for a musculoskeletal disorder? **Select all that apply.**
    1. Report adverse reactions, especially vision changes.
    2. Be alert to reactions such as skin rash, fever, cough, or easy bruising.
    3. Encourage liberal fluid intake and measure intake and output.
    4. Ask the client to compensate for missed dosages.
    5. Be attentive to providing emotional support in dealing with the condition.

8. A client is prescribed infliximab (Remicade) for the treatment of rheumatoid arthritis. In which of the following client conditions is the use of infliximab contraindicated?
   1. Peptic ulcer disease
   2. Renal disorders
   3. Hepatic disorders
   4. Cardiac disease

9. Which of the following classes of medications are used in the treatment of osteoporosis?
   1. Bisphosphonates
   2. DMARDs
   3. Uric acid inhibitors
   4. Skeletal muscle relaxants

10. Which of the following is an example of a skeletal muscle relaxant?
    1. Allopurinol
    2. Alendronate
    3. Baclofen
    4. Hydroxychloroquine

11. Which of the following bisphosphonate drugs may be given once a year?
    1. Zoledronic acid (Reclast)
    2. Alendronate (Fosamax)
    3. Ibandronate (Boniva)
    4. Risedronate (Actonel)

12. Which of the following is the most common adverse reaction to carisoprodol (Soma) that the nurse should discuss with the client?
    1. Dyspnea
    2. Drowsiness
    3. Hypertension
    4. Tachycardia

Drugs That Affect the Respiratory System

CHAPTER 30

Upper Respiratory System Drugs

Learning Objectives

- Compare and contrast the classes of medications used for upper respiratory system problems.
- Explain the uses, general drug actions, adverse reactions, contraindications, precautions, and interactions of intranasal steroids, antitussives, mucolytics, expectorants, antihistamines, and decongestants.
- Distinguish important preadministration and ongoing assessment activities that should be performed on the client receiving intranasal steroids, antitussive, mucolytic, expectorant, antihistamine, or decongestant.
- List nursing diagnoses particular to a client taking intranasal steroids, antitussive, mucolytic, expectorant, antihistamine, or decongestant.
- Examine ways to promote an optimal response to therapy, manage common adverse reactions, and educate the client about the use of intranasal steroids, antitussive, mucolytic, expectorant, antihistamine, or decongestant.

SECTION I: ASSESSING YOUR UNDERSTANDING

Activity A FILL IN THE BLANKS

1. The release of histamine produces a(n) _____ response.

2. A(n) _____ is a drug that aids in raising thick, tenacious mucus from the respiratory passages.

3. A(n) _____ is a drug that reduces the swelling of the nasal passages, which, in turn, opens clogged nasal passages and enhances drainage of the sinuses.

4. Nasal decongestants produce localized _____ of the small blood vessels of the nasal membranes.

5. A mucolytic is a drug that loosens _____ secretions.

Activity B DOSAGE CALCULATION

1. A client has been prescribed dextromethorphan syrup for the treatment of a cough. The nurse is teaching the client how to self-administer the drug using the 30-mL plastic cup provided with the drug. The syrup contains dextromethorphan 5 mg/5 mL. How many mL should the nurse show the client to pour into the cup if the dose is 15 mg?

_____

_____

2. A client with a persistent cough has been prescribed 10 mL of codeine syrup every 4 hr as needed for cough. The syrup contains codeine 15 mg/5 mL. How many milligrams of codeine will the client take in each dose?

_____

_____

3. A client with allergic rhinitis is prescribed a nasal spray for symptoms. The metered device administers fluticasone 50 µg per spray. How many micrograms of fluticasone will the client receive when each dose is two nasal sprays?

_____

_____

4. A child is prescribed an antihistamine for allergy symptoms. The oral solution contains cetirizine 5 mg/1 teaspoon. How many milligrams of cetirizine will the child receive in a 2-teaspoon dose?

_____

_____

5. If the child in question 4 was given 2 tablespoons of the antihistamine in error, how many milligrams of cetirizine did the child receive? (Note: 3 teaspoons = 1 tablespoon.)

_____

_____

Activity C MATCHING

1. Match the antitussive drugs in Column A with their uses in Column B.

Column A

____ 1. Codeine

____ 2. Guaifenesin

____ 3. Diphenhydramine

____ 4. Acetylcysteine

Column B

a. Reduce secretion viscosity

b. Increase respiratory secretions

c. Depress cough center in the brain

d. Reduce histamine reactions

2. Match the medications that interact with antihistaminic drugs in Column A with the effect of the interaction in Column B.

Column A

____ 1. Rifampin

____ 2. Monoamine oxidase inhibitor

____ 3. Beta blocker

____ 4. Opioid analgesic

____ 5. Aluminum-based antacid

Column B

a. Causes additive central nervous system (CNS) depressant effect

b. Increases the risk of cardiovascular effects

c. Reduces the absorption of certain antihistamines

d. Decreases the concentration of the antihistamine in the blood

e. Increases the anticholinergic and sedative effects of antihistamines

Activity D SHORT ANSWERS

A nurse's role in managing a client receiving an upper respiratory system drug involves monitoring and managing the client's needs after drug administration. The nurse also educates the client about use of the drug. Answer the following questions, which involve the nurse's role in the management of such situations.

1. A client with a persistent cough calls the clinic for advice about medications to reduce the symptoms. What assessments should the nurse perform over the telephone for this client?

_____

_____

2. A client with sinusitis is on a decongestant medication. He wants to know about the possible side effects of the medication. What should the nurse inform him regarding the possible side effects of this medication?

_____

_____

Activity E WORD FIND PUZZLE

Find five of the six drug classes that are used with upper respiratory system conditions (hint: "anti" has been removed from some drug classes). Which drug class is missing?

E	W	Q	R	K	S	G	M	T	H	D
X	H	J	P	U	I	R	U	K	Y	E
P	F	I	Y	T	D	L	C	H	W	C
E	V	L	S	C	S	K	O	F	T	O
C	Z	P	H	T	F	Q	L	J	I	N
T	R	T	W	K	A	C	Y	V	R	G
O	D	U	C	G	H	M	T	L	D	E
R	I	Y	F	J	D	U	I	P	G	S
A	G	W	L	R	T	S	C	N	J	T
N	J	K	Q	H	S	P	V	I	E	A
T	U	S	S	I	V	E	G	K	L	N
L	P	T	R	D	J	Y	F	Q	U	T

SECTION II: APPLYING YOUR KNOWLEDGE

Activity F CASE STUDY

Betty Peterson calls the primary health care provider (PHCP) regarding her cold symptoms. She has been taking a nasal decongestant for as long as she has been suffering from the cold symptoms. Betty tells you she is frustrated because it stopped working and she would like you to recommend a decongestant "that will really work this time."

1. As the telephone triage nurse, what assessment questions should you ask Betty?

_____

_____

2. In consultation with the PCHP, it is determined that Betty is suffering from decongestant rebound. As the telephone triage nurse, how will you explain this to Betty?

_____

_____

Now Map It Out! Use the templates provided in the appendix to add information and make client connections on a concept map.

Using information from the above scenario, map out Betty Peterson's drug prescriptions. Look for drug–drug interactions as the chapters build upon each other.

SECTION III: PRACTICING FOR NCLEX

Activity G NCLEX-STYLE QUESTIONS

Answer the following questions.

1. A long-term care client with a cough is prescribed an expectorant. What ongoing assessments should the nurse perform for this client? **Select all that apply.**
   1. Ask the client about ear infection.
   2. Assess the respiratory status of the client.
   3. Document the lung sounds of the client.
   4. Examine the pulse rate every 30 minutes.
   5. Document the consistency of sputum.

2. A home care nurse is preparing a teaching plan for a caregiver regarding an antitussive drug for an older client. Which of the following instructions should the nurse include in the teaching plan? **Select all that apply.**
   1. Take the medicine 1 hr before meals.
   2. Avoid irritants such as cigarettes, dust, or fumes.
   3. Avoid drinking fluids for 30 minutes after taking the drug.
   4. Take the medicine with milk to enhance absorption.
   5. Avoid chewing or breaking open the oral capsules.

3. A client has purchased a nasal decongestant for all members of the household to use. Which of the following instructions is a priority for the nurse to educate the client about the drug?

    1. Topical decongestants can sting or burn when used.
    2. Rebound congestion can occur with topical decongestants.
    3. Do not allow the tip to touch the nasal mucosa.
    4. Refrain from sharing the drug container with multiple users.

4. A nurse is assigned to care for a client who has been prescribed an antitussive. In which of the following conditions is the use of antitussives contraindicated?

    1. Asthma
    2. Liver dysfunction
    3. Cardiac problems
    4. Hypersensitivity

5. A client is prescribed a decongestant for allergic rhinitis. In which client conditions should the nurse administer the drug cautiously? **Select all that apply.**

    1. Hypertension
    2. Hyperthyroidism
    3. Conjunctivitis
    4. Nephropathy
    5. Glaucoma

6. A nurse is caring for a client with ineffective airway clearance. Which of the following is an appropriate nursing intervention to promote effective airway clearance?

    1. Suggest avoiding consumption of fruit juice.
    2. Encourage fluid intake of up to 2000 mL per day.
    3. Monitor fluid output of the client every 8 hr.
    4. Encourage taking antitussives after each coughing episode.

7. A nurse is caring for a client who has been using a eucalyptus product for the treatment of nasal congestion. What assessment question should the nurse ask the client about the use of this herbal medicine?

    1. Is the medicine taken on an empty stomach?
    2. Is the client pregnant?
    3. Is the drug used in a humidifier?
    4. Is the client warming the medicine before use?

8. A client experiencing a cough takes an OTC cough medicine. Under what conditions should the client consult the PHCP?

    1. Cough lasts more than 10 days.
    2. Cough is accompanied by dizziness.
    3. Frequency of coughing is 20 minutes.
    4. Cough is accompanied by vomiting.

9. A client with cystic fibrosis may use which medication to reduce the viscosity of respiratory secretions?

    1. Mucolytic
    2. Antitussive
    3. Expectorant
    4. Antihistamine

10. A client is taking levothyroxine 150 µg daily for hypothyroidism. Which of the following medications should be avoided in this client?

    1. Potassium iodide
    2. Dextromethorphan
    3. Codeine
    4. Benzonatate

11. A nurse is caring for a client in the hospital who is being discharged today with a prescription for benzonatate 200 mg orally three times daily. What would the nurse tell the client about this prescription during discharge counseling? **Select all that apply.**

   1. Benzonatate can cause GI upset and sedation.
   2. Benzonatate capsules should be sucked on like a lozenge.
   3. The client should drink plenty of fluids.
   4. Consumption of alcohol is permitted while taking benzonatate.
   5. Benzonatate can be taken more frequently than prescribed if needed.

12. Expectorants elicit their effect by which of the following mechanisms?

   1. Thinning respiratory secretions
   2. Breaking down thick mucus in the lower lungs
   3. Depressing the cough center in the brain
   4. Anesthetizing stretch receptors in the respiratory passages

31

Lower Respiratory System Drugs

Learning Objectives

- Explain the uses, general drug actions, general adverse reactions, contraindications, precautions, and interactions of the bronchodilators and antiasthma drugs.
- Distinguish important preadministration and ongoing assessment activities the nurse should perform on the client taking a bronchodilator or an antiasthma drug.
- List nursing diagnoses particular to a client taking a bronchodilator or an antiasthma drug.
- Examine ways to promote an optimal response to therapy, how to manage common adverse reactions, and important points to keep in mind when educating a client about the use of bronchodilators or an antiasthma drugs.

SECTION I: ASSESSING YOUR UNDERSTANDING

Activity A FILL IN THE BLANKS

1. Asthma is a chronic _____ disease causing spasmodic constriction of the bronchi.

2. When inflammation occurs in the lungs, a large amount of _____ is released from the mast cells.

3. In asthma, the airways become narrow and extra _____ clogs the smaller airways.

4. The asthma symptoms of wheezing and dyspnea cause the client to become _____.

5. _____ are the mainstay of treatment for many chronic pulmonary disorders.

Activity B **OUT IN THE COMMUNITY**

Return to your textbook and fill in the asthma action plan according to the plan established for Lillian Chase in Chapter 31. Answer the following questions according to the plan.

ASTHMA ACTION PLAN

For: _____ Doctor: _____ Date: _____

Doctor's Phone Number: _____ Hospital/Emergency Department Phone Number: _____

GREEN ZONE	**DOING WELL** • No cough, wheeze, chest tightness, or shortness of breath during the day or night • Can do usual activities **And, if a peak flow meter is used,** **Peak flow:** more than _____ (80 percent or more of my best peak flow) My best peak flow is: _____	**Daily Medications** Medicine _____ _____ _____ _____	How much to take _____ _____ _____ _____	When to take it _____ _____ _____ _____
	Before exercise	☐_____	☐2 or ☐4 puffs	5 minutes before exercise

YELLOW ZONE	**ASTHMA IS GETTING WORSE** • Cough, wheeze, chest tightness, or shortness of breath, or • Waking at night due to asthma, or • Can do some, but not all, usual activities –Or– **Peak flow:** _____ to _____ (50 to 79 percent of my best peak flow)

1st ➤ Add: quick-relief medicine—and keep taking your GREEN ZONE medicine.

_____ (quick-relief medicine)   _____ Number of puffs   Can repeat every _____ minutes
                                        or ☐Nebulizer, once   up to maximum of _____ doses

2nd ➤ **If your symptoms (and peak flow, if used) return to GREEN ZONE after 1 hour of above treatment:**
☐Continue monitoring to be sure you stay in the green zone.
        –Or–
If your symptoms (and peak flow, if used) do not return to GREEN ZONE after 1 hour of above treatment:
☐Take: _____ (quick-relief medicine)   _____ Number of puffs **or** ☐Nebulizer
☐Add: _____ mg per day For _____ (3-10) days
      (oral steroid)
☐Call the doctor ☐before/ ☐within_____ hours after taking the oral steroid.

RED ZONE	**MEDICAL ALERT!** • Very short of breath, or • Quick-relief medicines have not helped, • Cannot do usual activities, or • Symptoms are same or get worse after 24 hours in Yellow Zone –Or– **Peak flow:** less than _____ (50 percent of my best peak flow)

Take this medicine:
☐_____ (quick-relief medicine)   _____ Number of puffs **or** ☐Nebulizer
☐_____ mg
   (oral steroid)

Then call your doctor NOW. Go to the hospital or call an ambulance if:
• You are still in the red zone after 15 minutes AND
• You have not reached your doctor.

DANGER SIGNS   • **Trouble walking and talking due to shortness of breath**
                    • **Lips or fingernails are blue**

➤ • Take _____ puffs of _____ (quick relief medicine) AND
  • Go to the hospital or call for an ambulance _____ NOW!
                                                  (phone)

1. Lillian Chase needs to know the peak flow parameters for each of the three color zones. Calculate the peak flow ranges based on her personal best peak flow of 350.

_____

_____

2. Lillian Chase checked her peak flow and the reading was 295. What medication should she take at bedtime?

_____

_____

3. Before exercise, Lillian Chase is to take 2 puffs of albuterol. If the inhaler delivers albuterol 90 mcg/inhalation, how many micrograms of albuterol is in each dose?

_____

_____

Activity C MATCHING

1. Match the bronchodilator and antiasthmatic drugs given in Column A with their class given in Column B.

Column A

____ **1.** Albuterol

____ **2.** Theophylline

____ **3.** Flunisolide

____ **4.** Zafirlukast

____ **5.** Salmeterol

Column B

a. Leukotriene modifier

b. Long-acting beta$_2$-adrenergic (β_2-adrenergic)

c. Xanthine derivative

d. Short-acting beta$_2$-adrenergic

e. Inhaled corticosteroid

2. Match the drug in Column A with the likely interaction effect when combined with a sympathomimetic agent in Column B.

Column A

____ **1.** Adrenergic drugs

____ **2.** MAOI antidepressant

____ **3.** Methyldopa

____ **4.** Uterine stimulants

____ **5.** Theophylline

Column B

a. Increased pressor response

b. Possible additive effects

c. Possible severe hypotension

d. Increased risk of cardiotoxicity

e. Risk of severe headache and hypertensive crisis

Activity D SHORT ANSWERS

A nurse's role in managing clients who are being administered bronchodilators and antiasthma drugs involves monitoring and implementing interventions that aid in recovery. Answer the following questions, which involve the nurse's role in the management of such situations.

1. A client has been prescribed a Step Method for asthma control. What does that involve?

_____

_____

2. Why is it suggested that clients follow asthma action plans?

_____

_____

Activity E SUDOKU PUZZLE

Familiarize yourself with respiratory abbreviations.

PEV			LABA	SOB	MDI	EIB	SABA	
				COPD		PEV	SOB	
COPD		MDI			SABA			ICS
DPI			SABA					
MDI						LABA	DPI	
LABA	COPD	SOB		PEV			EIB	SABA
		PEV	SOB			COPD	MDI	
		LABA	COPD	MDI				DPI
	MDI	COPD		DPI	LABA	SABA	PEV	EIB

SECTION II: APPLYING YOUR KNOWLEDGE

Activity F CASE STUDY

Lillian Chase was diagnosed with asthma at age 8 years. Today she presents to the primary health care provider's office complaining of increased shortness of breath and coughing, especially at night, despite using an albuterol (Proventil) inhaler 1 or 2 inhalations every 4 to 6 hours as needed. Using the Step Method, the primary health care provider classifies Ms. Chase's asthma as Step 3.

1. What medications are recommended to treat Ms. Chase's asthma?

_____

_____

2. What environmental controls can Ms. Chase use to help control her asthma?

_____

_____

Now Map It Out! Use the templates provided in the appendix to add information and make client connections on a concept map.

Lillian's health care medication plan has been changed considerably due to some changes in her respiratory status. Make the notations on her concept map of the different changes in her asthma action plan. Once again review the other medications currently prescribed for Ms. Chase. Will the medication changes cause issues with any of the other drugs she is currently taking?

SECTION III: PRACTICING FOR NCLEX

Activity G NCLEX-STYLE QUESTIONS

Answer the following questions.

1. A client with asthma was recently diagnosed with glaucoma. Which of the following drugs should the nurse consider as relatively safe for this client?

   1. LABAs
   2. Xanthine derivatives
   3. SABAs
   4. Inhaled corticosteroids

2. A client is prescribed aminophylline for the symptomatic relief of bronchial asthma. The nurse is required to inform the client about other drugs that may interact with aminophylline. Which of the following drugs increases the effects of aminophylline?

   1. Ketoconazole
   2. Rifampin
   3. Loop diuretics
   4. Beta blockers

3. A client is prescribed aminophylline for emphysema. Which of the following factors should the nurse assess to check for the occurrence of any adverse effects?

   1. Electrocardiographic changes
   2. Fluid intake and output
   3. Consistency of the stool
   4. Changes in blood hemoglobin

4. A client is admitted to the ED with complaints of cough, difficulty breathing, and a wheezing sound during respiration. The client is diagnosed as having asthma. Which of the following additional symptoms might the nurse observe in the client?

   1. Decreased blood pressure
   2. Increased anxiety
   3. Decreased pulse rate
   4. Increased urination

5. A client is prescribed the antiasthmatic drug zafirlukast. The client's medical history indicates that the client is on aspirin for the pain relief of arthritis. Which of the following possible drug interactions should the nurse monitor for?

   1. Increased thrombolytic effect of aspirin
   2. Increased plasma levels of zafirlukast
   3. Decreased absorption of zafirlukast
   4. Decreased plasma levels of aspirin

6. Given below, in random order, are the steps involved in the progress of chronic inflammation seen in asthma. Arrange the steps in the correct order.

   1. Decreased airflow to the lungs
   2. Bronchospasm and inflammation
   3. Release of histamine from the mast cells
   4. Increased mucous production and edema of the airway
   5. Narrowing and clogging of the airways

7. A client with asthma has been prescribed a corticosteroid agent by inhalation for the long-term reduction of inflammation in the airways. Which of the following drugs are corticosteroid agents? **Select all that apply.**

   1. Cromolyn
   2. Flunisolide
   3. Beclomethasone
   4. Ipratropium
   5. Triamcinolone

8. A client with asthma has been prescribed the use of montelukast orally. What is the typical administration schedule for this drug?

   1. Once a day
   2. Twice a day
   3. Three times a day
   4. Four times a day

9. Which of the following is an example of a short-acting beta$_2$ (β_2) agonist (SABA)?
   1. Formoterol
   2. Salmeterol
   3. Albuterol
   4. Arformoterol

10. Which of the following may increase the risk of asthma-related death?
    1. Long-acting beta$_2$ agonists
    2. Inhaled corticosteroids
    3. Short-acting beta$_2$ agonists
    4. Mast cell stabilizers

11. Asthma exacerbations are usually preceded by an increase in which of the following symptoms? **Select all that apply.**
    1. Cough
    2. Chest tightness
    3. Nasal congestion
    4. Bradypnea
    5. Dyspnea

12. Xanthine derivatives elicit their effect by which of the following mechanisms?
    1. Stimulation of beta-adrenergic receptors
    2. Stimulation of the central nervous system
    3. Reduction of airway hyperresponsiveness
    4. Stabilization of mast cell membranes

Drugs That Affect the Cardiovascular System

Diuretics

- List the five general types of diuretics.
- Explain the uses, general drug actions, adverse reactions, contraindications, precautions, and interactions of the diuretics.
- Distinguish important preadministration and ongoing assessment activities that the nurse should perform on the client taking a diuretic.
- List nursing diagnoses particular to a client taking a diuretic.
- Examine ways to promote an optimal response to therapy, how to manage common adverse reactions, and important points to keep in mind when educating clients about the use of diuretics.

SECTION I: ASSESSING YOUR UNDERSTANDING

Activity A FILL IN THE BLANKS

1. Accumulation of excess fluid in the tissue or body is known as _____.

2. _____ anhydrase inhibition, which is the action of a diuretic drug, results in the excretion of sodium, potassium, bicarbonate, and water.

3. An increase in the _____ in the blood is known as hyperkalemia.

4. Extremity _____, meaning numbness, tingling, or flaccid muscles, may indicate hypokalemia, which is an adverse reaction to diuretics.

5. _____ reactions to diuretics involve rash and photosensitivity.

Activity B DOSAGE CALCULATION

1. A client with edema has been prescribed acetazolamide. The primary health care provider (PHCP) instructs the nurse to administer 250 mg of the drug every 4 hours. The drug is available in 500-mg tablets. How many tablets should the nurse administer to the client for each dose?

_____

_____

2. A client with edema due to cirrhosis of the liver has been prescribed 6 mg of bumetanide (Bumex) on a daily basis. The drug is available in 2-mg tablets. How many tablets should the nurse administer to the client every day?

_____

_____

3. A PHCP has prescribed 500 mg of chlorothiazide IV for a client to be given twice daily. The drug is available in a solution of 250 mg/5 mL. How many mL of the solution will be mixed into the IV secondary set for infusion?

_____

_____

4. A client has been ordered 200 mg of furosemide (Lasix) orally right now. Lasix 80-mg tablets are available in the Pyxis machine. How many tablets should the nurse administer to the client?

_____

_____

Activity C MATCHING

1. Match the diuretics in Column A with their uses in Column B.

Column A

____ **1.** Ethacrynic acid

____ **2.** Mannitol

____ **3.** Urea

____ **4.** Amiloride

____ **5.** Metolazone

Column B

a. Treatment of cerebral edema

b. Reduction of intracranial pressure

c. Prevention of polyuria with lithium use

d. Hypertension, edema due to CHF, cirrhosis, corticosteroid, and estrogen therapy

e. Short-term management of ascites caused by lymphedema

2. Match the interactant loop diuretics and their interactant drugs in Column A with the results given in Column B.

Column A

____ **1.** Loop diuretics + thrombolytics

____ **2.** Loop diuretics + lithium

____ **3.** Loop diuretics + aminoglycosides

____ **4.** Loop diuretics + digitalis

Column B

a. Increased risk of lithium toxicity

b. Increased risk of arrhythmias

c. Increased risk of bleeding

d. Increased risk of ototoxicity

Activity D SHORT ANSWERS

A nurse's role in managing clients who are prescribed a diuretic involves performing preadministrative and ongoing assessments during the course of the drug therapy. The nurse also monitors the clients administered diuretic drugs for the occurrence of any adverse reactions. Answer the following questions, which involve the nurse's role in the management of clients on diuretic drug therapy.

1. A client with edema is prescribed a diuretic drug. What preadministration assessments should the nurse perform before administration of this diuretic drug?

   _____

   _____

2. What is the nurse's role after the administration of a diuretic drug to a client?

   _____

   _____

Activity E CROSSWORD PUZZLE

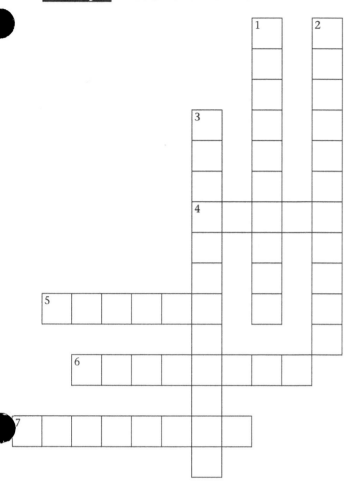

Across

4. Accumulation of excess water in the body
5. Cessation of urine production
6. Production of urine
7. Absence of urine production

Down

1. Low blood potassium level
2. Male breast enlargement
3. Increase in potassium levels in the blood

SECTION II: APPLYING YOUR KNOWLEDGE

Activity F CASE STUDY

Mrs. Moore is an 85-year-old woman. She is admitted to the hospital for treatment of significant edema associated with heart failure (HF). The PHCP has ordered furosemide (Lasix) IV 1 mg/kg every 6 hours.

1. If Mrs. Moore weighs 150 lb, how many mL should the nurse administer every 6 hours if furosemide (Lasix) is available in a 20-mg/mL vial?

_____

_____

2. During the administration of furosemide (Lasix), for what adverse reactions should the nurse observe Mrs. Moore?

_____

_____

Now Map It Out! Use the templates provided in the appendix to add information and make client connections on a concept map.

Review Mrs. Moore's concept map. She is taking a number of drugs and is a candidate for problems associated with polypharmacy. Add the client problem of nonadherence to your concept map as well as the addition of the drug from this chapter and determine what, if any, drug interactions exist with the medications taken now.

SECTION III: PRACTICING FOR NCLEX

Activity G **NCLEX-STYLE QUESTIONS**

Answer the following questions.

1. A nurse is caring for a client with edema. What assessments should the nurse perform on this client to promote an optimal response to therapy? **Select all that apply.**
   1. Measure and record client's weight daily.
   2. Check the pupils every 2 hours for dilation.
   3. Measure fluid intake and output every 8 hr.
   4. Assess respiratory rate every 4 hour.
   5. Check the client's response to light.

2. A nurse is caring for a client taking a diuretic. During assessment, the nurse observes that the client is experiencing GI upset after taking the prescribed drug. Which of the following interventions should the nurse perform when caring for this client?
   1. Ensure that the drug is taken on an empty stomach.
   2. Ensure that the drug is taken with food or milk.
   3. Instruct the client to reduce fluid intake.
   4. Avoid any consumption of fibrous food by the client.

3. A PHCP has prescribed a chlorothiazide drug to a client with hypertension. The client informs the nurse that they are also taking an antidiabetic drug for controlling diabetes. What interaction between these two drugs should the nurse monitor for in the client?
   1. Increased risk of ototoxicity
   2. Increased risk of hyperglycemia
   3. Increased hypersensitivity to antidiabetic
   4. Increased chlorothiazide effect

4. A nurse is preparing diet information for the client taking a diuretic. Which of the following foods should be included in a diet to replenish potassium lost from the diuretic? **Select all that apply.**
   1. Dried apricots
   2. Carrots
   3. Green beans
   4. Molasses

5. A nurse is caring for a client who complains of cramps and muscle pains. Assessment reveals that the client is also experiencing oliguria, hypotension, and GI disturbances. Which of the following conditions is the client experiencing?
   1. Exercise exhaustion
   2. Electrolyte imbalance
   3. Influenza
   4. HF

6. A client is prescribed amiloride, a potassium-sparing diuretic, by the PHCP. In which of the following conditions should the nurse discontinue the drug?
   1. If the client experiences gout attacks
   2. If the client's urine tests positive for glucose
   3. If client's serum potassium levels exceed 5.3 mEq/mL
   4. If excess fluid has been removed from the client's body

7. Which of the following is an example of a loop diuretic?
   1. Furosemide
   2. Hydrochlorothiazide
   3. Acetazolamide
   4. Spironolactone

8. Which of the following diuretics exerts its effect by inhibiting the enzyme carbonic anhydrase?
   1. Furosemide
   2. Acetazolamide
   3. Hydrochlorothiazide
   4. Spironolactone

9. Which of the following exerts its diuretic effects by increasing the density of the filtrate in the glomerulus?
   1. Mannitol
   2. Furosemide
   3. Hydrochlorothiazide
   4. Spironolactone

10. Which of the following exerts its diuretic effect by antagonizing the action of aldosterone?
   1. Spironolactone
   2. Furosemide
   3. Hydrochlorothiazide
   4. Acetazolamide

11. Which of the following exerts its effects by depressing the reabsorption of sodium in the collecting tubules, thereby increasing sodium and water excretion?
    1. Furosemide
    2. Hydrochlorothiazide
    3. Acetazolamide
    4. Triamterene

12. Which of the following exerts its diuretic effect by inhibiting the reabsorption of sodium and chloride ions in the early distal tubule of the nephron?
    1. Hydrochlorothiazide
    2. Acetazolamide
    3. Furosemide
    4. Spironolactone

33

Antihyperlipidemic Drugs

Learning Objectives

- Compare and contrast cholesterol, high-density lipoprotein (HDL), low-density lipoprotein (LDL), and triglyceride levels and how they contribute to the development of heart disease.
- Define therapeutic life changes (TLCs) and how they affect cholesterol levels.
- Explain the uses, general drug actions, general adverse reactions, contraindications, precautions, and interactions of antihyperlipidemic drugs.
- Distinguish important preadministration and ongoing assessment activities the nurse should perform on the client taking an antihyperlipidemic drug.
- List nursing diagnoses particular to a client taking an antihyperlipidemic drug.
- Examine ways to promote an optimal response to therapy, how to manage common adverse reactions, and important points to keep in mind when educating client about the use of antihyperlipidemic drugs.

SECTION I: ASSESSING YOUR UNDERSTANDING

Activity A FILL IN THE BLANKS

1. _____ is an increase in the lipids, which are a group of fats or fatlike substances in the blood.

2. Atherosclerosis is a disorder in which _____ deposits accumulate on the lining of the blood vessels.

3. High-density lipoproteins (HDLs) take cholesterol from the peripheral cells and transport it to the _____.

4. A substance that accelerates a chemical reaction without itself undergoing a change is called a _____.

5. _____ is a condition in which muscle damage results in the release of muscle cell contents into the bloodstream.

Activity B DOSAGE CALCULATION

1. A client with partial biliary obstruction has been prescribed 16 g of cholestyramine to be taken four times a day in equal doses. The drug is available in 4-g packets. How many packets would be required for one dose?

_____

_____

2. A client with hyperlipidemia has been prescribed 5 g of colestipol to be taken every day. Colestipol is available as 2.5-g tablets. How many tablets should be administered to the client in a day?

_____

_____

3. A client with hyperlipidemia has been prescribed 80 mg of atorvastatin per day. The drug is available in 40-mg tablets. How many tablets should the client take every day?

_____

_____

4. A client with dyslipidemia has been prescribed 60 mg of fluvastatin to be taken daily. The drug is available as 20-mg capsules. How many capsules should the client take in a day?

_____

_____

5. A client with hypercholesterolemia has been prescribed 40 mg of lovastatin per day. The drug is available in the form of 20-mg tablets. How many tablets should the client take daily?

_____

_____

Activity C MATCHING

1. Match the antihyperlipidemic drugs in Column A with their adverse reactions in Column B.

Column A

____ **1.** Rosuvastatin

____ **2.** Ezetimibe

____ **3.** Niacin

____ **4.** Gemfibrozil

Column B

a. Coughing

b. Tingling

c. Vertigo

d. Pharyngitis

2. Match the antihyperlipidemic drugs in Column A with their primary uses in Column B.

Column A

____ **1.** Cholestyramine

____ **2.** Atorvastatin

____ **3.** Fluvastatin

____ **4.** Lovastatin

Column B

a. Reduction of elevated serum triglyceride levels

b. Secondary prevention of cardiovascular events

c. Relief from partial biliary obstruction

d. Slowed progression of coronary artery disease

Activity D SHORT ANSWERS

A nurse's role in managing a client who has been prescribed an antihyperlipidemic drug involves performing preadministration and ongoing assessments during the course of the drug therapy. The nurse also monitors the clients for any occurrence of adverse reactions. Answer the following questions, which involve the nurse's role in the management of clients on antihyperlipidemic drug therapy.

1. A nurse is caring for a client with hyperlipidemia. What preadministration assessments should the nurse perform before the administration of a prescribed antihyperlipidemic drug?

_____

_____

2. What is the nurse's role after an antihyperlipidemic drug is administered to a client?

_____

_____

Activity E CROSSWORD PUZZLE

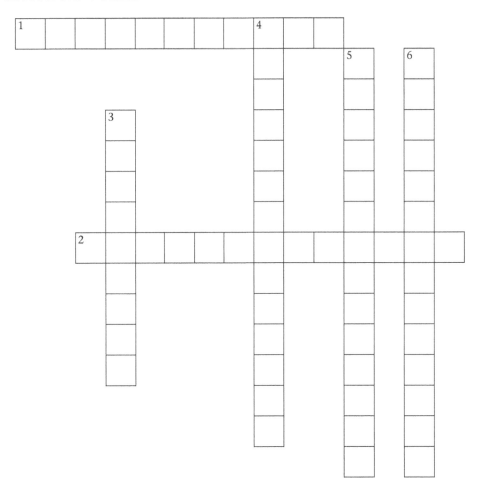

Across

1. Fatlike substance produced mostly in the liver of animals
2. Inflammation of the gallbladder

Down

3. Yellow deposits of cholesterol in tendons and soft tissues
4. Condition in which muscle damage results in the release of muscle cell contents into the bloodstream
5. Increase in the lipids in the blood
6. Stones in the gallbladder

SECTION II: APPLYING YOUR KNOWLEDGE

Activity F CASE STUDY

Alfredo Garcia's mother was admitted to the hospital after having a myocardial infarction. She has a history significant for diabetes, hypertension, and smoking (1 pack per day [ppd]). She is being discharged. The only new prescription she will be leaving with is pravastatin (Pravachol) 40 mg, with directions to take one tablet daily at bedtime. The physician has asked the nurse to go over discharge instructions with Mrs. Garcia. An interpreter is here to help you with the discharge counseling Mrs. Garcia requires about her new medication.

1. What class of antihyperlipidemic medication is pravastatin, and what should Mrs. Garcia be told about the medication?

_____

_____

2. What lifestyle modification should Mrs. Garcia be encouraged to follow?

_____

_____

Now Map It Out! Use the templates provided in the appendix to add information and make client connections on a concept map.

Alfredo is now concerned about his risk of heart disease. The Framingham Heart Study provides a tool to assess for heart attack risk. Mr. Garcia's record indicates a total cholesterol level of 242 and an HDL level of 36. Using the online tool, these cholesterol values, and other data from his concept map, determine Mr. Garcia's risk score.

SECTION III: PRACTICING FOR NCLEX

Activity G NCLEX-STYLE QUESTIONS

Answer the following questions.

1. A nurse is caring for a client prescribed the drug ezetimibe. What instruction should the nurse provide to the client if the drug is to be taken with cholestyramine, a bile acid sequestrant?
   1. Take the drug 2 hours before a bile acid sequestrant.
   2. Ensure a time gap of 1 hour between the intake of these two drugs.
   3. Take both drugs 30 minutes before meals.
   4. Take the bile acid sequestrant with warm water.

2. A nurse is caring for a client with primary hypercholesterolemia who is taking the drug ezetimibe. What adverse reaction to the drug should the nurse monitor for in the client?
   1. Vertigo
   2. Headache
   3. Cholelithiasis
   4. Arthralgia

3. A client is prescribed gemfibrozil drug therapy for high serum triglyceride levels. The client is also receiving an anticoagulant as a blood thinner. What interaction of these two drugs should the nurse monitor for in the client?
   1. Increased hypoglycemic effects
   2. Increased risk of severe myopathy
   3. Enhanced effect of the anticoagulant
   4. Increased risk of hypertension

4. In which of the following client aliments should the nurse exercise caution and monitor for exacerbation of problems while caring for clients who are taking HMG-CoA reductase inhibitors? **Select all that apply.**
   1. Peptic ulcer
   2. Acute infection
   3. Visual disturbances
   4. Unstable angina
   5. Endocrine disorders

5. A client tells the nurse they heard that garlic will lower serum cholesterol and triglyceride levels. This client is taking warfarin as an anticoagulant. What should the nurse tell the client is a potential adverse reaction when these are taken together?
   1. Bleeding
   2. Peptic ulcers
   3. Irritation
   4. Skin rashes

6. A nurse is caring for a client taking an antihyperlipidemic drug. The nurse observes an elevation of blood lipid levels rather than a decrease. What is a priority nursing intervention in this situation?
   1. Notify the PHCP for a different antihyperlipidemic drug.
   2. Collect blood samples for further examination.
   3. Administer next dose of the drug with milk.
   4. Record the fluid intake and output every hour.

7. A client informs the nurse that they have been taking a natural product—red yeast to improve blood lipid profile. Which toxic reaction associated with red yeast when taking a statin drug should the nurse relay to the client?
   1. Headache
   2. Dyspnea
   3. Muscle damage
   4. Dyspepsia

8. A nurse is caring for a client who has been prescribed colestipol for the treatment of hyperlipidemia. This drug is known to cause constipation. What instructions should the nurse provide to the client to help prevent constipation? **Select all that apply.**

   1. Exercise daily.
   2. Consume foods high in dietary fiber.
   3. Take the drug 1 hr after meals.
   4. Increase fluid intake.
   5. Take oral vitamin K supplements.

9. Increased levels of low-density lipoprotein (LDL) combined with certain risk factors can lead to the development of which medical condition?

   1. Diabetes
   2. Glaucoma
   3. Benign prostatic hyperplasia
   4. Heart disease

10. Which of the following herbal products have been promoted by the natural food industry to lower serum cholesterol and triglycerides? **Select all that apply.**

    1. Ginseng
    2. Red yeast rice
    3. Garlic
    4. Feverfew
    5. Black cohosh

11. Which of the following classes of medications are used to treat hyperlipidemia? **Select all that apply.**

    1. HMG-CoA reductase inhibitors
    2. Fibric acid derivatives
    3. Bile acid resins
    4. Calcium channel blockers
    5. Angiotensin II receptor blockers

12. Bile acid resins can decrease serum levels of several medications, primarily via which mechanism?

    1. Inhibition of hepatic enzymes
    2. Decreased gastrointestinal absorption
    3. Modifying liver metabolism
    4. Increased renal excretion

CHAPTER 34

Antihypertensive Drugs

Learning Objectives

- Compare and contrast the various types of hypertension and risk factors involved.
- Identify normal and abnormal blood pressure levels for adults.
- List the various types of drugs used to treat hypertension.
- Explain the general drug actions, uses, adverse reactions, contraindications, precautions, and interactions of the antihypertensive drugs.
- Distinguish important preadministration and ongoing assessment activities the nurse should perform for the client taking an antihypertensive drug.
- Explain why blood pressure determinations are important during therapy with an antihypertensive drug.
- List nursing diagnoses particular to a client taking an antihypertensive drug.
- Examine ways to promote an optimal response to therapy, how to manage adverse reactions, and important points to keep in mind when educating clients about the use of an antihypertensive drug.

SECTION I: ASSESSING YOUR UNDERSTANDING

Activity A FILL IN THE BLANKS

1. Angiotensin I is converted to angiotensin II, which is a powerful _____.

2. Furosemide and hydrochlorothiazide are examples of _____ agents used in the treatment of hypertension.

3. Diazoxide and nitroprusside are drugs used in the management of _____ emergencies.

4. Aldosterone promotes the retention of _____ and water, which contributes to the rise in blood pressure.

5. Electrolyte imbalance such as _____, which is a low blood sodium level, occurs with diuretic usage.

Activity B DOSAGE CALCULATION

1. A hypertensive client's daily dose of captopril is 200 mg, in two divided doses. It is available as 50-mg tablets. How many tablets should the client take in each dose?

2. A client is prescribed 40 mg of hydralazine IV to be given for hypertensive emergency management. Each ampule contains 20 mg/mL of hydralazine. How many ampules will the nurse use to give the required dosage?

3. A client is prescribed 100 mg of losartan daily for hypertension. The tablets are available in 50-mg strength. How many tablets should the client take daily?

4. A nurse is to give 150 mg of atenolol to a client with hypertension. The tablets are available in 50-mg strength. How many tablets should the nurse administer?

_____

_____

5. A doctor prescribes 2 mg of doxazosin daily for hypertension. The drug is available in 2- or 4-mg tablets. Which tablet should be dispensed to prevent errors?

_____

_____

Activity C MATCHING

1. Match the terms associated with hypertension given in Column A with their correct description given in Column B.

Column A

____ **1.** Hypertension

____ **2.** Primary hypertension

____ **3.** Hypertensive emergency

____ **4.** Secondary hypertension

____ **5.** Prehypertension

Column B

a. Blood pressure rise with no known, discernible cause; has been associated with certain risk factors such as diet and lifestyle

b. When a direct cause of the hypertension can be identified

c. Defined as a blood pressure of 130/80 mm Hg or higher

d. Rise in blood pressure where the systolic pressure is between 120 and 129 mm Hg with a diastolic pressure at or below 80 mm Hg

e. Rise in blood pressure to extremely high levels, which can lead to damage of target organs such as kidney, eye, and heart if not lowered

2. Using the Summary Drug Tables in your textbook, look for patterns in how drugs are named, and match the antihypertensive drug ending (suffix) in Column A with the drug class in Column B.

Column A

____ **1.** -lol

____ **2.** -sin

____ **3.** -ine

____ **4.** -pril

____ **5.** -tan

Column B

a. Angiotensin-converting enzyme inhibitor (ACEI)

b. Beta-adrenergic (β-adrenergic) blocking drug

c. Angiotensin II receptor antagonist

d. Alpha-adrenergic (α-adrenergic) blocking drug

e. Calcium channel blocker

Activity D SHORT ANSWERS

A nurse's role in managing clients who are being administered antihypertensive drugs involves monitoring and implementing interventions that aid in the recovery of the clients. Answer the following questions, which involve the nurse's role in the management of such situations.

1. A client has been prescribed captopril for hypertension. During the course of the therapy, what assessments should the nurse carry out?

_____

_____

2. A client is prescribed metoprolol for hypertension. What points should the nurse include in the client teaching plan?

_____

_____

Activity E CROSSWORD PUZZLE

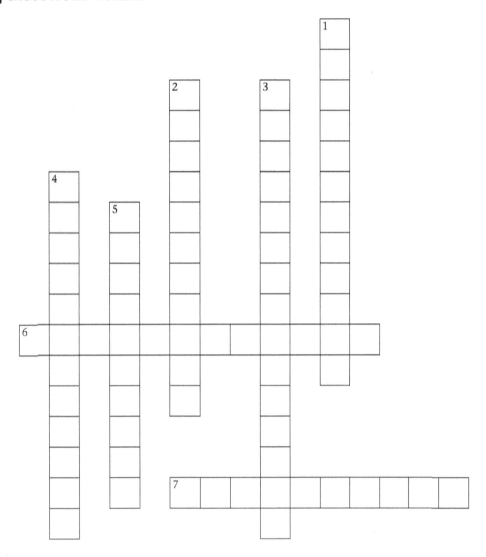

Across

6. Increase in the diameter of the blood vessels that, when widespread, results in a drop in blood pressure

7. Pertaining to something that normally occurs or is produced within the organism

Down

1. High blood pressure that stays elevated over time

2. Decrease in blood pressure occurring after standing in one place for an extended period

3. Systolic blood pressure between 120 and 129 mm Hg

4. Low blood sodium level

5. Localized wheals or swelling in subcutaneous tissues or mucous membranes, which may be due to an allergic response; also called angioneurotic edema

SECTION II: APPLYING YOUR KNOWLEDGE

Activity F CASE STUDY

Alfredo Garcia is a 55-year-old man, who came to the clinic with upper respiratory symptoms. His vital signs during triage are as follows: BP 172/120 mm Hg, HR 96 bpm, temperature 98.5°F, weight 97.7 kg (215 lb), and height 5 ft 6 in. He currently has no other diagnosed medical conditions. The primary health care provider gives Mr. Garcia a prescription for Lopressor HCT, one tablet by mouth daily in the morning.

1. In which stage of hypertension would you place Mr. Garcia? Is this an appropriate medication choice?

   _____

   _____

2. What lifestyle modification should Mr. Garcia be encouraged to follow?

   _____

   _____

Now Map It Out! Use the templates provided in the appendix to add information and make client connections on a concept map.

Review Mr. Garcia's concept map. He is taking a number of drugs and is a candidate for problems associated with polypharmacy. Add the drugs for hypertension to your concept map and look at the other defined problems and drugs used in order to determine what, if any, drug interactions exist with the medications now added.

SECTION III: PRACTICING FOR NCLEX

Activity G NCLEX-STYLE QUESTIONS

Answer the following questions.

1. When assessing a 40-year-old client, the nurse observes an increase in the client's blood pressure. Which of the following changes in blood pressure is indicative of prehypertension?
   1. Systolic pressure between 120 and 129 mm Hg
   2. Systolic pressure between 100 and 119 mm Hg
   3. Systolic pressure between 80 and 99 mm Hg
   4. Systolic pressure between 60 and 79 mm Hg

2. A client is diagnosed with renal impairment and hypertension. Which of the following drugs is contraindicated in renal impairment?
   1. Doxazosin
   2. Captopril
   3. Hydralazine
   4. Minoxidil

3. A nurse is monitoring a client admitted to the emergency department in a hypertensive emergency. Which of the following drugs should be administered in such situations?
   1. Amlodipine
   2. Acebutolol
   3. Diltiazem
   4. Nitroprusside

4. A nurse is monitoring a client on minoxidil for hypertension. Which of the following findings should the nurse report immediately to the primary health care provider when the client is taking minoxidil? **Select all that apply.**
   1. Swelling of the face
   2. Pulse rate increase of more than 5 beats per minute
   3. Weight gain of 1 lb
   4. Difficulty breathing
   5. Angina and severe indigestion

5. A nurse is caring for a client receiving captopril for hypertension. Which of the following precautions should the nurse take when administering captopril?
    1. Administer captopril 1 hour before or 2 hours after food.
    2. Rub the client's back before administering captopril.
    3. Ensure that the client exercises before administering captopril.
    4. Take captopril along with antacids.

6. A client receiving terazosin for hypertension complains of dizziness when sitting up. Which of the following instructions should the nurse give the client? **Select all that apply.**
    1. Rise slowly from a sitting or lying position.
    2. Increase fluid intake.
    3. Apply a cool cloth over the forehead.
    4. Rest on the bed for 1 or 2 minutes before rising.
    5. Stand still for a few minutes after rising.

7. A client asks the nurse about natural supplements to help reduce blood pressure. The nurse knows some products will interact with hypertensive medications. Which of the following would the nurse identify as having possible interactions? **Select all that apply.**
    1. Hawthorn tea
    2. St. John's wort
    3. Orange juice
    4. Grapefruit

8. A nurse checks a client's blood pressure and finds it to be 128/80 mm Hg. This client should be classified as having which stage of hypertension?
    1. Prehypertension
    2. Stage 1 hypertension
    3. Stage 2 hypertension
    4. Normotensive

9. Which of the following lowers blood pressure primarily via suppression of the rennin–angiotensin–aldosterone system?
    1. Verapamil
    2. Diltiazem
    3. Lisinopril
    4. Furosemide

10. Hypertension increases a person's risk for which of the following? **Select all that apply.**
    1. Heart failure
    2. Tuberculosis
    3. Hearing loss
    4. Kidney disease
    5. Liver disease

11. Once a client develops primary hypertension, therapy should last for how long?
    1. Until blood pressure is 120/80 mm Hg
    2. 1 year
    3. For life
    4. 5 years

12. Select the cause of secondary hypertension.
    1. Weight gain
    2. Kidney disease
    3. Smoking
    4. Hip fractures

35

Antianginal and Vasodilating Drugs

- Describe the two types of antianginal drugs.
- Explain the general actions, uses, adverse reactions, contraindications, precautions, and interactions of antianginal and vasodilating drugs.
- Distinguish important preadministration and ongoing assessment activities the nurse should perform on the client taking an antianginal or vasodilating drug.
- List nursing diagnoses particular to a client taking an antianginal or vasodilating drug.
- Examine ways to promote an optimal response to therapy, how to manage common adverse reactions, and important points to keep in mind when educating clients about the use of antianginal or vasodilating drugs.

SECTION I: ASSESSING YOUR UNDERSTANDING

Activity A FILL IN THE BLANKS

1. Antianginal drugs relieve chest pain by dilating _____ arteries and thereby increasing the blood supply to the cardiac musculature.

2. The contractions of cardiac and vascular smooth muscles depend on the movement of extracellular _____ ions through specific ion channels.

3. Nitrates act by relaxing the _____ muscle layer of the blood vessels.

4. Contact _____ may occur with the use of transdermal nitrate.

5. A client who uses nitrates should not take _____ drugs.

Activity B DOSAGE CALCULATION

1. A nurse has to administer 40 mg of isosorbide orally to a client for the treatment of angina. The tablet is available in 20-mg strength. How many tablets should the nurse administer to the client?

   _____

   _____

2. A client is prescribed 10 mg of amlodipine for Prinzmetal angina. The tablet is available in 5-mg strength. How many tablets should the client take to relieve his angina?

   _____

   _____

3. A client has been prescribed 12.5 mg of IV diltiazem for atrial fibrillation. Each ampule contains 5 mL of solution in the strength of 5 mg/mL. What amount of the solution should the nurse draw from the ampule to give the correct dosage?

   _____

   _____

4. A client requires 50 mg of nifedipine daily for the treatment of chronic stable angina. The drug is available in the strength of 25 mg per tablet. How many tablets should the client consume daily?

_____

_____

Activity C MATCHING

1. Match the antianginal and vasodilator drugs in Column A with their appropriate uses in Column B.

Column A

____ **1.** Verapamil

____ **2.** Nifedipine

____ **3.** Bosentan

____ **4.** Nitroglycerin, intravenous

Column B

a. Used to control blood pressure in perioperative hypertension associated with surgical procedures

b. Used in the treatment of cardiac arrhythmias

c. Used to treat PAH

d. Used in the treatment of Prinzmetal variant angina

2. Match the terms associated with angina in Column A with their correct descriptions in Column B.

Column A

____ **1.** Atherosclerosis

____ **2.** Angina

____ **3.** Ischemia

Column B

a. Condition in which there is reduced blood supply to an area

b. Characterized by the presence of fatty plaque deposits on the inner wall of the arteries

c. Characterized by chest pain occurring as a result of decreased oxygen supply to the heart muscles

Activity D SHORT ANSWERS

A nurse's role in managing clients who are being administered antianginal drugs involves monitoring and implementing interventions that aid in the client's recovery. Answer the following questions, which involve the nurse's role in the management of such situations.

1. A client has been admitted to the ED with a severe anginal attack. Sublingual nitroglycerin is prescribed and the client will be discharged to home with family. What instructions should the nurse provide the client on discharge?

_____

_____

2. The adult child who accompanied the client with angina to the ED wants to know how frequently the sublingual nitroglycerin can be given. What should the nurse tell the client's child?

_____

_____

Activity E **CROSSWORD PUZZLE**

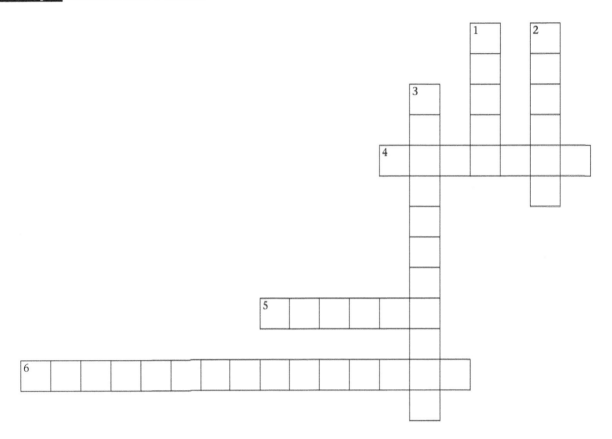

Across

4. Pertaining to a substance applied directly to the skin by patch, ointment, gel, or other formulation

5. Acute pain in the chest resulting from decreased blood supply to the heart muscle

6. Disease characterized by deposits of fatty plaques on the inner walls of arteries

Down

1. Under the tongue

2. Space in the mouth between the gum and the cheek in either the upper or lower jaw

3. Prevention

SECTION II: APPLYING YOUR KNOWLEDGE

Activity F **CASE STUDY**

Mrs. Moore is being discharged from the hospital today and was given a prescription for nitroglycerin (Nitrostat) tablets.

1. Mrs. Moore asks the nurse, "What is this new tablet for?"

_____

_____

2. How should Mrs. Moore be instructed to use the nitroglycerin sublingual tablets?

_____

_____

Now Map It Out! Use the templates provided in the appendix to add information and make client connections on a concept map.

Time for a medicine reconciliation for Mrs. Moore. Read the case studies here and in Chapter 35 of the textbook and you will see how confused this client is with drug administration. Additionally, she has medications added to her routine, which are contradictory. Can you find them?

SECTION III: PRACTICING FOR NCLEX

Activity G **NCLEX-STYLE QUESTIONS**

Answer the following questions.

1. A nurse caring for a client who has been prescribed a nitrate for anginal attacks should assess which of the following before creating a written teaching plan?
   1. What fruit juices does the client like to drink
   2. A through pain assessment
   3. Health literacy level
   4. Insurance coverage

2. Which activity is most likely to precipitate an angina attack?
   1. Watching TV late at night
   2. Cutting vegetables at a sink
   3. Sitting in a boat
   4. Climbing a flight of stairs

3. A nurse is educating a group of nursing students on the various effects of calcium channel blockers on the heart. Which of the following are the effects of calcium channel blockers on the heart? **Select all that apply.**
   1. Increase the heart rate
   2. Slow the conduction velocity
   3. Depress myocardial contractility
   4. Cause rapid atrial muscle contraction
   5. Dilate the coronary arteries

4. A client is admitted to a telemetry unit for angina management and is started on IV diltiazem. Which of the following adverse reactions should the nurse monitor for in the client? **Select all that apply.**
   1. Hypertension
   2. Tachycardia
   3. Rash
   4. Headache
   5. Dizziness

5. A client taking transdermal nitrates lives with his daughter and two small grandchildren. What should the nurse teach the family as a safe method to dispose of the transdermal patches?
   1. Cut into small pieces before disposal.
   2. Fold the adhesive sides together when removing.
   3. Flush them immediately in the toilet.
   4. Put in a plastic bag.

6. Pulmonary arterial hypertension (PAH) is associated with autoimmune diseases. Which of the following client panels should the primary health care provider routinely screen for PAH?
   1. Systemic lupus erythematosus
   2. Sarcoidosis
   3. Scleroderma
   4. Sjögren syndrome

7. Nitrates are available in which of the following dosage forms? **Select all that apply.**
   1. Sublingual
   2. Transdermal
   3. Parenteral
   4. Rectal
   5. Aerosol spray

8. Which of the following laboratory tests should be done before a client starts drug therapy for PAH?
   1. Hepatic enzymes
   2. Thyroid-stimulating hormone (TSH) level
   3. IGRA tuberculosis test
   4. Pregnancy test

9. Nitrates can result in which of the following adverse reactions? **Select all that apply.**

1. Headache
2. Flushing
3. Diarrhea
4. Hypotension
5. Blurred vision

10. Nitrates should not be used in clients with which of the following?

1. Closed-angle glaucoma
2. Asthma
3. Diabetes
4. Hypertension

36

Anticoagulant and Thrombolytic Drugs

Learning Objectives

- Describe hemostasis and thrombosis.
- Explain the uses, general drug actions, adverse reactions, contraindications, precautions, and interactions of anticoagulant, antiplatelet, and thrombolytic drugs.
- Distinguish important preadministration and ongoing assessment activities the nurse should perform on the client taking an anticoagulant, antiplatelet, or thrombolytic drug.
- List nursing diagnoses particular to a client taking an anticoagulant, antiplatelet, or thrombolytic drug.
- Examine ways to promote an optimal response to therapy, how to manage common adverse reactions, and important points to keep in mind when educating clients about the use of anticoagulant, antiplatelet, and thrombolytic drugs.

SECTION I: ASSESSING YOUR UNDERSTANDING

Activity A FILL IN THE BLANKS

1. _____ is essential for the clotting of blood.

2. Venous _____ can develop as the result of venous stasis, injury to the vessel wall, or altered blood coagulation.

3. _____ thrombosis can occur because of atherosclerosis or arrhythmias.

4. Drugs that help to eliminate clots are known as _____.

5. Deep vein thrombosis typically occurs in the lower _____ and is the most common type of venous thrombosis.

Activity B DOSAGE CALCULATION

1. A client with atrial fibrillation has been prescribed 10,000 units of dalteparin per day. The drug is available in 10,000 units/0.4 mL. How many mL of solution should the nurse administer to the client each day?

   _____

   _____

2. A client has been prescribed 7.5 mg of warfarin per day for the prophylaxis of venous thrombosis. On-hand availability of the drug is 2.5-mg tablets. How many tablets should the nurse administer to the client every day?

   _____

   _____

3. A client with intermittent claudication has been prescribed 100 mg of cilostazol to be administered orally twice a day. The drug is available in the form of 50-mg tablets. How many tablets should be administered to the client per dose?

   _____

   _____

4. A client has been prescribed a single loading dose containing 300 mg of clopidogrel for treatment of acute coronary syndrome. The drug is available in 75-mg tablets. How many tablets should the nurse administer to the client in the loading dose?

_____

_____

5. A client undergoing treatment for thrombotic stroke is prescribed the drug ticlopidine. The primary health care provider has instructed the nurse to administer 250 mg of ticlopidine twice a day to the client. The drug is available in 250-mg tablets. How many tablets should the nurse remove from the automated dispensing machine for each dose?

_____

_____

Activity C MATCHING

1. Match the drugs in Column A with their adverse reactions in Column B.

Column A

____ **1.** Heparin

____ **2.** Cilostazol

____ **3.** Ticlopidine

____ **4.** Dalteparin

Column B

a. Dyspepsia

b. Rash

c. Heart palpitations

d. Chills

2. Match the antiplatelet drugs in Column A with their uses in Column B.

Column A

____ **1.** Clopidogrel

____ **2.** Ticlopidine

____ **3.** Cilostazol

____ **4.** Fondaparinux

Column B

a. Intermittent claudication

b. Recent myocardial infarction

c. DVT prophylaxis

d. Thrombotic stroke

Activity D SHORT ANSWERS

A nurse's role in managing clients who are being administered anticoagulant and thrombolytic drugs involves monitoring the clients and implementing interventions that aid in their recovery. Answer the following questions, which involve the nurse's role in the management of such situations.

1. A nurse has been caring for a client with deep venous thrombosis (DVT). Posttreatment, the nurse has to evaluate the effectiveness of the treatment plan. What factors should the nurse consider to determine the success of the treatment plan?

_____

_____

2. A nurse is caring for a client who has been administered alteplase for an acute brain attack. What should the nurse monitor in the GI and urinary system for the indication of bleeding?

_____

_____

Activity E CROSSWORD PUZZLE

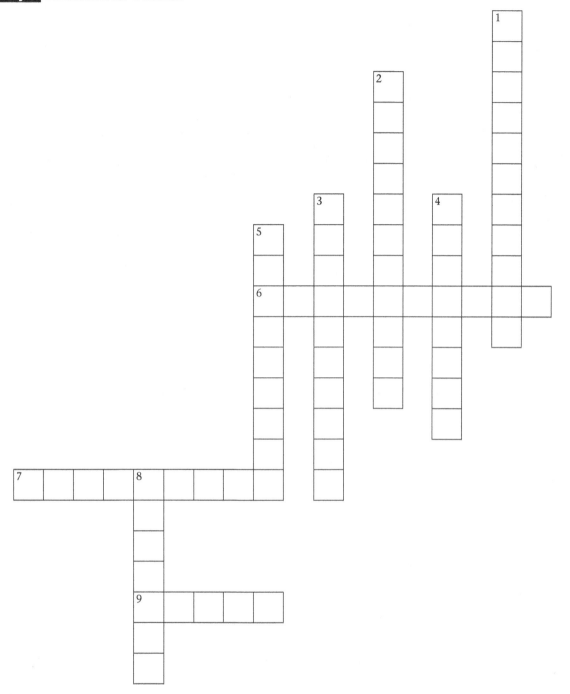

Across

6. Formation of a blood clot
7. Clumping of blood elements
9. Dissolution or destruction of cells

Down

1. Complex process by which fibrin forms and blood clots
2. Substance that is essential for the clotting of blood
3. Drug that dissolves clots already formed within blood vessel walls
4. Blood clot
5. Pinpoint-sized red hemorrhagic spots on the skin
8. Thrombus that detaches from a blood vessel wall and travels through the bloodstream

SECTION II: APPLYING YOUR KNOWLEDGE

Activity F CASE STUDY

Mr. Phillip is being discharged from the hospital today after an episode of atrial fibrillation. He is being discharged with a prescription for warfarin 5 mg with directions to take one tablet daily at 5 p.m. The primary health care provider has asked the nurse to complete discharge counseling with Mr. Phillip.

1. How often will Mr. Phillip need a PT/INR drawn?

   _____

   _____

2. What are the signs of warfarin overdose?

   _____

   _____

Now Map It Out! Use the templates provided in the appendix to add information and make client connections on a concept map.

Review Mr. Phillip's concept map. He is taking a number of drugs and is a candidate for problems associated with polypharmacy. Look at the other defined problems and drugs used to determine what, if any, drug interactions exist with the medications now added.

SECTION III: PRACTICING FOR NCLEX

Activity G NCLEX-STYLE QUESTIONS

Answer the following questions.

1. Alteplase has been administered to a client with acute ischemic stroke. Which of the following adverse reactions associated with the drug administration should the nurse monitor for in the client? **Select all that apply.**
   1. Gingival bleeding
   2. Erythema
   3. Epistaxis
   4. Ecchymosis
   5. Anemia

2. A nurse is caring for a client who has been prescribed abciximab during coronary angioplasty. The client is also taking aspirin for pain relief. What effects of the interaction between these two drugs should the nurse observe for in the client?
   1. Decreased effectiveness of aspirin
   2. Increased effectiveness of abciximab
   3. Increased risk of bleeding
   4. Decreased absorption of abciximab

3. A client says he must refuse the anticoagulant due to a religious objection to pork products. Which of the following drugs is not derived from pork?
   1. Warfarin
   2. Fondaparinux
   3. Enoxaparin
   4. Dalteparin

4. A nurse is caring for a client taking antiplatelet drugs. What instruction should the nurse include in the teaching plan for this client?
   1. Use a soft toothbrush.
   2. Take foods low in vitamin K.
   3. Take medication with food.
   4. Take the drug at a different time each day.

5. A client is undergoing warfarin drug therapy. After taking the drug, the client develops signs of GI bleeding. Which of the following tasks is the best intervention to monitor bleeding by the nurse?
   1. Inspect urine for red-orange color.
   2. Monitor vital signs every 4 hours.
   3. Inspect for bright red to black stools.
   4. Monitor client's fluid intake and output.

6. A nurse is required to administer heparin subcutaneously to a client. What should the nurse do to avoid the possibility of the development of local irritation, pain, or hematoma?
   1. Avoid application of firm pressure after the injection.
   2. Avoid administration sites such as buttocks and lateral thighs.
   3. Use an area within 2 in of the umbilicus for drug administration.
   4. Avoid intramuscular (IM) administration of the drug.

7. A nurse is caring for a client receiving parenteral anticoagulant drug therapy. The nurse suspects the client may have an overdose of the drug. What intervention should the nurse perform if administration of this drug is necessary?
   1. Measure the client's body temperature every hour.
   2. Monitor the client's pulse rate every 2 hours.
   3. Observe the client for new evidence of bleeding.
   4. Administer the drug to the client via the IV route.

8. A client is administered a thrombolytic drug. The drug is known to cause bleeding. Which of the following symptoms of internal bleeding should the nurse monitor for in the client? **Select all that apply.**
   1. Black, tarry stools
   2. Hematuria
   3. Leg cramps
   4. Petechiae
   5. Coffee-ground emesis

9. Which of the following is used to treat a warfarin overdose?
   1. Protamine
   2. Urokinase
   3. Phytonadione
   4. Alteplase

10. Use of St. John's wort during warfarin therapy can result in which of the following?
    1. Increased risk of bleeding
    2. Increased risk of thrombus formation
    3. Increase blood pressure
    4. Increased platelet count

11. When is it indicated to administer a 300-mg dose of clopidogrel (Plavix) to a client, instead of the 75-mg oral dose?
    1. As a maintenance dose
    2. In treatment of myocardial infarction
    3. In treatment of stroke
    4. As a loading dose

12. Thrombolytic drugs are contraindicated in which of the following? **Select all that apply.**
    1. Active bleeding
    2. History of stroke
    3. Active infection
    4. History of aneurysm
    5. Recent abdominal surgery

37

Cardiotonic and Antiarrhythmic Drugs

- Compare and contrast heart failure in relationship to left ventricular failure, right ventricular failure, neurohormonal activity, and treatment options.
- Describe the different types of cardiac arrhythmias.
- Explain the uses, general drug actions, general adverse reactions, contraindications, precautions, and interactions of the cardiotonic and antiarrhythmic drugs.
- Discuss the use of other drugs with positive inotropic action.
- Distinguish important preadministration and ongoing assessment activities the nurse should perform on the client taking a cardiotonic or antiarrhythmic drug.
- List nursing diagnoses particular to a client taking a cardiotonic or antiarrhythmic drug.
- Identify the symptoms of digitalis toxicity.
- Examine ways to promote an optimal response to therapy, how to manage common adverse reactions, and important points to keep in mind when administering cardiotonic and antiarrhythmic drugs.

SECTION I: ASSESSING YOUR UNDERSTANDING

Activity A FILL IN THE BLANKS

1. _____ ventricular dysfunction results in pulmonary symptoms, which include dyspnea and moist cough.

2. All antiarrhythmic drugs may cause new arrhythmias or worsen existing arrhythmias, even though they are administered to resolve an existing arrhythmia. This phenomenon is called the _____ effect.

3. The antiarrhythmic drugs are classified according to their effects on the _____.

4. The procedure of starting a client on digoxin drug therapy and establishing a constant blood level is called _____.

Activity B DOSAGE CALCULATION

1. A primary health care provider prescribes 0.25 mg of digoxin to a client with heart failure. The available digoxin tablet is 0.125 mg. How many tablets should the nurse administer to the client?

   _____

   _____

2. A primary health care provider has prescribed 1.25 mg of digoxin as the loading dose for a client with atrial fibrillation. Each 5 mL ampule contains digoxin 0.25 mg/mL. How many ampules of digoxin should the nurse administer?

   _____

   _____

3. A client weighing 55 kg has been prescribed 1 mg/kg IV of ibutilide for atrial fibrillation. How milligrams of the drug should the nurse administer to the client?

_____

_____

4. A primary health care provider has prescribed 0.75 mg of digoxin to be given IV for a client with atrial flutter. Each digoxin ampule contains 2 mL of solution in the strength of 0.25 mg/mL. How many ampules of digoxin will the nurse need for this IV injection?

_____

_____

5. A client with hypertension has been prescribed the drug acebutolol 390 mg/day in two equally divided doses orally. How many milligrams of the drug will be administered in each dose?

_____

_____

Activity C MATCHING

1. Match the drugs that interact with the cardiotonics in Column A with the effect of their interaction in Column B.

Column A

____ 1. Amiodarone

____ 2. Antacid

____ 3. Thyroid hormone

____ 4. Loop diuretic

Column B

a. Decreases serum digitalis levels

b. Results in electrolyte imbalance

c. Increases serum digitalis levels

d. Decreases effectiveness of digoxin

2. Match the terms associated with heart failure in Column A with their description in Column B.

Column A

____ 1. Cardiac hypertrophy

____ 2. Nocturia

____ 3. Heart failure

____ 4. Cardiotonics

Column B

a. Inability of the heart to pump sufficient quantities of blood to meet tissue demands

b. Enlargement of cardiac musculature

c. Agents that bring about an increase in heart contraction

d. A need to urinate frequently at night

Activity D SHORT ANSWERS

A nurse's role in managing clients who are being treated with digoxin involves careful monitoring and implementing interventions that aid in recovery. Answer the following questions, which involve the nurse's role in the management of such situations.

1. A client is diagnosed with heart failure and requires digoxin therapy. What physical assessment should a nurse carry out in a client before starting digoxin?

_____

_____

2. A client had rapid digitalization for heart failure and is required to continue taking digitalis for a prolonged period. What teaching plan should the nurse implement for clients taking digitalis?

_____

_____

Activity E CROSSWORD PUZZLE

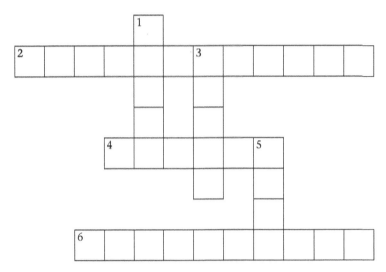

Across

2. Class of drugs that increase the efficiency and improve the contraction of the heart muscle
4. This type of fibrillation is a cardiac arrhythmia that results in an irregular and often rapid ventricular rate
6. Type of heart failure in which the heart cannot pump enough blood to meet the tissue needs of the body

Down

1. This side of heart failure presents with fluid backup in the body such as distended neck veins, peripheral edema, and hepatic engorgement
3. Normal doses of a cardiotonic drug can still cause these effects
5. This side of heart failure leads to pulmonary symptoms such as dyspnea and moist cough

SECTION II: APPLYING YOUR KNOWLEDGE

Activity F CASE STUDY

 Mrs. Moore was hospitalized for heart failure when unable to tolerate a beta blocking drug. The primary health care provider orders a loading dose of digoxin 0.75 mg to be given IV. The digoxin is available in a solution of 0.5 mg/mL.

1. How many milliliters should the nurse prepare?

_____

_____

2. What should the nurse do before administering the IV dose?

_____

_____

Now Map It Out! Use the templates provided in the appendix to add information and make client connections on a concept map.

Review Mrs. Moore's concept map. A beta blocker drug was a good choice because of the risk for multiple drug interactions. Now that she is being switched to digoxin, what drug interactions do you identify with her current medication routine?

SECTION III: PRACTICING FOR NCLEX

Activity G NCLEX-STYLE QUESTIONS

Answer the following questions.

1. A client arrives at an urgent care center complaining of dyspnea and a hacking cough. The nurse assessing the client notes that there are distended jugular veins, edema of the extremities, and reduced ejection fraction. Which of the following conditions do these symptoms indicate?
   1. Heart failure
   2. Glomerulonephritis
   3. Pulmonary disease
   4. Hypothyroidism

2. When caring for a client on digoxin, the nurse observes that the client's pulse rate is 56 bpm. The client is also complaining of nausea and vomiting. Which of the following is the most appropriate intervention in this situation?
   1. Administer milrinone.
   2. Increase the rate of digoxin infusion.
   3. Perform gastrointestinal suction.
   4. Withhold the drug and notify the PHCP.

3. A client has been admitted for heart failure and is on digoxin. The nurse monitoring the client notes that the serum digoxin level is 2.5 mg/mL. Which of the following signs would validate a case of digoxin toxicity? **Select all that apply.**
   1. Anorexia
   2. Headache
   3. Weakness
   4. Blurred vision
   5. Vomiting

4. A client with a cardiac arrhythmia is prescribed an antiarrhythmic agent. The client comes to an urgent care facility feeling ill. Which of the following adverse reactions are possible with the use of an antiarrhythmic agent? **Select all that apply.**
   1. Weakness
   2. Hypertension
   3. Insomnia
   4. Arrhythmias
   5. Lightheadedness

5. A nurse is caring for a client on digitalis. The client complains of nausea and vomiting after 2 days of digitalis administration. Which of the following is the appropriate nursing intervention in this situation? **Select all that apply.**
   1. Ensure that the client takes double the drug dosage.
   2. Ensure that the client consumes small, frequent meals.
   3. Ensure that the client consumes fluids 1 hour before meals.
   4. Ensure that the client rinses their mouth after the consumption of meals.
   5. Restrict fluid consumption at meal times.

6. A client is admitted to an ED with atrial flutter. The client complains of headache after the first dose of digitalis is administered. Which of the following additional adverse effects of digitalis should a nurse assess for in such a situation? **Select all that apply.**
   1. Hepatotoxicity
   2. Angina
   3. Drowsiness
   4. Vomiting
   5. Arrhythmia

7. A nurse is required to monitor the vital signs of a client with paroxysmal atrial tachycardia who is on an antiarrhythmic agent. Which of the following pulse rates should the nurse report immediately to the primary health care provider?
   1. 82 bpm
   2. 92 bpm
   3. 102 bpm
   4. 142 bpm

8. A client with heart failure has been advised to continue digoxin therapy. Prior to discharge, the nurse teaches the steps of calculating the pulse. Arrange the steps involved in calculating the pulse in the correct order.
   1. Record the number of times the pulse beats in a minute.
   2. Place the nondominant arm on a table or armchair.
   3. Place index and third fingers of the other hand on wrist bone.
   4. Feel for the beating or pulsing sensation, which is the pulse.
   5. If pulse rate is more than 100 bpm, notify the primary health care provider.

9. A nurse is caring for an 86-year-old client on antiarrhythmic drugs. Which of the following signs, if present, indicates the development of heart failure in the client?
   a. Decrease in weight
   b. Shortness of breath
   c. Increased volume of urine
   d. Chills and fever

10. Which of the following symptoms would most likely be present in a client with right ventricular dysfunction? **Select all that apply.**
    1. Peripheral edema
    2. Neck vein distention
    3. Orthopnea
    4. Weight loss
    5. Nocturia

11. Which of the following classes of medications are currently used as first-line treatments of heart failure? **Select all that apply.**
    1. Angiotensin-converting enzyme inhibitors (ACEIs)
    2. Loop diuretics
    3. Cardiotonics
    4. Beta blockers
    5. Angiotensin II receptor blockers (ARBs)

12. When educating a group of nursing students on antiarrhythmic drugs, the nurse cites which of the following as an example of a class IA antiarrhythmic drug?
    1. Lidocaine
    2. Disopyramide
    3. Propafenone
    4. Amiodarone

Drugs That Affect the Gastrointestinal System

Upper Gastrointestinal System Drugs

Learning Objectives

- Explain the general drug actions, uses, adverse reactions, contraindications, precautions, and interactions of drugs used to treat conditions of the upper gastrointestinal (GI) system.
- Distinguish important preadministration and ongoing assessment activities the nurse should perform with the client receiving a drug used to treat conditions of the upper GI system.
- List nursing diagnoses particular to a client receiving a drug used to treat conditions of the upper GI system.
- Examine ways to promote an optimal response to therapy, how to manage adverse reactions, and important points to keep in mind when educating clients about the use of drugs to treat conditions of the upper GI system.

SECTION I: ASSESSING YOUR UNDERSTANDING

Activity A FILL IN THE BLANKS

1. The _____ system is a long tube within the body where ingested food and fluids are prepared for absorption and ultimate replenishment of nutrients to the cells.

2. The _____ connects the mouth to the stomach where food is mixed with acids and enzymes to become a solution for absorption.

3. Forceful expulsion of gastric contents through the mouth is known as _____.

4. _____ is a medically available cannabinoid prescribed for antiemetic use.

5. Proton pump inhibitors are particularly important in the treatment of *Helicobacter pylori* in clients with active _____ ulcers.

Activity B DOSAGE CALCULATION

1. A primary health care provider has prescribed 2.5 mg of dronabinol to a client as an HIV appetite stimulant, to be taken twice a day. The client is being given a pass for a 3-day trip. The drug is available in the form of 2.5-mg capsules at the facility's pharmacy. How many capsules should the nurse obtain for the client to take on the trip?

_____

_____

2. A primary health care provider has prescribed 40 mg of esomeprazole to a client daily for the treatment of erosive esophagitis. The drug is available as 20-mg capsules at the local pharmacy. How many capsules will the client take per dose?

_____

_____

3. A client has been prescribed 800 mg of cimetidine in four equally divided doses for the treatment of suspected gastric ulcers. The drug is available as 200-mg tablets. How many tablets should the client take at the bedtime dose?

_____

_____

4. A long-term care client has been prescribed 300 mg of nizatidine per dose for the treatment of GERD. The drug is available as 150-mg tablets. How many tablets should the nurse administer to the client in each dose?

_____

_____

5. A client has been prescribed lansoprazole 30 mg once daily for the treatment of GI malabsorption related to cystic fibrosis. The drug is available as 15-mg capsules. How many capsules should the nurse administer to the client for a daily dose?

_____

_____

Activity C MATCHING

1. Using the Summary Drug Tables in your textbook, look for patterns in how drugs are named, and match the upper GI drug ending (suffix) in Column A with the drug class in Column B.

Column A

____ 1. -inum

____ 2. -dine

____ 3. -zole

____ 4. -zine

____ 5. -tron

Column B

a. Proton pump inhibitors

b. Antidopaminergic drugs

c. Acid neutralizers

d. 5-HT3 receptor antagonists

e. Histamine H_2 antagonists

2. Match the drug in Column A with the likely interaction effect when combined with an antacid in Column B.

Column A

____ 1. Chlorpromazine

____ 2. Tetracycline

____ 3. Corticosteroids

____ 4. Salicylates

____ 5. Amphetamines

Column B

a. Decreased effectiveness of anti-inflammatory properties

b. Decreased absorption of the interactant drug

c. Decreased effectiveness of anti-infective

d. Interactant drug is excreted slowly from the urine

e. Pain reliever is excreted rapidly from the urine

Activity D SHORT ANSWERS

A nurse's role in managing clients receiving a drug for an upper GI disorder involves assisting the client through preadministration assessment. The nurse also monitors the client for the occurrence of any adverse reactions. Answer the following questions, which involve the nurse's role in the management of such situations.

1. A client with severe nausea and vomiting has been prescribed an antiemetic drug. What preadministration assessments should the nurse perform for this client?

_____

_____

2. After the preadministration assessment, the client is administered an antiemetic drug. What is the nurse's role after administration of the drug?

_____

_____

LABELING

Label the different parts of the gastrointestinal system in the figure provided.

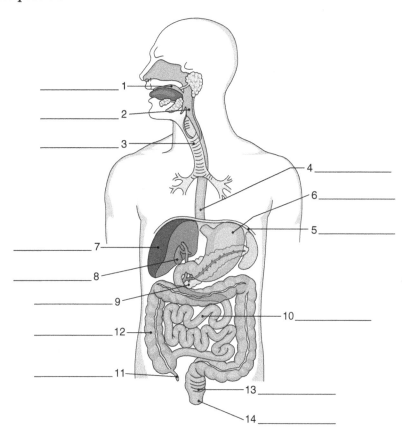

1 _____
2 _____
3 _____
4 _____
6 _____
5 _____
7 _____
8 _____
9 _____
10 _____
12 _____
11 _____
13 _____
14 _____

SECTION II: APPLYING YOUR KNOWLEDGE

CASE STUDY

Janna Wong presents to the primary health care provider's office for her sports physical. While in the office, she mentions she is going on a cruise for spring break next week. Last time she was on a boat she suffered a bout of motion sickness and asks the nurse what she can do to prevent it.

1. What product can be used prophylactically to prevent motion sickness?

_____

_____

2. The primary health care provider writes Janna a prescription for scopolamine (Transderm Scop). How should the nurse instruct Janna to use the patch?

_____

_____

Now Map It Out! Use the templates provided in the appendix to add information and make client connections on a concept map.

This mapping exercise is going to take some creative investigating on your part. Janna Wong's prescribed medication for motion sickness can have a direct effect upon some of the other symptoms and problems she has experienced as you have followed her case study in the textbook and study guide. See if you can find this medication in greater depth of another chapter, then plot out on your map of Janna where this interaction will happen.

SECTION III: PRACTICING FOR NCLEX

Activity G NCLEX-STYLE QUESTIONS

Answer the following questions.

1. A client has been prescribed dronabinol for fibromyalgia pain. Which of the following adverse reactions should the nurse teach the client to monitor for?
   1. Gastric upset
   2. Hypoxia
   3. Euphoria
   4. Asthenia

2. A nurse is caring for a client who has been administered antacids for the treatment of heartburn or regurgitation. The client informs the nurse that they are also taking aspirin for pain relief. What effect of the interaction between the two drugs should the nurse assess for in the client?
   1. Reduced pain relief
   2. Decreased white blood cell count
   3. Increased risk of bleeding
   4. Increased risk of dehydration

3. A primary health care provider has asked a nurse to start promethazine administration for a client with nausea. For which of the following client conditions should the nurse administer the drug with caution? **Select all that apply.**
   1. Hypertension
   2. Sleep apnea
   3. Renal disease
   4. Epilepsy
   5. Viral illness

4. A client with an episode of vertigo is recommended an antiemetic for motion sickness as part of the discharge plan at the urgent care facility. What should the nurse include in the teaching plan for the client?
   1. Increase frequency of dose if symptoms worsen.
   2. Avoid direct exposure to sunlight.
   3. Take other drugs 1 hour before taking the antiemetic.
   4. Avoid performing detailed activities when taking the drug.

5. A client who has undergone surgery is prescribed IV acid-reducing drugs. What is the priority assessment the nurse should monitor during administration of the drug to the client?
   1. Rate of IV infusion
   2. Body temperature every hour
   3. Irritation due to drug administration
   4. Blood pressure every 2 hours

6. A nurse is caring for a client undergoing antacid drug therapy. The client complains of diarrhea after taking the drug. What intervention should the nurse perform in this case?
   1. Remove items with strong odor.
   2. Change to a different antacid.
   3. Record the client's temperature every hour.
   4. Record the client's fluid intake and output.

7. A nurse is caring for a client undergoing antiemetic drug therapy to prevent nausea. The client reports loss of appetite due to nausea. What should the nurse do to enhance the client's appetite?
   1. Suggest consumption of milk products.
   2. Suggest physical exercises.
   3. Remove items with strong smell and odor.
   4. Avoid giving frequent oral rinses to the client.

8. Which of the following drugs treat heartburn by neutralizing the acidity of the stomach and by combining with hydrochloric acid (HCl) and increasing the pH of the stomach acid?
   1. Omeprazole (Prilosec)
   2. Famotidine (Pepcid)
   3. Magaldrate (Riopan)
   4. Metoclopramide (Reglan)

9. The nurse should warn a client taking magnesium- and sodium-containing antacids about which of the following adverse effects?
   1. Diarrhea
   2. Constipation
   3. Dehydration
   4. Flatulence

10. The nurse should warn a client taking aluminum- and calcium-containing antacids about which of the following adverse effects?
    1. Diarrhea
    2. Dehydration
    3. Flatulence
    4. Constipation

11. Which of the following antacids is contraindicated in clients with heart failure?
    1. Sodium bicarbonate (Bell-Ans)
    2. Calcium carbonate (Tums)
    3. Magnesium hydroxide (Milk of Magnesia)
    4. Aluminum hydroxide (ALternaGEL)

12. Which of the following medications loses its effectiveness even when administered 2 hours before an antacid?
    1. Quinidine
    2. Digoxin
    3. Dextroamphetamine
    4. Simvastatin

Lower Gastrointestinal System Drugs

- Describe how inflammatory bowel disease alters function of the lower gastrointestinal (GI) system.
- List the types of drugs prescribed or recommended for lower GI disorders.
- Explain the uses, general drug actions, general adverse reactions, contraindications, precautions, and interactions associated with lower GI drugs.
- Distinguish important preadministration and ongoing assessment activities the nurse should perform on the client taking a lower GI drug.
- List nursing diagnoses particular to a client taking a lower GI drug.
- Examine ways to promote an optimal response to therapy, how to manage common adverse reactions, and important points to keep in mind when educating clients about the use of lower GI drugs.

SECTION I: ASSESSING YOUR UNDERSTANDING

Activity A FILL IN THE BLANKS

1. Transit of contents rapidly through the bowel is called _____.

2. The herb _____ is used for treatment of digestive upsets, menstrual cramps, and stomach ulcers.

3. For short-term relief or prevention of constipation, a _____ is prescribed.

4. Charcoal may be used in the prevention of nonspecific _____ associated with kidney dialysis treatment.

5. The drug class _____ are used to treat Crohn disease and ulcerative colitis.

Activity B DOSAGE CALCULATION

1. The nurse is instructing a client with ulcerative colitis to set up a daily medication box. Balsalazide is supplied in 750-mg capsules and the daily dose of balsalazide is 2250 mg. How many capsules are needed to load the medication box for a 7-day period?

_____

_____

2. A client with rectal inflammation has been prescribed mesalamine. The primary health care provider has prescribed 200 mg of mesalamine to be taken four times a day. The drug is available in 200-mg tablets. How many tablets should the client take for each dose?

_____

_____

3. A client undergoing radiation therapy of the lower abdomen has been prescribed one Lomotil tablet after every loose stool for 2 days. When returning to the clinic, the client reports taking five tablets. If each tablet of Lomotil contains 5 mg of diphenoxylate, how much diphenoxylate has been taken in 2 days?

_____

_____

4. A nurse caring for a client with renal disease is to administer 30 mL of mineral oil to the client at bedtime. The mineral oil comes in 15-mL disposable containers. How many containers will the nurse provide to the client at bedtime?

_____

_____

5. A primary health care provider has prescribed 10 mg of bisacodyl on a daily basis to a client for the relief of constipation. The drug is available as 5-mg tablets. How many tablets should the client take every day?

_____

_____

Activity C MATCHING

1. Match the drugs in Column A with their uses in Column B.

Column A

____ **1.** Loperamide

____ **2.** Simethicone

____ **3.** Lactulose

____ **4.** Psyllium

Column B

a. Prevention of the formation of gas pockets in the intestine

b. Added fiber for irritable bowel syndrome

c. Treatment of chronic diarrhea associated with IBD

d. Reduction of blood ammonia levels in hepatic encephalopathy

2. Match the drugs used in managing lower GI disorders in Column A with their adverse reactions in Column B.

Column A

____ **1.** Infliximab

____ **2.** Difenoxin

____ **3.** Charcoal

____ **4.** Sulfasalazine

Column B

a. Black stools

b. Constipation

c. Anorexia

d. Sore throat

Activity D SHORT ANSWERS

A nurse's role in managing clients who have been prescribed drugs for lower GI disorders involves performing preadministrative and ongoing assessments during the course of drug therapy. The nurse also monitors the clients for the occurrence of any adverse reactions after administration of the drug. Answer the following questions, which involve the nurse's role in the management of such situations.

1. A client with dyspepsia has been prescribed simethicone. What preadministration assessments should the nurse perform before administration of the simethicone drug?

_____

_____

_____

2. What is the nurse's role after administering the drug to the client?

_____

_____

_____

Activity E **CROSSWORD PUZZLE**

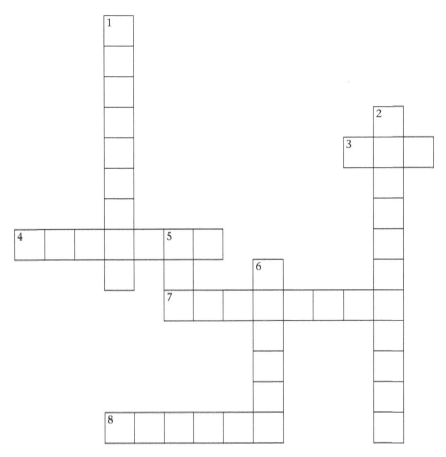

Across

3. Abbreviation for irritable bowel syndrome
4. Type of ulcerative disease that causes inflammation in the intestines
7. A loose, watery stool
8. Another term for gas

Down

1. Term for fullness or epigastric discomfort
2. A watery stool leakage around a hard fecal impaction
5. Abbreviation for inflammatory bowel disease
6. A type of inflammatory bowel disease

SECTION II: APPLYING YOUR KNOWLEDGE

Activity F **CASE STUDY**

Betty Peterson presents to the primary health care provider's office for a follow-up appointment. Her chief complaint today is hard stools and straining to have a bowel movement. Her current medications include amitriptyline (Elavil) 25 mg bedtime for mood, ferrous sulfate (Feosol) 325 mg TID for fatigue, and lisinopril/HCTZ (Prinzide) 20/25 mg daily for high blood pressure.

1. Which of Ms. Peterson's medications may be contributing to the constipation?

_____

_____

2. What nonpharmacologic steps can Ms. Peterson take to relieve constipation?

_____

_____

Now Map It Out! Use the templates provided in the appendix to add information and make client connections on a concept map.

In this chapter of the study guide and the textbook, you have been given a number of medications that Betty Peterson is currently taking. As a result she is experiencing some uncomfortable constipation. Pull out your concept map on Betty Peterson. Add the drugs taken and determine what can be added without disturbing the balance of the medications taken now.

SECTION III: PRACTICING FOR NCLEX

Activity G NCLEX-STYLE QUESTIONS

Answer the following questions.

1. A nurse is caring for a client with proctosigmoiditis. The primary health care provider has prescribed mesalamine to the client. The client informs the nurse that they are also taking antidiabetic drugs for the management of diabetes mellitus. What condition should the nurse monitor for in this client as a result of the interaction of the two drugs?
   1. Increased effect of hypoglycemic drugs
   2. Increased risk of bleeding
   3. Increased blood glucose level
   4. Reduced effect of mesalamine

2. A nurse is caring for a client with acute diarrhea who has been prescribed loperamide. Which of the following adverse reactions to the drug should the nurse monitor for in the client?
   1. Excessive urination
   2. Constipation
   3. Anorexia
   4. Sore throat

3. A primary health care provider has prescribed bismuth to a client with abdominal cramps. For which of the following conditions in the client should the nurse administer the drug with caution?
   1. *Salmonella* diarrhea
   2. Severe diarrhea
   3. Inflammatory bowel disease
   4. Irritable bowel syndrome

4. A client is prescribed simethicone for indigestion upon discharge from the urgent care facility. What instruction should the nurse offer the client regarding self-administration of the drug at home?
   1. Take the drug early in the morning.
   2. Chew the tablets thoroughly.
   3. Drink a glass of water after taking the drug.
   4. Take the drug with a glass of juice.

5. A nurse is caring for a client with chronic diarrhea. The primary health care provider has prescribed diphenoxylate to the client. What intervention should the nurse perform when caring for this client?
   1. Encourage the client to drink extra fluids.
   2. Avoid the use of commercial electrolytes.
   3. Encourage the client to eat foods high in fiber.
   4. Encourage the client to exercise.

6. A nurse is to instruct a client on renal dialysis in the right method of administering mineral oil for constipation. Which of the following should the nurse instruct the client for optimal response to therapy?
   1. Take it half an hour after a meal.
   2. Take it before breakfast.
   3. Take it at bedtime after dinner.
   4. Take it on an empty stomach in the evening.

7. A nurse is caring for an outpatient undergoing laxative therapy. Which of the following is an effect of the prolonged use of a laxative that the nurse should inform the client about?
   1. Agranulocytosis
   2. Electrolyte imbalances
   3. Bone density changes
   4. Renal impairment

8. A nurse needs to start antidiarrheal drug therapy for a client. For which of the following client conditions is an antidiarrheal contraindicated?
   1. Constipation
   2. Nausea
   3. Obstructive jaundice
   4. Abdominal distention

9. Clients with a sulfonamide allergy should avoid the use of which of the following to treat an ulcerative colitis flare?
    1. Infliximab
    2. Famotidine
    3. Mesalamine
    4. Metoclopramide

10. Which of the following herbal products has been used to treat digestive upset and stomach ulcers?
    1. Chamomile
    2. Kava
    3. Saw palmetto
    4. Valerian

11. Which of the following is an antidiarrheal that decreases intestinal peristalsis?
    1. Loperamide (Imodium)
    2. Sodium bicarbonate (Bell-Ans)
    3. Diphenoxylate (Lomotil)
    4. Omeprazole (Prilosec)

12. Which of the following over-the-counter medications is used to treat flatulence?
    1. Loperamide (Imodium)
    2. Simethicone (Mylicon)
    3. Olsalazine (Dipentum)
    4. Psyllium (Metamucil)

UNIT **10**

Drugs That Affect the Endocrine System

Antidiabetic Drugs

Learning Objectives

- Describe the two types of diabetes mellitus.
- Explain the types, uses, general drug actions, adverse reactions, contraindications, precautions, and interactions of the antidiabetic drugs.
- Distinguish important preadministration and ongoing assessment activities the nurse should perform with the client taking an antidiabetic drug.
- List nursing diagnoses particular to a client taking an antidiabetic drug.
- Examine ways to promote an optimal response to therapy, how to manage common adverse reactions, and important points to keep in mind when educating clients about the use of antidiabetic drugs.

SECTION I: ASSESSING YOUR UNDERSTANDING

Activity A FILL IN THE BLANKS

1. Diabetes mellitus is a chronic disorder characterized by insufficient _____ production by the beta cells of the pancreas.

2. Increased urination is termed _____.

3. An elevated blood glucose or sugar level is termed _____.

4. When blood glucose levels are high, glucose molecules attach to _____ in the red blood cells.

5. Diabetic _____ is a potentially life-threatening deficiency of insulin.

Activity B DOSAGE CALCULATION

1. A long-term care client with type 2 diabetes has been prescribed 30 mg of pioglitazone by a primary health care provider (PHCP). The drug is sent from the pharmacy in 15-mg tablets. How many tablets should the nurse administer to the client for each dose?

   _____

   _____

2. A client is prescribed 30 units NPH insulin mixed with 15 units of regular insulin. What is the total insulin dosage?

   _____

   _____

3. A client at a long-term care facility has been prescribed nateglinide 180 mg (Starlix) to be divided into three equal doses before meals. The drug is available in 60-mg tablets. How many tablets should the nurse administer to the client per dose?

   _____

   _____

4. A client has been prescribed 2550 mg of metformin daily to be taken in three equally divided doses a day shortly before meals. The metformin is dispensed in 850-mg tablets. How many tablets should the client take in each dose?

   _____

   _____

5. A client with type 2 diabetes has been prescribed the drug miglitol. The nurse is to teach the caregiver to administer 50 mg of the drug three times a day with meals. The drug is available in 50-mg tablets. How many tablets should the nurse instruct the caregiver to administer to the client with each meal?

_____

_____

1. Match the antidiabetic drugs in Column A with their uses in Column B.

Column A

____ **1.** Metformin

____ **2.** Glargine

____ **3.** Glucagon

Column B

a. Hypoglycemia

b. Type 2 diabetes

c. Basal insulin

2. Match the antidiabetic drugs in Column A with their adverse reactions in Column B.

Column A

____ **1.** Rosiglitazone

____ **2.** Repaglinide

____ **3.** Metformin

____ **4.** Canagliflozin

Column B

a. Increased flatulence

b. Genital yeast infections

c. Weight gain

d. Respiratory symptoms

A nurse's role in managing clients who are being administered oral antidiabetic drugs involves monitoring the clients and implementing interventions that aid in their recovery. Answer the following questions, which involve the nurse's role in the management of such situations.

1. A nurse has analyzed assessment data and selected the following nursing diagnoses for the client:

- **Acute confusion** related to hypoglycemia effects on mentation
- **Anxiety** related to uncertainty of diagnosis, testing own glucose levels, self-injection, dietary restrictions, other factors (specify)

How will the nurse evaluate the effectiveness of the treatment plan?

_____

_____

2. A nurse has been caring for a client with type 2 diabetes. What instructions should the nurse offer to the client and client's family to increase adherence and empower self-care strategies by the client?

_____

_____

Activity E CROSSWORD PUZZLE

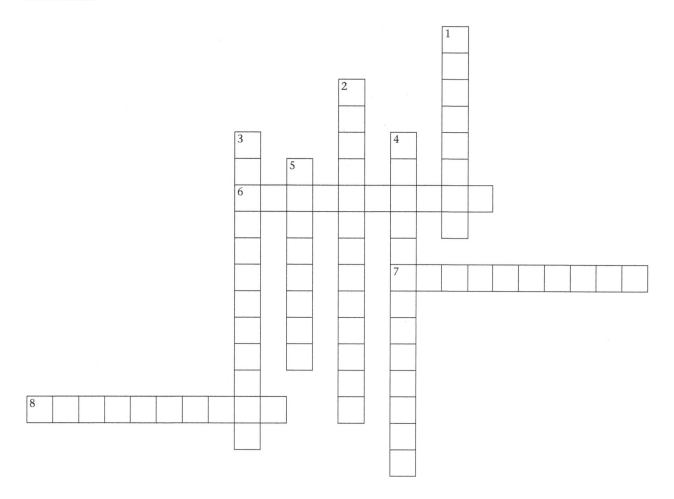

Across

6. Excessive thirst

7. Device to monitor blood glucose level

8. Eating large amounts of food

Down

1. Increased urination

2. Atrophy of subcutaneous fat

3. Low blood glucose (sugar) level

4. High blood glucose (sugar) level

5. Hormone secreted by the alpha (α) cells of the pancreas that increases the concentration of glucose in the blood

SECTION II: APPLYING YOUR KNOWLEDGE

Activity F CASE STUDY

 Emma Arthur is a client on the nurse's home health assignment. When the nurse reaches her home, the neighbor, Betty Peterson, is trying to help Mrs. Arthur with her blood glucose testing. Mrs. Arthur has a number of chronic illnesses. Her current medications include glyburide/metformin (Glucovance) 5/500 mg 2 tabs BID, pioglitazone 45 mg every morning, simvastatin 20 mg QHS, and losartan/HCTZ (Hyzaar) 100/25 mg daily. Looking at the electronic record, the nurse notes that her hospital blood glucose readings were 250–350 mg/dL 2 hours after meals and 130–160 mg/dL fasting.

1. The nurse has determined diabetic management to be an overwhelming task for Mrs. Arthur, yet Betty tells the nurse she is willing to help out. Looking at the situation, the nurse determines that she will start with reviewing home blood glucose monitoring. A positive experience is important; therefore, the nurse asks them to teach back the set up and perform this skill. What steps are critical in this process for the women to know?

_____

_____

2. The women look more at ease, and the nurse decides to see if any of Mrs. Arthur's medications would interact with each other and cause hypo- or hyperglycemia. Look at the drugs she is taking and consult your textbook to see what interactions may occur.

_____

_____

Now Map It Out! Use the templates provided in the appendix to add information and make client connections on a concept map.

Food intake is not the sole cause of hyperglycemia. In the textbook case study in Chapter 40, Mr. Phillip has seen a rise in his blood sugar and is distressed about this outcome. See if you can identify other factors that may be contributing to Mr. Phillip's rise in blood glucose from your concept map.

SECTION III: PRACTICING FOR NCLEX

Activity G NCLEX-STYLE QUESTIONS

Answer the following questions.

1. A client at a long-term care facility has been prescribed pioglitazone for the treatment of type 2 diabetes. Which of the following medical diagnoses would contradict the use of this drug?
   1. Heart failure
   2. Osteoarthritis
   3. Hyperlipidemia
   4. Hypertension

2. A nurse is caring for a client with gestational diabetes. The client asks the nurse during which stage of pregnancy the need for insulin is greatest. Which of the following should the nurse reply?
   1. Immediately after conception
   2. First trimester of pregnancy
   3. Third trimester of pregnancy
   4. Immediately after delivery

3. A nurse is assigned to administer a bolus dose of regular insulin to a client with type 1 diabetes mellitus. What care should be taken by the nurse before administering insulin?
   1. Administer 15 minutes before a meal.
   2. Administer 30–60 minutes before a meal.
   3. Administer once at bedtime via subcutaneous route.
   4. Administer within 5–10 minutes of a meal.

4. A nurse is to administer an insulin mixture of lispro and long-acting insulin. What care should the nurse take with regard to preparing the solution?
   1. Confirm with the PHCP whether the solution can be mixed in the solution vial.
   2. Draw up lispro first in the syringe while preparing the solution.
   3. Confirm if the ratio of insulin to be administered is 70/30.
   4. Keep the mixture for 1 hour if the client has difficulty controlling diabetes.

5. A nurse is preparing a teaching plan for a client who has been prescribed alpha-glucosidase (α-glucosidase) inhibitors. What instruction should the nurse include in the teaching plan for this client?
   1. Double drug dose in case of a skipped meal.
   2. Report respiratory distress or muscular aches to the PHCP.
   3. Keep a source of glucose tablets ready for signs of low blood glucose.
   4. Take the drug at different times each day.

6. A nurse is required to administer insulin to a client who has undergone a renal transplantation. Which method of insulin delivery should the nurse anticipate will be ordered for the client?
   1. Needle and syringe method
   2. Jet injection system method
   3. Syringe with prefilled cartridge
   4. Insulin pump method

7. A nurse at a long-term care facility is preparing an insulin solution to be administered to a client with diabetes. What precaution should the nurse take before withdrawing the syringe from the insulin vial?
   1. Eliminate air bubbles from the syringe barrel.
   2. Shake the vial vigorously just before withdrawal.
   3. Ensure the vial has been undisturbed for an hour.
   4. Use a syringe labeled with a higher concentration.

8. Glycosylated hemoglobin measures average blood glucose over what time period?
   1. Past 12–24 hours
   2. Past 7–10 days
   3. Past 1–2 months
   4. Past 3–4 months

9. Insulin is produced by which organ in the human body?
   1. Pancreas
   2. Spleen
   3. Liver
   4. Kidney

10. Which of the following is an example of rapid-acting insulin product?
    1. Lispro (Humalog)
    2. Glargine (Lantus)
    3. Detemir (Levemir)
    4. Isophane insulin suspension (Humulin N)

11. Which of the following is an example of long-acting insulin product?
    1. Lispro (Humalog)
    2. Glargine (Lantus)
    3. Aspart (Apidra)
    4. Isophane insulin suspension (Humulin N)

12. During insulin teaching, when should the nurse advise the client to administer aspart (Apidra)?
    1. Immediately before a meal
    2. At bedtime
    3. 30–60 minutes before a meal
    4. Immediately after a meal

41

Pituitary and Adrenocortical Hormones

- List the hormones produced by the pituitary gland and the adrenal cortex.
- Explain general actions, uses, adverse reactions, contraindications, precautions, and interactions of the pituitary and adrenocortical hormones.
- Distinguish important preadministration and ongoing assessment activities the nurse should perform with a client taking a pituitary or adrenocortical hormone.
- List nursing diagnoses particular to a client taking a pituitary or adrenocortical hormone.
- Examine ways to promote an optimal response to therapy, how to manage common adverse reactions, and important points to keep in mind when educating clients about the use of pituitary and adrenocortical hormones.

SECTION I: ASSESSING YOUR UNDERSTANDING

Activity A FILL IN THE BLANKS

1. ACTH stimulates the adrenal cortex to secrete the _____.

2. The anterior pituitary hormone _____ is the only hormone that is not used medically.

3. Follicle-stimulating hormone and luteinizing hormone are called _____ because they influence the organs of reproduction.

4. The _____ mechanism is used by glands to signal the need for or cessation of hormonal production.

5. The posterior pituitary gland produces two hormones: _____ and _____.

Activity B DOSAGE CALCULATION

1. A primary health care provider has prescribed 20 mg of somatropin daily via injection to a client for decreased pituitary function. The drug is available as 10 mg/mL. How many mL will the client self-inject per dose?

   _____

   _____

2. A client is prescribed 1 mg of cabergoline twice weekly for the treatment of acromegaly. The drug is available as 0.5-mg tablets. How many tablets should the nurse instruct the client to take per dose?

   _____

   _____

3. A nurse is caring for a client with a severe allergy. The primary health care provider has prescribed a loading dose of 8 mg of dexamethasone in an IM injection. The dexamethasone is available as 4 mg/mL. How many mL will the nurse prepare of the solution for injection?

_____

_____

4. A primary health care provider has prescribed a tapered dose of dexamethasone orally for the client to take at home: four 0.75-mg tablets on day 2, same for day 3, two 0.75-mg tablets on day 4, and one 0.75-mg tablet on days 5 through 7. How many tablets will the nurse need to fill the medication dispenser box for a week of medication administration for this client?

_____

_____

5. A nurse is caring for a client with psoriatic arthritis. The primary health care provider has prescribed 20 mg of prednisone on a daily basis. The drug is available as 10-mg tablets. How many tablets should the nurse administer to the client for each dose?

_____

_____

Activity C MATCHING

1. Match the drugs in Column A with their uses in Column B.

Column A

____ **1.** Desmopressin

____ **2.** Bromocriptine

____ **3.** Budesonide

____ **4.** Fludrocortisone

Column B

a. Treatment of Parkinson disease

b. Treatment of nocturnal enuresis

c. Therapy for Addison disease

d. Treatment of Crohn disease

2. Match the drugs in Column A with their adverse reactions in Column B.

Column A

____ **1.** Octreotide

____ **2.** Vasopressin

____ **3.** Somatropin

____ **4.** Clomiphene

Column B

a. Ovarian enlargement

b. Arthralgia

c. Sinus bradycardia

d. Tremor

Activity D SHORT ANSWERS

A nurse's role in managing clients receiving growth hormones involves assisting them in order to promote an optimal response to growth hormone therapy. The nurse also helps clients by educating them and their families about the successful implementation of therapy. Answer the following questions, which involve the nurse's role in the management of such situations.

1. A 10-year-old client has enrolled in a growth hormone program. What are the steps the nurse should teach a family member regarding daily subcutaneous injection of the growth hormone therapy?

_____

_____

2. What is the nurse's role in educating the client and his family about the growth hormone therapy?

_____

_____

Activity E **CROSSWORD PUZZLE**

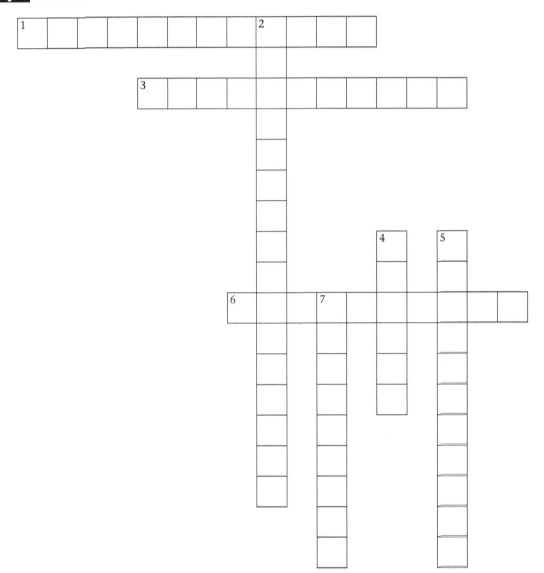

Across

1. Failure of the testes to descend into the scrotum
3. Regulates the reabsorption of fluid by the kidney
6. Group of symptoms (including moon face, buffalo hump) due to the disease caused by the overproduction of endogenous glucocorticoids

Down

2. Syndrome in which sudden ovarian enlargement is caused by overstimulation
4. Glands responsible for sexual activity and characteristics
5. A menstrual cycle in which ovulation (release of egg) does not occur
7. Excess growth of facial and body hair in women

SECTION II: APPLYING YOUR KNOWLEDGE

Activity F CASE STUDY

 Janna Wong's friend wants to tell her classmates about diabetes insipidus and administration of desmopressin. The mother of the child is a nurse and comes to help explain the disease to the students.

1. The students in class ask what they can do to help her from getting sick or what they should do if she has a problem. What should the nurse tell them?

   _____

   _____

2. What adverse reactions might she experience with the drug?

   _____

   _____

Now Map It Out! Use the templates provided in the appendix to add information and make client connections on a concept map.

Lillian Chase experiences asthma symptoms on a yearly basis. Looking at the concept map for Lillian, how many interactions can you identify that may potentially result if a glucocorticoid is added to her medication routine for asthma symptoms?

SECTION III: PRACTICING FOR NCLEX

Activity G NCLEX-STYLE QUESTIONS

Answer the following questions.

1. A nurse is caring for a client with diabetes insipidus on extended bedrest in an acute care facility. The primary health care provider has prescribed vasopressin for the client. Scanning the electronic health record (EHR), the nurse notes that the client is also taking oral anticoagulants. What effect should the nurse anticipate due to the interaction of these two drugs?
   1. Increased risk of hypokalemia
   2. Increased need for antidiabetic medication
   3. Decreased muscle function
   4. Decreased antidiuretic effect

2. A primary health care provider has prescribed a glucocorticoid to the client with acute thyroiditis. What intervention should the nurse perform as part of ongoing assessment during the course of treatment?
   1. Record the client's abdominal girth.
   2. Monitor for a rise in blood glucose level.
   3. Measure the specific gravity of the urine.
   4. Monitor bone age periodically.

3. A primary health care provider prescribes hydrocortisone injection to a client with an arthritic knee. Which of the following instructions should the nurse teach the client regarding activity?
   1. Line dancing can be resumed as soon as you get home.
   2. The pain may stop, but do not overuse the joint.
   3. Do not drink any fluids for 8 hour after the injection.
   4. If pain resumes, take a long walk to make it feel better.

4. A client with adrenocortical deficiency is prescribed fludrocortisone by a primary health care provider. Which of the following adverse reactions would indicate the dose of the drug is not enough?
   1. Joint pain
   2. Hypothyroidism
   3. Hypotension
   4. Insulin resistance

5. A primary health care provider has prescribed ganirelix to a client to stimulate ovulation. During the course of the treatment, the client calls to complain of visual disturbances. Which of the following precautionary measures should the nurse take?
   1. Discontinue the drug therapy
   2. Administer the drug with food
   3. Perform a CBC test
   4. Assess skin integrity

6. A client in a long-term care facility is prescribed glucocorticoids for systemic lupus erythematosus (SLE). Which nursing diagnosis is most appropriate for the client?
    1. Pain related to abdominal distention
    2. Deydration related to inability to replenish fluid intake
    3. Disturbed body image related to drug adverse reactions
    4. Infection risk related to masking of signs of infection

7. A postsurgical client is prescribed vasopressin for a diagnostic abdominal roentgenography. Which of the following tasks should the nurse perform during implementation of the procedure?
    1. Give enema before first dose of vasopressin.
    2. Check stools for evidence of bleeding.
    3. Monitor client for rash, urticaria, and hypotension.
    4. Provide daily oral drug doses before 9 a.m.

8. A nurse is caring for a client undergoing long-term glucocorticoid therapy. Which of the following symptoms is the nurse most likely to observe in the client as a result of cushingoid effects? **Select all that apply.**
    1. Dehydration
    2. Buffalo hump
    3. Muscle strength
    4. Moon face
    5. Weight loss

9. Which of the following hormones is secreted by the posterior pituitary gland?
    1. Vasopressin
    2. Gonadotropin
    3. Somatropin
    4. Adrenocorticotropic hormone (ACTH)

10. Diabetes insipidus is treated with replacement of which of the following hormones?
    1. Gonadotropin
    2. Somatropin
    3. Vasopressin
    4. ACTH

11. Which of the following hormones is responsible for the regulation of reabsorption of water by the kidneys?
    1. Vasopressin
    2. Gonadotropin
    3. Somatotropin
    4. ACTH

12. Which of the following medications binds to estrogen receptors, decreasing the amount of available estrogen receptors and causing the anterior pituitary to increase secretion of FSH and LH?
    1. Clomiphene (Clomid)
    2. Medroxyprogesterone (Provera)
    3. Estradiol (Estrace)
    4. Estropipate (Ogen)

CHAPTER 42

Thyroid and Antithyroid Drugs

Learning Objectives

- Identify the hormones produced by the thyroid gland.
- Explain the uses, general drug actions, adverse reactions, contraindications, precautions, and interactions of thyroid and antithyroid drugs.
- Distinguish important preadministration and ongoing assessment activities the nurse should perform with the client taking a thyroid or antithyroid drug.
- Examine ways to promote an optimal response to therapy, how to manage adverse reactions, and important points to keep in mind when educating clients about the use of thyroid and antithyroid drugs.

SECTION I: ASSESSING YOUR UNDERSTANDING

Activity A FILL IN THE BLANKS

1. _____ is an increase in the amount of thyroid hormones manufactured and secreted.

2. Thyroid hormones are used as replacement therapy when the client is _____.

3. _____ is a substance that is quickly absorbed by the thyroid gland.

4. When a normal thyroid gland is functioning, this is called the _____ state.

5. _____ drugs inhibit the manufacture of thyroid hormones.

Activity B DOSAGE CALCULATION

1. A primary health care provider (PHCP) has prescribed 40 mcg/day of levothyroxine. The drug is available as 20-mcg tablets. How many tablets should the client take per dose?

2. A client is prescribed methimazole for the treatment of hyperthyroidism. The PHCP instructs the nurse to administer 10 mg of the drug in 8-hour intervals daily. The available tablets are 5 mg. How many tablets should the nurse administer to the client in a dose?

3. A client is prescribed 300 mg of propylthiouracil daily in three equally divided doses at 8-hour intervals. The drug is available in the form of 100-mg tablets. How many tablets should the nurse administer to the client in each dose?

4. A long-term care client with hypothyroidism is prescribed thyroid USP. The PHCP has prescribed 30 mg of the drug initially each day to the client. The drug is available in 15-mg tablets. How many tablets should the nurse administer to the client per day?

5. A PHCP prescribes 0.2 mg Levothroid daily to the client for treatment of hypothyroidism. How many micrograms of Levothroid is in this dose?

_____

_____

1. Match the drugs in Column A with their adverse reactions in Column B.

Column A

____ **1.** Levothyroxine (T_4)

____ **2.** Methimazole

____ **3.** Sodium iodide (^{131}I)

Column B

a. Hives

b. Palpitations

c. Agranulocytosis

2. Match the interactant drugs in Column A with the effect of their interaction with the thyroid hormones in Column B.

Column A

____ **1.** Digoxin

____ **2.** Insulin

____ **3.** Oral anticoagulant

____ **4.** Antidepressants

Column B

a. Increased risk of hypoglycemia

b. Decreased effectiveness of thyroid drug

c. Decreased effectiveness of cardiac drug

d. Prolonged bleeding

A nurse's role in managing clients who are being administered thyroid hormones involves monitoring the clients and implementing interventions that aid in their recovery. Answer the following questions, which involve the nurse's role in the management of such situations.

1. A client undergoing thyroid hormone replacement therapy is discharged. What information should the nurse provide to the client and family emphasizing the importance of taking the replacement therapy?

_____

_____

2. A nurse is caring for a client undergoing thyroid hormone therapy. Post therapy, the nurse needs to evaluate the effectiveness of the therapy. What factors should the nurse consider to determine the success of the therapy?

_____

_____

Activity E CROSSWORD PUZZLE

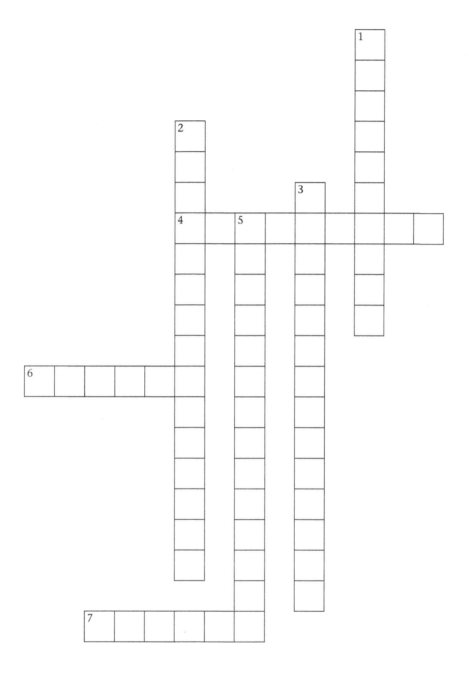

Across

4. Normal thyroid function

6. Enlargement of the thyroid gland causing a swelling in the front part of the neck, usually caused by hyperthyroidism

7. Autoimmune disorder leading to overactivity of the thyroid gland

Down

1. Autoimmune disease attacking the thyroid, typically resulting in hypothyroid function

2. Overactive thyroid function

3. Underactive thyroid function

5. Severe hyperthyroidism characterized by high fever, extreme tachycardia, and altered mental status

SECTION II: APPLYING YOUR KNOWLEDGE

Activity F **CASE STUDY**

 While Janna Wong is in to see the PHCP today, the clinic nurse is troubled by Janna's mother's appearance. She states it is just hard to keep up with all of Janna's activities. Mrs. Wong notes that she has noticed some weight gain, cold intolerance, sleepiness, and dry skin. The PHCP checks her TSH and diagnoses Mrs. Wong with hypothyroidism. She is given a prescription for levothyroxine (Synthroid) 50 mcg daily.

1. How should the nurse instruct Mrs. Wong to take the levothyroxine (Synthroid)?

_____

_____

2. How long can it take for Mrs. Wong to see the effects of the levothyroxine (Synthroid)?

_____

_____

Now Map It Out! Use the templates provided in the appendix to add information and make client connections on a concept map.

Before the physician confirms a medical diagnosis of dementia for Mrs. Moore, a TSH blood level is ordered. Using her concept map, identify the factors that warrant ruling out thyroid disease.

SECTION III: PRACTICING FOR NCLEX

Activity G **NCLEX-STYLE QUESTIONS**

Answer the following questions.

1. A client is administered methimazole for the treatment of hyperthyroidism. Which of the following adverse reactions to the drug should the nurse notify the PHCP about immediately?
   1. Tachycardia
   2. Agranulocytosis
   3. Weight loss
   4. Fatigue

2. A nurse is caring for a client receiving thyroid hormones. The client is also taking digoxin for a cardiac problem. What effect of drug interaction should the nurse observe for in the client?
   1. Decreased effectiveness of the cardiac drug
   2. Increased risk of prolonged bleeding
   3. Decreased effectiveness of the thyroid drug
   4. Increased potential for bleeding

3. A nurse is caring for a client undergoing thyroid hormone therapy. What signs of therapeutic response should the nurse monitor for after the thyroid hormone is administered to the client?
   1. Agranulocytosis
   2. Headache
   3. Mild diuresis
   4. Loss of hair

4. A client with cardiovascular disease is administered thyroid hormones. The occurrence of which symptom would justify reducing the client's dosage of thyroid hormones by the PHCP?
   1. High fever
   2. Chest pain
   3. Sweating
   4. Headache

5. A client is administered an antithyroid drug by the PHCP. Which of the following signs indicate the client could be suffering from thyroid storm?
   1. Somnolence
   2. Decreased pulse rate
   3. Anger
   4. Altered mental status

6. A client is prescribed thyroid hormone therapy. In which of the following client conditions is the drug contraindicated?
   1. Agranulocytosis
   2. Adrenal cortical insufficiency
   3. Granulocytopenia
   4. Hypoprothrombinemia

7. A health care provider administers thyroid hormone therapy to a client. Which of the following signs of hyperthyroidism should the nurse teach the client to report to the PHCP before the next dose is due? **Select all that apply.**
    1. Moist skin
    2. Easy bruising
    3. Moderate hypertension
    4. Increased appetite
    5. Sore throat

8. Which of the following is an inflammatory disease causing hypothyroidism?
    1. Euthyroid goiter
    2. Hashimoto thyroiditis
    3. Cold nodule
    4. Autoimmune hyperthyroidism

9. Which of the following is the drug of choice for hypothyroidism because it is relatively inexpensive, requires once-a-day dosing, and has a more uniform potency than do other thyroid hormone replacement drugs?
    1. Propylthiouracil (PTU)
    2. Methimazole (Tapazole)
    3. Levothyroxine (Synthroid)
    4. Liotrix (Thyrolar)

10. A nurse should be cautious not to administer levothyroxine (Synthroid) to a client who has recently had which of the following?
    1. Myocardial infarction
    2. Cataract surgery
    3. Seizure
    4. Hypoglycemic episode

11. Levothyroxine (Synthroid) is classified in which pregnancy category?
    1. Category A
    2. Category B
    3. Category C
    4. Category X

43 •

Male and Female Hormones

Learning Objectives

- Explain the medical uses, actions, adverse reactions, contraindications, precautions, and interactions of the male and female hormones.
- Distinguish important preadministration and ongoing assessment activities the nurse should perform with the client taking male or female hormones.
- List nursing diagnoses particular to a client taking male or female hormones.
- Examine ways to promote an optimal response to therapy, how to manage adverse reactions, and important points to keep in mind when educating the client about the use of male or female hormones.

SECTION I: ASSESSING YOUR UNDERSTANDING

Activity A FILL IN THE BLANKS

1. The age of onset of first menstruation is called _____.

2. Hormones produced by the body are called _____ hormones.

3. _____ is called reverse tissue-depleting processes of the body.

4. Sex hormones play a vital role in the development and maintenance of _____ _____.

5. Testosterone and its derivatives are collectively called _____.

Activity B DOSAGE CALCULATION

1. A client with advanced breast cancer is prescribed fluoxymesterone 20 mg/day in two equally divided doses. Fluoxymesterone is available in 10-mg tablets. How many tablets will the client take per dose?

_____

_____

2. A client with anorexia and anemia weighing 30 kg has been prescribed 5 mg/kg of Anadrol-50 (oxymetholone) orally per day. Anadrol-50 is available as 50-mg tablets. How many tablets should the client take each day?

_____

_____

3. A client with primary ovarian failure has been prescribed 1.5 mg of estropipate as a daily dose. How many of the estropipate tablets (0.75 mg) should the nurse instruct the client to take daily?

_____

_____

4. A client with endometriosis has been prescribed Aygestin (norethindrone) to be taken at a dose of 5 mg/day for the first 2 weeks and 7.5 mg/day for the next 2 weeks. How many of the 5-mg tablets should the nurse instruct the client to take per dose during the third and the fourth week?

_____

_____

5. A client has been prescribed 200 mg of oral progesterone daily for the prevention of endometrial hyperplasia. How many of the 100-mg progesterone capsules should the client take daily?

_____

_____

Activity C MATCHING

1. Match the hormones/drugs in Column A with the conditions they are used for in Column B.

Column A

____ **1.** Androgens

____ **2.** Anabolic steroids

____ **3.** Estrogens

____ **4.** Progestins

Column B

a. Anemia of renal insufficiency

b. Endometriosis

c. Male hypogonadism

d. Atrophic vaginitis

2. Match the hormones/drugs in Column A with the adverse reactions in Column B.

Column A

____ **1.** Anabolic steroids

____ **2.** Progestins

____ **3.** Estrogens

____ **4.** Androgens

Column B

a. Erectile dysfunction

b. Gynecomastia

c. Menstrual spotting

d. Thromboembolism

Activity D SHORT ANSWERS

A nurse's role in managing clients who are receiving hormone therapy involves monitoring and implementing interventions that aid in recovery. Answer the following questions, which involve the nurse's role in the management of such situations.

1. A nurse is caring for a client who is on androgen therapy. What assessments should the nurse implement when monitoring for excess fluid volume in the client?

_____

_____

2. A nurse is educating a client who plans to take oral contraceptives as a method of birth control. What points should the nurse include in the teaching plan when educating the client regarding oral contraceptives?

_____

_____

Activity E CROSSWORD PUZZLE

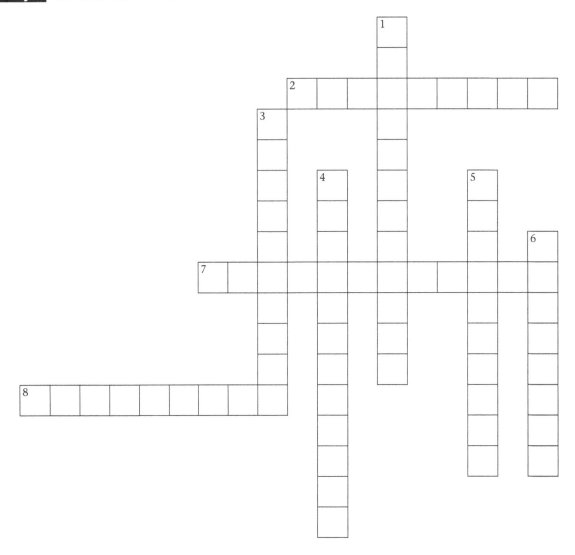

Across

2. Male hormone, testosterone and its derivatives

7. Female hormone produced by the corpus luteum that works in the uterus (along with estrogen) to prepare the uterus for possible conception

8. Tissue-building process

Down

1. Acquisition of male sexual characteristics by a woman

3. Tissue-depleting process

4. Male breast enlargement

5. Pertaining to something that normally occurs or is produced within the organism

6. Age of onset of first menstruation

SECTION II: APPLYING YOUR KNOWLEDGE

Activity F CASE STUDY

 Janna Wong presents to the free health clinic to obtain emergency contraception after contraceptive failure. She has no medical conditions and takes no medications.

1. It is important for the nurse to question a client seeking emergency contraception about when the unprotected intercourse or contraceptive failure occurred, as emergency contraception needs to be taken soon after the event. How long after unprotected intercourse or contraceptive failure occurs should high-dose levonorgestrel (Plan B) be administered?

_____

_____

2. How should levonorgestrel (Plan B) be taken?

_____

_____

Now Map It Out! Use the templates provided in the appendix to add information and make client connections on a concept map.

Using the concept map for Janna Wong, add the medication request from the case study above. How does this now affect the map for interactions?

SECTION III: PRACTICING FOR NCLEX

Activity G NCLEX-STYLE QUESTIONS

Answer the following questions.

1. A client has been prescribed androgen therapy. Which of the following conditions should the nurse consider to be an indication for such a prescription?
   1. Adrenal cortical cancer
   2. Testosterone deficiency
   3. Benign prostatic hypertrophy
   4. Male pattern baldness

2. Following a major road accident and disability 2 years ago, a client experienced profound weight loss. The client tells the nurse that they had been prescribed a drug to promote weight gain during that time. Which class of drugs is most likely to be prescribed for weight gain after a significant loss?
   1. Androgen hormones
   2. Progestins
   3. Conjugate estrogens
   4. Anabolic steroids

3. A client with obesity is receiving anticoagulant therapy as a prophylaxis for thromboembolism following an appendectomy. Which of the following interactions may be seen when androgens or androgen hormone inhibitors are used at the same time in this client?
   1. Increased antidiuretic effect
   2. Decreased anticoagulant effect
   3. Increased risk of hypoglycemia
   4. Increased risk of paranoia

4. A nurse caring for a male client with hypogonadism who has been prescribed androgen therapy is required to educate the client about the use of the drug and its possible adverse effects. Which of the following is an adverse effect of androgen therapy?
   1. Enlargement of testes
   2. Gynecomastia
   3. Virilization
   4. Frequent urination

5. The male hormone testosterone aids in the development of secondary sex characteristics. Which of the following are secondary sex characteristics in a male? **Select all that apply.**
   1. Facial hair
   2. Pigmentation of areolae
   3. Fallopian tube development
   4. Deepening voice
   5. Muscle development

6. The use of anabolic steroids is associated with psychological disturbances when taken by healthy males. Which of the following severe mental changes may be seen by a client taking anabolic steroids for a prolonged time?
   1. Clear focal attentiveness
   2. Severe depression
   3. Autism
   4. Schizophrenia

7. A 20-year-old woman taking oral contraceptives is anxious that she has missed 1 day's dose. Which of the following instructions should the nurse offer the client?
   1. Discontinue the drug and use another form of birth control until the next cycle.
   2. Take two tablets for the next 2 days and continue with the normal schedule.
   3. Remember to take one tablet the next day and forget about the missed dose.
   4. Take the missed dose as soon as remembered or take two tablets the next day.

8. When educating a group of nursing students regarding the various female hormones, the nurse identifies which of the following hormones as a synthetic estrogen that is available only as a drug?
   1. Estradiol
   2. Estrone
   3. Estriol
   4. Estropipate

9. The nurse is working with a woman taking a male hormone for advanced cancer. Which is the best nursing intervention to offer for the adverse reaction of virilization?
   1. Provide magazines with trendy-dressed models.
   2. Suggest head coverings and concealing makeup.
   3. Instruct in graceful walking and sitting.
   4. Refer to a gym for exercises.

10. Which of the following is an example of an androgen that can be used to treat hypogonadism?
    1. Fluoxymesterone
    2. Nandrolone
    3. Dutasteride
    4. Oxymetholone

11. Which of the following medications can be used to treat anemia?
    1. Fluoxymesterone
    2. Oxymetholone
    3. Finasteride
    4. Dutasteride

12. Which of the following is an example of an anabolic steroid?
    1. Nandrolone
    2. Fluoxymesterone
    3. Testosterone
    4. Dutasteride

44

Uterine Drugs

Learning Objectives

- Explain the actions, uses, adverse reactions, contraindications, precautions, and interactions of drugs acting on the uterus.
- Distinguish important preadministration and ongoing assessment activities the nurse should perform with the client taking an oxytocic or tocolytic drug.
- List some nursing diagnoses particular to a client taking an oxytocic or tocolytic drug.
- Examine ways to promote an optimal response to therapy, how to manage adverse reactions, and important points to keep in mind when educating clients about the use of an oxytocic or tocolytic drug.

SECTION I: ASSESSING YOUR UNDERSTANDING

Activity A FILL IN THE BLANKS

1. Oxytocic drugs are used antepartum to induce uterine _____.

2. Oxytocin is an endogenous hormone produced by the _____ pituitary gland.

3. A complication of pregnancy characterized by convulsive seizures and coma is known as _____.

4. The prevention of preterm labor (PTL) is called _____.

5. Large doses of oxytocin lead to water intoxication due to its _____ effect.

Activity B DOSAGE CALCULATION

1. A doctor prescribes a client 10 units of oxytocin IM following a delivery. The drug is available as 10 units/1 mL in a 3-mL vial. How many mL will the nurse draw up to administer to the client?

_____

_____

2. A client in PTL has been prescribed nifedipine 20 mg orally every 4 hours. Each tablet of nifedipine contains 10 mg. How many tablets should the nurse administer to the client in each dose?

_____

_____

3. A client with postpartum bleeding has been prescribed 0.2 mg of methylergonovine orally twice a day. The available methylergonovine tablet is 0.2 mg. How many tablets should the nurse administer to the client per dose?

_____

_____

4. A doctor prescribes 50 mg of indomethacin oral suspension to a client in PTL. The available solution contains 25 mg of indomethacin per 5 mL. What volume of the solution should the nurse administer to the client?

_____

_____

5. A doctor prescribes 0.25 mg of Brethine (terbutaline) subcutaneous injection to a client in PTL. Each ampule contains 1 mg of Brethine per 1 mL of solution. What volume of the available solution should the nurse administer to the client?

_____

_____

6. A client with postpartum bleeding has been prescribed 5 units of oxytocin. The available 1-mL ampule contains 10 units of oxytocin. What volume of the solution should the nurse administer to the client?

_____

_____

Activity C MATCHING

1. Match the drugs acting on the uterus in Column A with their adverse reactions in Column B.

Column A	Column B
___ 1. Indomethacin	a. Diplopia
___ 2. Oxytocin	b. Cardiac arrhythmias
___ 3. Magnesium	c. Heartburn
___ 4. Nifedipine	d. Hypokalemia
___ 5. Terbutaline	e. Nasal congestion

2. Match the drugs acting on the uterus in Column A with their contraindications in Column B.

Column A	Column B
___ 1. Tocolytics	a. Before delivery of placenta
___ 2. Oxytocin	b. Eclampsia
___ 3. Methyler-gonovine	c. Cephalopelvic disproportion
___ 4. Magnesium	d. With nonsteroidal anti-inflammatory drugs (NSAIDs)
___ 5. Indomethacin	e. Myocardial damage

Activity D SHORT ANSWERS

A nurse's role in managing clients who are being administered drugs acting on the uterus involves monitoring and implementing interventions that aid in recovery. Answer the following questions, which involve the nurse's role in the management of such situations.

1. A nurse is required to monitor the uterine contractions of a client who is receiving an oxytocin infusion. What conditions would alert the nurse to discontinue the oxytocin infusion?

_____

_____

2. What ongoing assessment should the nurse engage in when caring for a client receiving tocolytic drugs?

_____

_____

Activity E **CROSSWORD PUZZLE**

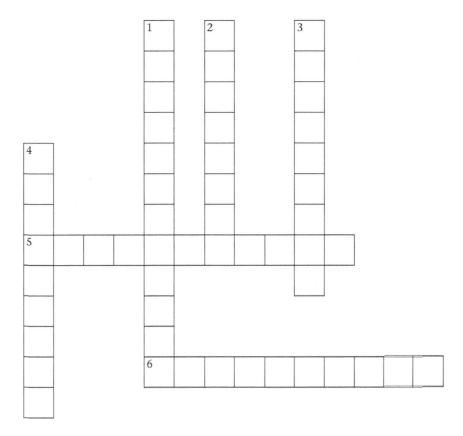

Across

5. Excessive protein in the urine
6. The time during pregnancy before childbirth

Down

1. A condition in pregnancy, near term, when the woman becomes hypertensive and excess protein is found in her urine
2. An endogenous hormone produced by the posterior pituitary gland that has uterus-stimulating properties
3. To prevent PTL
4. A condition where seizures and possible coma happen in pregnancy after 20 weeks in a woman who has become hypertensive and excess protein is found in the urine

SECTION II: APPLYING YOUR KNOWLEDGE

Activity F **CASE STUDY**

Betty Peterson's daughter, Stella, is admitted to the labor and delivery floor of the hospital to give birth to her first child. She is post term and the physician has ordered her to receive oxytocin (Pitocin) IV to induce labor.

1. Before the nurse starts the IV oxytocin (Pitocin), what information should be obtained from Stella?

_____

_____

2. Once the oxytocin (Pitocin) is started IV, for which adverse effects should the nurse monitor Stella?

_____

_____

SECTION III: PRACTICING FOR NCLEX

Activity G NCLEX-STYLE QUESTIONS

Answer the following questions.

1. Which of the following is an indication to prescribe oxytocin to begin labor?
   1. Placenta previa
   2. PTL
   3. Gestational diabetes
   4. Uterine atony

2. A client is to receive methylergonovine after expulsion of the placenta following childbirth. Which is the preferred route of administration?
   1. Vaginally
   2. IM injection
   3. IV injection
   4. Orally

3. A pregnant client in her 26th week of gestation is admitted to an antepartum unit with PTL. In which of the following conditions is magnesium sulfate most appropriate?
   1. Cephalopelvic disproportion
   2. Hypertension
   3. Total placenta previa
   4. Eclampsia with convulsions

4. A 31-year-old client in her 28th week of gestation is experiencing PTL. The client has been administered IV magnesium sulfate to prolong the pregnancy. Which of the following drugs are administered to mature fetal organs in utero?
   1. Growth hormones
   2. Pediatric vitamins
   3. Corticosteroids
   4. Bronchodilators

5. A 32-year-old pregnant woman is admitted to the hospital with labor pains. The client is prescribed carboprost during the third stage of labor after the placenta has been delivered. In which of the following conditions is the reason this drug is chosen over other oxytocic drugs?
   1. Renal disease
   2. During lactation
   3. Heart disease
   4. Hypertension

6. A nurse is given an order to administer methylergonovine to a postpartum client who is hemorrhaging. Which of the following nursing interventions should the nurse implement when administering the drug? Select all that apply.
   1. Monitor vital signs at least every 4 hours.
   2. Discontinue the drug if the client develops abdominal cramping.
   3. Notify the health care provider if abdominal cramping is severe.
   4. Note character and amount of vaginal bleeding.
   5. Place the client in a lateral position.

7. The nurse observes signs of excess fluid volume in the laboring client. Which of the following drugs leads to the danger of an excessive fluid volume (water intoxication)?
   1. Oxytocin
   2. Nifedipine
   3. Magnesium sulfate
   4. Terbutaline

8. A client in her 28th week of gestation is experiencing PTL and is prescribed magnesium sulfate. Which of the following is a property of magnesium sulfate?
   1. It is a calcium antagonist.
   2. It blocks the production of prostaglandins.
   3. It has an antidiuretic action.
   4. It acts as a uterine stimulant.

9. Which of the following is used antepartum to induce uterine contractions?
   1. Oxytocin
   2. Ritodrine
   3. Indomethacin
   4. Terbutaline

10. Oxytocin is an endogenous hormone produced by which of the following?
    1. Adrenal gland
    2. Posterior pituitary gland
    3. Uterus
    4. Corpus luteum

11. How would the client self-administer oxytocin (Pitocin) to stimulate the milk ejection reflex?
    1. Intranasally
    2. Topically
    3. Subcutaneously
    4. Orally

12. A nurse should monitor a client receiving oxytocin (Pitocin) for which of the following adverse effects?
    1. Cardiac arrhythmias
    2. Hypotension
    3. Headache
    4. Dizziness

Drugs That Affect The Urinary System

CHAPTER 45

Menopause and Andropause Drugs

Learning Objectives

- Describe changes occurring in the urinary and reproductive systems because of aging.
- Explain the uses, general drug actions, adverse reactions, contraindications, precautions, and interactions of the drugs used to treat symptoms associated with menopause and andropause.
- Distinguish important preadministration and ongoing assessment activities the nurse should perform with the client taking a drug for a change resulting from menopause or andropause.
- List nursing diagnoses for a client taking a drug for a change resulting from menopause or andropause.
- Examine ways to promote an optimal response to therapy, how to manage adverse reactions, and important points to keep in mind when educating clients about the use of drugs to treat a change resulting from menopause or andropause.

SECTION I: ASSESSING YOUR UNDERSTANDING

Activity A FILL IN THE BLANKS

1. As hormonal influence lessens in women, this period of life is called _____.

2. Aging women have an increased risk for _____ disease with the use of estrogen replacement therapy (ERT).

3. Effects of childbirth and loss of muscle tone in pelvic structures leads to _____ incontinence.

4. Aging changes in the male reproductive system occur primarily in the _____.

5. The development of the _____ gland is dependent on the potent androgen 5-alpha (5-α)-dihydrotestosterone (DHT).

Activity B DOSAGE CALCULATION

1. A client with metastatic breast cancer has been prescribed a daily dose of tamoxifen 40 mg orally in two equally divided doses per day. Tamoxifen is available in a 10-mg tablet. How many tablets do they need to take in a single dose?

_____

_____

2. A client is prescribed 0.6 mg Premarin (conjugated estrogen) orally for menopausal symptoms. Premarin is available as 0.3-mg tablets. How many tablets should the client take each day?

_____

_____

3. Fesoterodine 8 mg orally has been prescribed for a client with overactive bladder symptoms. The client was started on a lower dose initially and has the drug in 4-mg tablet strength. Seven tablets are left in the bottle. How many complete doses are available to the client before refilling the prescription?

_____

_____

4. A client with benign prostatic hyperplasia (BPH) has been prescribed silodosin 8 mg once orally with a meal. Silodosin is available in 4-mg capsules. How many capsules should the client take daily?

_____

_____

5. A client with ED is prescribed sildenafil 50-mg tablets. If the recommended dose is no more than 100 mg of sildenafil daily, how many tablets can the client use?

_____

_____

Activity C MATCHING

1. Using the Summary Drug Tables in your textbook, look for patterns in how drugs are named, and match the andropause drug ending (suffix) in Column A with the drug class in Column B.

Column A

____ **1.** -teride

____ **2.** -afil

____ **3.** -sin

Column B

a. Phosphodiesterase type 5 inhibitors for erectile dysfunction

b. Peripherally acting antiadrenergic drug

c. AHI for BPH

2. Match the drugs used in hormonal therapy for cancer in Column A with their common adverse effects in Column B.

Column A

____ **1.** Bicalutamide

____ **2.** Testolactone

____ **3.** Goserelin

____ **4.** Leuprolide

Column B

a. Bone pain

b. Hot flashes

c. Extremity edema

d. Breast atrophy

Activity D SHORT ANSWERS

A nurse's role in managing clients who are receiving therapy for menopause involves monitoring and implementing interventions that aid in recovery. Answer the following questions, which involve the nurse's role in the management of such situations.

1. A nurse is caring for a client who is seen for menopausal symptoms. The client brings a copy of a study about health risks associated with ERT. What action should the nurse implement with regard to her concerns about ERT therapy?

_____

_____

2. The client decides to start ERT using the transdermal system to dispense estrogen. What points should the nurse include in the teaching plan when educating the client regarding the use of transdermal estrogen?

_____

_____

Activity E

Familiarize yourself with genitourinary abbreviations.

BPH	GU		ED					HRT
HRT	OBS	AHI	UTI	GU			ED	DHT
ERT	UTI		BPH				AHI	
AHI		GU				OBS	BPH	
ED				ERT	BPH	HRT		AHI
	BPH		HRT	AHI	GU	ED	DHT	
	AHI	HRT	GU	BPH				
	ED		ERT		HRT	AHI	OBS	
	ERT					UTI		BPH

SECTION II: APPLYING YOUR KNOWLEDGE

Activity F CASE STUDY

 Mr. Phillip is prescribed finasteride for BPH symptoms. His daughter, who is aged 42 years, comes to visit with her two young children. While at the house, the visiting nurse has stopped in to check Mr. Phillip's medications and he remembers that he did not take his morning medications yet.

1. The daughter gets up to go get his pills. What precaution should the nurse tell the daughter before she handles the daily medications?

_____

_____

2. The daughter returns with the various morning pills, and she tells the nurse her dad looks like he is feeling better and even a little bit younger, and it seems his hair is getting thicker. What could be causing this to happen?

_____

_____

Now Map It Out! Use the templates provided in the appendix to add information and make client connections on a concept map.

Mr. Phillip's issues with aging urinary symptoms have been discussed in both the textbook and study guide for Chapter 45. Using the concept map for Mr. Phillip, add the information to the map regarding his symptoms, treatment options, and results.

SECTION III: PRACTICING FOR NCLEX

Activity G NCLEX-STYLE QUESTIONS

Answer the following questions.

1. A nurse is caring for a client with an overactive bladder who has been prescribed darifenacin (Enablex). The drug is known to cause dry mouth. What instructions should the nurse offer the client to get relief from dry mouth?
   1. Suck on sugarless lozenges.
   2. Refrain from consuming hard candy.
   3. Consume foods rich in fiber.
   4. Always take the drug with milk.

2. A nurse is caring for a client receiving solifenacin for the treatment of an overactive bladder. What adverse reaction to the drug should the nurse monitor for in the client?
   1. Headache
   2. Dry eyes
   3. Pruritus
   4. Rash

3. A client has been prescribed an androgen hormone inhibitor. Which of the following conditions should the nurse consider to be an indication for such a prescription?
   1. Adrenal cortical cancer
   2. Testosterone deficiency
   3. BPH
   4. Menopause

4. A nurse is to start a client on antispasmodic drug therapy. For which of the following conditions is the use of antispasmodics contraindicated?
   1. Convulsive disorders
   2. Cerebral arteriosclerosis
   3. Myasthenia gravis
   4. Hepatic impairment

5. A woman is experiencing symptoms of menopause and decides to try black cohosh, a herbal remedy, to alleviate these symptoms. Which of the following possible adverse reactions might the client experience while taking the herb?
   1. Low blood pressure
   2. Ringing in the ears
   3. Impaired vision
   4. Weight loss

6. A nurse is caring for a client receiving flavoxate for the treatment of urinary problems. During assessment, the client complains of constipation. What intervention should the nurse suggest when caring for this client?
   1. Increase the client's intake of fluids.
   2. Increase the client's intake of citrus fruits.
   3. Decrease the client's consumption of milk products.
   4. Administer the drug to the client with tepid water.

7. Aging causes a number of changes in the female reproductive system. Which of the following conditions occurs as a result of fat atrophy and hormonal changes?
   1. Pelvic floor muscles become stronger.
   2. The vaginal pH becomes more acidic.
   3. Vaginal walls increase in size and elasticity.
   4. Increased time for sexual arousal is needed.

8. If a premenopausal female has her ovaries removed, which of the following methods of administration is preferred for estrogen replacement?
   1. Oral
   2. Transdermal
   3. Vaginal
   4. Injectable

9. Kidneys reduce in size and blood flow diminishes to the organ as a person ages. How much is renal function reduced due to the normal aging process?
   1. 10 times
   2. 400 mL/min
   3. 50%
   4. By a factor of 7

10. Which of the following is an example of an androgen hormone inhibitor that is used to treat clients with BPH?
    1. Dutasteride (Avodart)
    2. Oxymetholone (Anadrol-50)
    3. Oxandrolone (Oxandrin)
    4. Methyltestosterone (Testred)

11. Which of the following is an example of a drug used for advanced prostatic cancer?
    1. Tamoxifen
    2. Flutamide
    3. Megestrol
    4. Letrozole

12. Which of the following interventions is used with urge incontinence and not typically with stress incontinence?
    1. Behavioral interventions
    2. Pessaries
    3. Oral medications
    4. Surgery

Urinary Tract Anti-infectives and Other Urinary Drugs

- Explain the uses, general drug actions, adverse reactions, contraindications, precautions, and interactions of the drugs used to treat infections and symptoms associated with urinary tract infections.
- Distinguish important preadministration and ongoing assessment activities the nurse should perform with the client taking a drug for a urinary tract infection.
- List nursing diagnoses particular to a client taking a drug for a urinary tract infection.
- Examine ways to promote an optimal response to therapy, how to manage adverse reactions, and important points to keep in mind when educating clients about the use of drugs to treat urinary tract infections.

SECTION I: ASSESSING YOUR UNDERSTANDING

Activity A FILL IN THE BLANKS

1. The most common structure affected by urinary tract infection (UTI) is the
   _____.

2. Women are at greater risk for UTIs because the _____ is considerably shorter in females than in males.

3. Urgency, frequency, pressure, burning, and pain on urination are the clinical findings of bladder inflammation or _____.

4. Drugs that slow or retard the multiplication of bacteria are called _____.

5. Drugs that kill or destroy bacteria are called
   _____.

Activity B DOSAGE CALCULATION

1. A client with an acute bacterial UTI has been prescribed 50 mg of nitrofurantoin to be administered four times a day. Macrodantin 50-mg capsules are dispensed to the client. How many capsules should the client take for each dose?

   _____

   _____

2. A client with acute cystitis has been prescribed a single 6 g dose of fosfomycin to be taken with food. The drug is available in 3-g powder packets. How many packets should the client prepare for her dose?

   _____

   _____

3. A client is seen in an urgent care facility for lower abdominal pain and has been prescribed phenazopyridine 200 mg orally three times a day for bladder irritation. The drug is available in 200-mg tablets and the treatment is only to be used for 2 days. How many tablets should the pharmacy at the clinic dispense to the client?

_____

_____

4. A client in a long-term care facility has been prescribed nitrofurantoin for an acute bacterial UTI. The primary health care provider (PHCP) has prescribed 50 mg of the drug to be taken four times a day. The drug is available in an oral suspension, nitrofurantoin 25 mg/5 mL. How many mL should the nurse administer to the client in each dose?

_____

_____

Activity C MATCHING

Match the urinary drugs in Column A with their uses in Column B.

Column A

____ 1. Amoxicillin

____ 2. Nitrofurantoin

____ 3. Phenazopyridine

Column B

a. Chronic bacterial UTIs

b. Acute bacterial UTIs

c. Bladder analgesic

Activity D SHORT ANSWERS

A nurse's role in managing clients who are being administered urinary tract anti-infectives, antispasmodics, and other urinary drugs involves monitoring the clients and implementing interventions that aid in their recovery. Answer the following questions, which involve the nurse's role in the management of such situations.

1. A nurse is to instruct a group of new mothers about infant care. The nurse tells the group that *Escherichia coli* from the bowel is a bacterium that causes UTIs. One young mother asks, "If both baby girls and boys poop, why would little girls be more likely to get bacterial infections?" How should the nurse respond to this question?

_____

_____

2. The young mother wants to know what steps she can take to prevent UTI in her baby daughter. What instructions should the nurse offer the client as UTI prevention strategies for the newborn?

_____

_____

Activity E LABELING

Label the different parts of the genitourinary system.

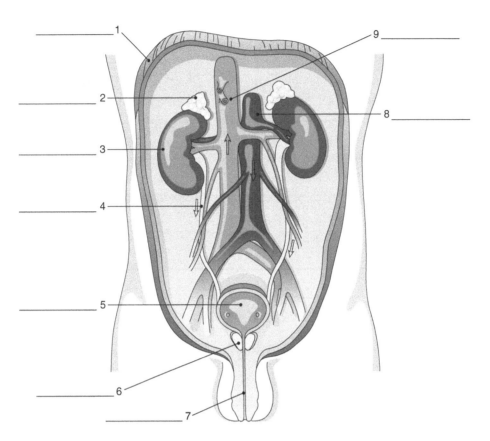

1 _____

2 _____

3 _____

4 _____

5 _____

6 _____

7 _____

9 _____

8 _____

SECTION II: APPLYING YOUR KNOWLEDGE

Activity F CASE STUDY

Janna Wong presents to the PHCP's office with complaints of dysuria, oliguria, and increased frequency. After examining Janna and interpreting her urinalysis, the PHCP diagnoses her with a UTI. The PHCP gives her a prescription for nitrofurantoin (Macrobid) 50 mg × 7 days.

1. Prior to leaving the office, what adverse reactions should the nurse discuss with Janna?

    _____

    _____

    _____

2. What age-specific nonpharmacologic measures should the nurse discuss with Janna?

    _____

    _____

Now Map It Out! Use the templates provided in the appendix to add information and make client connections on a concept map.

Janna Wong has been treated for a number of issues in both the textbook and in the study guide. As you add her UTI and medication to her map, check to see if there are any drug—drug interactions you would be concerned with at this time.

SECTION III: PRACTICING FOR NCLEX

Activity G NCLEX-STYLE QUESTIONS

Answer the following questions.

1. If the anti-infectives used for UTIs have little value with systemic infections, why are they used to treat UTIs?
    1. Inexpensive compared to other drugs.
    2. Action occurs in the urine.
    3. Metabolism is different.
    4. Bladder cannot absorb them.

2. A nurse is caring for a client receiving nitrofurantoin drug therapy for the treatment of a bladder infection. What adverse reaction to the drug should the nurse monitor for in the client?
    1. Pulmonary reaction
    2. Jaundice
    3. Cardiac damage
    4. Renal impairment

3. A client with an acute bacterial urinary tract infection is undergoing sulfamethoxazole drug therapy. The client is also receiving an oral anticoagulant as a blood thinner. What condition should the nurse monitor for in this client as a result of the interaction of the two drugs?
    1. Increased risk of bleeding
    2. Urinary tract excretion of the anti-infective
    3. Delay in gastric emptying
    4. Decreased effect of sulfamethoxazole

4. A nurse is caring for a client who has been prescribed a urinary anti-infective. What interventions should the nurse perform when administering the drug to decrease the pain experienced by the client on voiding?
    1. Administer the drug strictly with milk.
    2. Administer the drug after meals.
    3. Administer the drug with cranberry juice.
    4. Ensure drug administration with warm water.

5. A nurse is caring for a client receiving a phenazopyridine drug for the treatment of irritation of the lower genitourinary tract. The client is also receiving an antibacterial drug for UTI. What consideration should the nurse note when administering phenazopyridine in combination with an antibacterial drug?
    1. Encourage client to drink at least 2000 mL of fluid daily.
    2. Administer the drug with cranberry or prune juice.
    3. Limit administering phenazopyridine to no more than 2 days.
    4. Administer phenazopyridine 2 hours before giving the antibacterial drug.

6. A nurse is caring for a client receiving a nitrofurantoin urinary tract anti-infective at a long-term care facility. What nursing intervention should the nurse perform to prevent irritation in the stomach?
    1. Administer the drug with apple juice.
    2. Administer the drug with milk.
    3. Administer the drug at bedtime.
    4. Administer the drug 1 hour before meals.

7. A nurse is caring for a client who has been prescribed a urinary tract anti-infective for the treatment of UTI. What preadministration assessments should the nurse perform when caring for the client? **Select all that apply.**
    1. Question the client regarding symptoms of infection.
    2. Assess the client for urinary frequency and bladder distention.
    3. Take and record the vital signs of the client.
    4. Constantly monitor the client's body temperature.
    5. Assist in performing a repeat urinalysis and culture test.

8. Which of the following drugs used to treat UTIs is not from the antibiotic or sulfonamide classes of anti-infective medications?
    1. Amoxicillin
    2. Fluoroquinolones
    3. Nitrofurantoin
    4. Trimethoprim

9. Which of the following exerts a topical analgesic effect on the lining of the urinary tract?
   1. Phenazopyridine
   2. Flavoxate
   3. Amoxicillin
   4. Methenamine

10. The use of nitrofurantoin has been known to cause acute and chronic reactions in which of the following systems?
    1. Cardiovascular
    2. Digestive
    3. Respiratory
    4. Nervous

11. Cranberry juice is used to reduce UTIs. What other benefit does this herbal product have?
    1. Prevents dental plaque
    2. Stops rheumatoid arthritis flares
    3. Reduces depression
    4. Diminishes asthma symptoms

12. It is important for the nurse to obtain an allergy history before administering an anti-infective because clients who are allergic to tartrazine should not take which of the following?
    1. Amoxicillin
    2. Methenamine
    3. Ciprofloxacin
    4. Nitrofurantoin

Drugs that Affect the Immune System

47

Vaccines

- Discuss humoral immunity and cell-mediated immunity.
- Compare and contrast the different types of immunity.
- Explain the use of vaccines, toxoids, immune globulins, and antivenins to provide immunity against disease.
- Distinguish preadministration and ongoing assessments the nurse should perform with the client receiving an immunologic agent.
- Identify nursing diagnoses particular to a client receiving an immunologic agent.
- Examine ways to promote an optimal response, management of common adverse reactions, special considerations, and important points to keep in mind when educating a client taking an immunologic agent.

SECTION I: ASSESSING YOUR UNDERSTANDING

Activity A FILL IN THE BLANKS

1. When salicylates are administered with varicella vaccine, there is an increased risk of developing _____ syndrome.

2. _____ acquired active immunity occurs when an individual is given a weakened antigen, which stimulates the formation of antibodies.

3. _____ injection is administered as an additional dose of vaccine to enhance the production of antibodies so that the desired level of immunity is maintained.

4. _____ refers to the ability of the body to identify and resist microorganisms that are potentially harmful.

5. _____-mediated immunity depends on the actions of the T lymphocytes.

Activity B DOSAGE CALCULATION

1. A primary health care provider prescribes an immunizing dose of 0.5 mL of meningococcal vaccine to a client as part of a routine immunization program. After reconstitution, the solution becomes 0.8 mL. What amount of reconstituted solution is left in the vial after injecting the prescribed dose to the client?

   _____

   _____

2. A single vial of Pneumovax 23 contains 3 mL of the vaccine solution. The nurse administers 0.5 mL of the solution subcutaneously to each client. How many clients can be vaccinated using a single vial?

   _____

   _____

3. The diluent needed for a single dose of *Haemophilus influenzae* vaccine is 0.6 mL. How many mL of diluent is necessary to prepare five doses of *H. influenzae* vaccine?

   _____

   _____

4. A nurse has been asked to reconstitute a hepatitis B vaccine solution. The diluent supplied is 1 mL, and when mixed with the vaccine powder the solution is increased by 50%. How many mL of the reconstituted solution is in the prescribed dose?

———————————————————————

———————————————————————

5. A primary health care provider prescribes 0.5 mL of a single-dose poliovirus vaccine for each client to be given IM. The available vaccine solution after reconstitution is 4 mL. How many injections can be given from the vial?

———————————————————————

———————————————————————

Activity C MATCHING

Match the terms associated with immunity in Column A with their definitions in Column B.

Column A

____ **1.** Active immunity

____ **2.** Passive immunity

____ **3.** Toxin

____ **4.** Vaccine

____ **5.** Globulins

Column B

a. Injection of ready-made antibodies

b. Attenuated or killed antigen

c. Protein present in blood serum or plasma

d. Poisonous substance produced by some bacteria

e. Use of agents to stimulate antibody formation

Activity D SHORT ANSWERS

A nurse's role in managing clients receiving an immunologic agent involves diagnosis, planning, and implementation. Answer the following questions, which involve the nurse's role in the management of such cases.

1. Access the following website: http://www2a.cdc.gov/nip/adultimmsched/.

Take the quiz and determine if you have the recommended immunizations. Compare your answers with fellow students.

———————————————————————

———————————————————————

2. How do the recommendations differ if you take the quiz as a non–health care student or if you add information about overseas travel?

———————————————————————

———————————————————————

Activity E SUDOKU PUZZLE

Familiarize yourself with immunization abbreviations.

HEP B	DTaP		CMI					IGIV
IGIV	MMR	CDC	IPV	DTaP			CMI	FLU
IgA	IPV		HEP B				CDC	
CDC		DTaP				MMR	HEP B	
CMI				IgA	HEP B	IGIV		CDC
	HEP B		IGIV	CDC	DTaP	CMI	FLU	
	CDC	IGIV	DTaP	HEP B				
	CMI		IgA		IGIV	CDC	MMR	
	IgA				CMI	IPV		HEP B

SECTION II: APPLYING YOUR KNOWLEDGE

Activity F CASE STUDY

Jimmy Peterson is a 4-month-old boy. He is at the clinic with his mother; she hurried out of the house and forgot to bring Jimmy's immunization book to the well-child visit.

1. According to the recommended schedule of immunization, which ones are due for Jimmy at this clinic visit?

_____

_____

2. Betty Peterson is at home and found the immunization book. When called she notes that Jimmy missed the second Hep B and Hib injections. Which of any of these can be "caught up" this month?

_____

_____

Now Map It Out! Use the templates provided in the appendix to add information and make client connections on a concept map.

Passive immunity can be obtained by a series of injections and exposure to the antigen. Using the concept map for Janna Wong, can you identify a medical problem that would benefit from passive immunity?

SECTION III: PRACTICING FOR NCLEX

Activity G NCLEX-STYLE QUESTIONS

Answer the following questions.

1. A group of student nurses is studying immunity principles. Which type of immunity protects the body from bacterial and viral infections?
   1. Cell-mediated
   2. Passive
   3. Humoral
   4. Active

2. Which of the following is the best description of a vaccine?
   1. A molecule that binds with protein
   2. Weakened or killed antigen
   3. Immune response of the body
   4. Resistance to infection

3. When educating clients on immunologic agents, the nurse identifies which of the following white blood cells that plays a major role in maintaining humoral immunity?
   1. Neutrophil
   2. Eosinophil
   3. Lymphocyte
   4. Basophil

4. When educating nursing students about vaccines, the nurse explains that in which of the following cases can vaccines be administered to humans? **Select all that apply.**
   1. Routine immunization of infants and children
   2. Adults at high risk for certain diseases
   3. Immunization of pregnant women against rubella
   4. Immunization of adults against tetanus
   5. Immunization of children and adults with leukemia

5. A client was rushed to the hospital following a rattlesnake bite. The nurse assesses the time of the bite before injecting the antivenin. Antivenin injections should be administered within which of the following time periods to yield the most effective response?
   1. Within 24 hours
   2. Within 12 hours
   3. Within 4 hours
   4. Within 1 hour

6. A nurse is caring for a client with chickenpox. Which of the following is a late complication of the chickenpox virus?
   1. Reye syndrome
   2. Acute renal failure
   3. Herpes zoster
   4. Hepatitis

7. When educating a group of nursing students on vaccines, the nurse identifies which of the following conditions may vaccines be administered with caution rather than contraindicated?
   1. Lactation
   2. Lymphoma
   3. Nonlocalized cancer
   4. Leukemia

8. Cell-mediated immunity depends on which of the following?
   1. The action of B lymphocytes
   2. Antigen–antibody response
   3. The action of T lymphocytes
   4. Globulin production

9. Which of the following is responsible for a delayed-type immune response?
   1. B lymphocytes
   2. Macrophages
   3. Antibodies
   4. T lymphocytes

CHAPTER 47 VACCINES 255

10. The administration of immunizations to a client is a form of what type of immunity?

1. Artificial active immunity
2. Naturally active immunity
3. Passive active immunity
4. Attenuated active immunity

11. The administration of immune globulins or antivenins to a client is a form of what type of immunity?

1. Artificial immunity
2. Natural immunity
3. Passive immunity
4. Attenuated immunity

12. The nurse must administer which of the following to a client prior to exposure to the disease-causing organism in order for the client to be protected against the disease?

1. Toxoids
2. Immune globulins
3. Antivenins
4. Antibodies

CHAPTER 48

Immunostimulants and Immunomodulators

Learning Objectives

- Describe how immunity-related cells communicate to each other in the body.
- Explain how interferons are used to treat multiple sclerosis.
- Describe the function of the different types of blood cells.
- List the drugs used in the treatment of anemia and bleeding and prevention of infection.
- Explain the actions, uses, general adverse reactions, contraindications, precautions, and interactions of the agents used in the treatment of anemia and bleeding and prevention of infection.
- Distinguish important preadministration and ongoing assessment activities the nurse should perform on a client receiving an agent used in the treatment of anemia and bleeding and prevention of infection.
- Identify nursing diagnoses particular to a client receiving an agent used in the treatment of anemia and bleeding and prevention of infection.
- Examine ways to promote an optimal response to therapy and important points to keep in mind when educating clients about the use of an agent used in the treatment of anemia and bleeding and prevention of infection.

SECTION I: ASSESSING YOUR UNDERSTANDING

Activity A FILL IN THE BLANKS

1. _____ are a group of proteins involved in cell-to-cell communication.

2. _____ is the process of making RBCs in the body.

3. _____ is a condition caused by an insufficient amount of hemoglobin delivering oxygen to the tissues.

4. _____ supply our cells with oxygen from the lungs to the tissues.

Activity B DOSAGE CALCULATION

1. A client had chemotherapy yesterday and comes to the outpatient chemotherapy clinic to begin filgrastim injections. The initial dose will be filgrastim 5 mcg/kg, and the client weighs 60 kg. How many mcg will the nurse prepare for the initial dose?

_____

_____

2. Filgrastim is supplied as 300 mcg/1 mL. On the second day of colony-stimulating factor (CSF) treatment, the client is to receive filgrastim 4 mcg/kg and weighs 58 kg. How many mL will be in this injection?

_____

_____

3. The home health nurse is helping a client set up a weekly pill container. The client is prescribed 90 mg of oral Feosol in two equally divided doses per day. Feosol is available as tablets of 45 mg. How many tablets would the client require for a week?

_____

_____

4. A primary health care provider (PHCP) prescribes 6000 units of epoetin alfa per day for a client with chronic renal failure–associated anemia. Epoetin alfa is supplied in vials of 3000 units/1 mL. How many mL of epoetin alfa solution will the nurse have to administer to the client per day?

_____

_____

5. A PHCP prescribes 135 mcg of peginterferon alfa per day for a client with chronic hepatitis. Peginterferon alfa is supplied in vials of 180 mcg/1 mL. How many mL of peginterferon alfa solution will the nurse have to administer to the client per injection?

_____

_____

Activity C MATCHING

1. Match the types of anemia in Column A with their corresponding descriptions in Column B.

Column A

____ **1.** Iron deficiency anemia

____ **2.** Anemia in chronic renal failure

____ **3.** Pernicious anemia

____ **4.** Folic acid deficiency anemia

Column B

a. Anemia occurring because of a dietary lack of folic acid, a component necessary in the formation of RBCs

b. Anemia resulting from lack of secretions by the gastric mucosa of the intrinsic factor essential to the formation of RBCs and the absorption of vitamin B_{12}

c. Anemia resulting from a reduced production of erythropoietin, a hormone secreted by the kidney that stimulates the production of RBCs

d. Anemia characterized by an inadequate amount of iron in the body to produce hemoglobin

2. Match the drugs in Column A with their corresponding treatment uses in Column B.

Column A

____ **1.** Filgrastim

____ **2.** Darbepoetin alfa

____ **3.** Oprelvekin

____ **4.** Feosol

Column B

a. Iron deficiency anemia

b. Thrombocytopenia

c. Chronic anemia

d. Neutropenia

Activity D SHORT ANSWERS

A nurse's role in managing clients who are being administered drugs for the treatment of iron deficiency anemia involves monitoring them and implementing interventions that aid in their recovery. Answer the following questions, which involve the nurse's role in the management of such situations.

1. A client with iron deficiency anemia has been recommended a ferrous (iron) tablet. What should a nurse assess for in the client before administering the first dose of ferrous tablets?

_____

_____

2. A client is administered ferric (iron) tablets for the treatment of iron deficiency anemia. The nurse is to counsel the client regarding dietary choices to improve the iron content of their diet. What foods will increase iron intake?

_____

_____

Activity E WORD FIND PUZZLE

Find the eight types of cells that are produced in the blood and lymph systems.

K	A	D	M	L	Y	M	P	H	O	C	Y	T	E
B	G	F	H	B	N	L	Q	Y	S	W	D	T	O
P	N	S	W	N	A	R	H	Z	A	L	Y	F	S
E	D	L	K	T	E	D	B	G	K	C	J	G	I
F	K	M	E	Q	D	U	P	J	O	R	J	B	N
T	B	L	V	Y	F	M	T	Y	D	F	N	A	O
A	E	J	A	H	K	L	R	R	Q	Y	H	S	P
T	K	Q	G	P	R	A	N	K	O	B	L	O	H
L	P	R	Z	J	K	D	S	V	W	P	Q	P	I
M	W	S	D	A	K	B	F	G	U	A	H	H	L
V	Y	N	G	L	Q	H	J	M	L	G	K	I	M
C	R	E	D	B	L	O	O	D	C	E	L	L	L
R	M	O	N	O	C	Y	T	E	J	S	B	Q	G

SECTION II: APPLYING YOUR KNOWLEDGE

Activity F CASE STUDY

 Antonia Lopez is a cousin of Alfredo Garcia; she is aged 43 years. Mrs. Lopez was recently diagnosed with cancer and she has started chemotherapy. As the nurse, you have called to tell her she will be receiving filgrastim (Neupogen) to treat neutropenia during chemotherapy.

1. Mrs. Lopez is concerned about coming in for more treatments. How would you explain this segment of her therapy?

   _____

   _____

   _____

2. The nurse should obtain a thorough medical history prior to the administration of filgrastim (Neupogen) as it should be used cautiously in clients with what medical conditions?

   _____

   _____

   _____

SECTION III: PRACTICING FOR NCLEX

Activity G NCLEX-STYLE QUESTIONS

Answer the following questions.

1. A client with chronic pancreatitis has severe folic acid deficiency (megaloblastic) anemia and is administered a folic acid injection. What adverse reactions should the nurse monitor for in this client?
   1. Anorexia
   2. Allergic hypersensitivity
   3. Arthralgia
   4. Adrenal hyperplasia

2. Which of the following anemias must be treated parenterally due to the lack of ability to absorb vitamins in the gut?
   1. Folic acid deficiency
   2. Iron deficiency
   3. Vitamin B_{12} deficiency
   4. Platelet deficiency

3. A nurse is caring for a client with Parkinson disease who will start iron supplements. The nurse checks the EHR to see if they are taking methyldopa. Which of the following conditions should the nurse monitor for in the client as a result of the interaction between the two drugs once the iron drug regimen begins?
   1. Decreased blood pressure
   2. Increased heart rate
   3. Increased Parkinson symptoms
   4. Increased absorption of iron

4. A nurse is teaching a nutrition class, and a question is asked about who may have vitamin B_{12} deficiency since it is associated with intrinsic factor. Which of the following people need to supplement their diets to fulfill their nutritional needs and prevent a deficiency of vitamin B_{12}?
   1. Heavy smokers
   2. Pregnant women
   3. Those with a strict vegan lifestyle
   4. Chronic alcoholics

5. A client receiving ferrous tablets for the treatment of anemia is to be discharged shortly. What should the nurse include in the client teaching plan when providing care on an outpatient basis?
   1. May take with antacids
   2. May take with meals if you have GI upset
   3. Drink the liquid iron preparation out of a glass
   4. Take with an iron-fortified multivitamin

6. A nurse is caring for a client receiving CSFs for the treatment of neutropenia. Which of the following adverse reactions should the nurse monitor for when caring for the client? **Select all that apply.**
   1. Bone pain
   2. Hypertension
   3. Insomnia
   4. Skin rash
   5. Nausea

7. What information should the nurse offer the client regarding adverse reactions to oral iron supplements?
   1. The color of the stools will be black.
   2. Expect an increase in palpitations.
   3. Weight will increase.
   4. A rash may develop.

8. A nurse is caring for a client receiving iron supplements. Which of the following foods should the client avoid consuming when taking the supplement as it would interfere with the absorption of iron?
   1. Milk
   2. Poultry
   3. Meat
   4. Fish

9. Which of the following types of cells supply our body with oxygen from the lungs?
   1. Leukocytes
   2. Megakaryocytes
   3. Erythrocytes
   4. Neutrophils

10. Which of the following types of cells fragment and become particles that control the bleeding from microscopic to major tears in our tissues?
    1. Megakaryocytes
    2. Erythrocytes
    3. Leukocytes
    4. Neutrophils

11. For which of the following issues is a client at the highest risk for, if they become neutropenic as a result of antineoplastic therapy?
    1. Vomiting
    2. GI bleeding
    3. Venous thromboembolism
    4. Infection

12. Anemia can result in which of the following?
    1. Increased platelet production
    2. Decreased neutrophil production
    3. Decreased platelet production
    4. Increased neutrophil production

13. The process by which the body is stimulated to make more of a specific type of blood cell is known as which of the following?
    1. Hematopoiesis
    2. Metabolism
    3. Neogenesis
    4. Regeneration

CHAPTER 49

Immune Blockers

Learning Objectives

On completion of this chapter, the student will:

- List the classes of immune blockers used in the immunosuppressive treatment of diseases.
- Explain the uses, general drug actions, general adverse reactions, contraindications, precautions, and interactions of the immune blocker drugs.
- Distinguish important preadministration and ongoing assessment activities the nurse should perform with the client receiving immune blocker drugs.
- List nursing diagnoses particular to a client receiving immunotherapy drugs.
- Examine ways to promote an optimal response to therapy, how to manage common adverse reactions, and important points to keep in mind when educating clients about the use of an immune blocker drug.

SECTION I: ASSESSING YOUR UNDERSTANDING

Activity A FILL IN THE BLANKS

1. _____ immunity involves the lymphatic system and the T lymphocytes (T cells).

2. Humoral immunity involves _____ creation.

3. Passive immunity requires _____ dosing.

4. _____ drugs are used to treat autoimmune diseases and reduce organ rejection in transplant clients.

5. Drugs ending in _____ are derived from mouse tissue and have the highest risk for hypersensitive reaction.

Activity B DOSAGE CALCULATION

1. A client with asthma has been prescribed dupilumab for self-injection at home. The drug is available in 300 mg/2 mL single dose prefilled pens. If the client is to self-administer the drug every 2 weeks, how many syringes are needed to fill the prescription on a monthly basis?

   _____

   _____

2. A client who is 1 day posttransplant is weighed; the scale reads 156.5 pounds. How many kilograms does this client weigh?

   _____

   _____

3. On Day 1 posttransplant, the above client is to receive belatacept by IV infusion. The drug is dosed 10 mg/kg of body weight. How many milligrams of belatacept will be in the IV infusion?

   _____

   _____

4. A client with MS has been prescribed monomethyl fumarate (Bafiertam). The PHCP orders 95 mg orally BID. The drug is available in 95 mg delayed-release capsules. How many capsules should the client self-administer per dose?

   _____

   _____

5. If a client taking Bafiertam 95 mg orally BID is to travel for 14 days, how many capsules do they need to have on hand so as to not miss a dose?

_____

_____

1. Match the type of T cell in Column A with their corresponding actions in Column B.

Column A

_____ **1.** Helper T cells

_____ **2.** Cytotoxic T cells

_____ **3.** Memory T cells

_____ **4.** Natural killer cells

_____ **5.** Suppressor T cells

Column B

a. Suppresses the immune response once the threat is gone

b. Attack cells directly by altering the cell membrane and causing cell lysis (destruction)

c. Will recognize previous contact with antigens and activate an immune response

d. Coordinates the immune response and increase B-lymphocyte antibody production

e. Recognizes specific antigens, then attack and kill the cell

Activity D SHORT ANSWERS

A nurse's role in managing clients who have been administered monoclonal antibodies (mAbs) for the treatment of multiple sclerosis involves monitoring them and implementing interventions that aid in their recovery. Answer the following questions, which involve the nurse's role in the management of such situations.

1. A client has a friend who received mAb treatment for cancer. They said that person had a really bad reaction to the treatment. The friend's treatment involved a chimeric drug, whereas your client will receive an mAb made strictly from human tissue. How can you explain the differences in reactions experienced?

_____

_____

2. What is the nurse's role in monitoring for hypersensitive reactions during mAb infusions?

_____

_____

Activity E EXPLAIN THE DRUG NAME

Using the information in Box 49.1 of the textbook, determine the tissue used to make the following monoclonal antibodies:

1. Dupilumab

2. Eptinezumab

3. Adalimumab

4. Infliximab

5. Rituximab

SECTION II: APPLYING YOUR KNOWLEDGE

Activity F CASE STUDY

Mr. Park, like many lay persons, sees drug therapy advertised on television. Why do you think drug companies are advertising drugs like immunotherapy on TV? What is the benefit to the pharmaceutical company?

SECTION III: PRACTICING FOR NCLEX

Activity G NCLEX-STYLE QUESTIONS

Answer the following questions.

1. Which body system is suppressed to prevent organ rejection following an organ transplant?
   1. Cardiovascular
   2. Gastrointestinal
   3. Immune
   4. Respiratory

2. A nurse is asking assessment questions to a client receiving mAbs for the first time. Which of the following historical question(s) are important to ask? **Select all that apply.**

1. "Have you been to a cardiologist recently?"
2. "How many children have you had?"
3. "Have you traveled to a country requiring immunization?"
4. "Have you ever had viral hepatitis?"

3. A client receiving immunotherapy is complaining of an itchy back rash. Which of the following is the best explanation of for this adverse reaction?

1. Reaction of drug to food being consumed
2. Soap must have too much perfume in it
3. A sun reaction
4. Inflammatory response to the therapy

4. A client in the ambulatory clinic is scheduled for a drug that is likely to cause an infusion reaction. Which of the following drugs are used as a premedication regime intended to reduce the reaction?

1. Acetaminophen and diphenhydramine
2. Corticosteroids and diphenhydramine
3. Meperidine and corticosteroids
4. Acetaminophen and meperidine

5. A client has been prescribed glatiramer for self-administration. Which of the following points should the nurse include in the teaching program?

1. Monitoring for bone marrow suppression will be done weekly.
2. Do not put sunscreen on if you develop a skin reaction.
3. Do not substitute 2 of the 20 mg drug for the 40 mg drug.
4. Flush the toilet frequently to prevent cross contamination.

6. A drug that works by passive immunity needs to be which of the following?

1. Given only by injection
2. Be administered repeatedly for protection
3. Administered multiple times daily for effectiveness
4. Taken for at least a year for immunity to work

7. As the nurse is interviewing a client new to the clinic, they state "I'm too tired to get up and do anything." Which is the best statement to make at this time?

1. "That's okay, you have plenty of time later."
2. "Fatigue requires that you rest more."
3. "Try a short walk, a balance of rest and activity helps."
4. "Cold or salty foods will give you energy."

8. Proteins which help the immune system identify foreign antigens is called?

1. An autoimmune condition
2. A T-cell lymphocyte
3. An antibody
4. A monoclonal antibody

9. Which of the actions occur with immunosuppressive drugs? **Select all that apply.**

1. Inhibit the inflammatory response
2. Inhibit B-cell activity
3. Inhibit T-cell activation
4. Reduce antibody formation

10. Flu-like symptoms (an adverse reaction to monoclonal antibody administration) are characterized by the following symptoms?

1. Chills, fever, headache
2. Malaise, diarrhea, muscle pains
3. Infusion pain, edema, cough
4. Nausea, sore throat, reduced appetite

11. A generalized immune response can result from immunotherapy. Which class of drugs is typically given to diminish this response?

1. Steroids
2. Pain relievers
3. Antihistamines
4. Antivirals

12. Biosimilar drugs have an additional four-digit suffix to indicate the difference from a biologic drug. How is this suffix generated?

1. Based on tissue of origin
2. Randomly
3. Selected by manufacturer
4. Disease treating specificity

Drugs That Fight Cancer

Traditional Chemotherapy

- List the types of drugs used in the treatment of neoplastic diseases.
- Explain the uses, general drug actions, general adverse reactions, contraindications, precautions, and interactions of the traditional chemotherapy drugs.
- Distinguish important preadministration and ongoing assessment activities the nurse should perform with the client taking traditional chemotherapy drugs.
- List nursing diagnoses particular to a client taking traditional chemotherapy drugs.
- Examine ways to promote an optimal response to therapy, how to manage common adverse reactions, and important points to keep in mind when educating clients about the use of an traditional chemotherapy drug.

SECTION I: ASSESSING YOUR UNDERSTANDING

Activity A FILL IN THE BLANKS

1. The term _____ typically refers to therapy with antineoplastic drugs.

2. Decreased production of new cells by the bone marrow is called _____.

3. Clients with _____ have a decreased resistance to infection.

4. When cancer spreads from the primary tumor to other areas of the body, this is termed as _____.

5. _____ drugs are given with traditional chemotherapy to protect certain normal tissue or body organs.

Activity B SEQUENCING

Write the correct sequence of the phases of the cell cycle in the boxes provided.

1. Actual splitting into two cells—mitotic phase

2. Dormant or resting phase

3. Preparation for cell division phase

4. RNA and protein-building phase

5. DNA synthesis phase

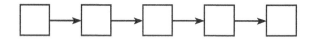

Activity C MATCHING

1. Match the terms in Column A with their corresponding meaning in Column B.

Column A	Column B
____ **1.** Alopecia	**a.** Relief of symptoms
____ **2.** Metastasis	**b.** Loss of hair
____ **3.** Palliation	**c.** Capable of soft-tissue necrosis
____ **4.** Vesicant	**d.** Inflammation of the mouth
____ **5.** Stomatitis	**e.** Spread of cancer to other sites

2. Match the equipment items in Column A with their corresponding protective use in Column B.

Column A	Column B
____ **1.** Gloves	**a.** Reduce spillage onto clothing
____ **2.** Gowns	**b.** Prevent inhalation of drug particles
____ **3.** Goggles	**c.** Prevent absorption by the skin
____ **4.** Masks	**d.** Reduce splashes to eyes

Activity D SHORT ANSWERS

A nurse's role in managing clients undergoing traditional chemotherapy involves not just the treatment or the cause for treatment but also managing the effects produced by a particular adverse reaction due to the treatment. Answer the following questions, which involve the nurse's role in caring for a client undergoing traditional chemotherapy.

1. A nurse is caring for a male client who will begin oral chemotherapy. What are important concepts to teach to prevent exposure to others as the chemotherapy is eliminated from the body?

_____

_____

2. A client living in a small rural town is to start chemotherapy in a large health care facility a number of miles from home. When asked why this is happening, how should the nurse explain the need to go to a different facility to receive chemotherapeutic drugs?

_____

_____

Activity E CROSSWORD PUZZLE

Chemotherapeutic Drug Activity

Across

1. This class of drugs delays or inhibits cell division and blocks the reproductive ability of malignant cells

4. An alkaloid agent that interferes with amino acid production in the S phase

5. What antimetabolite drugs do to RNA and DNA synthesis

Down

2. These agents manipulate the body's ability to recognize and fight the cancer cells

3. The alkylating agents change the cell environment from acid to this, which in turn damages the cell

SECTION II: APPLYING YOUR KNOWLEDGE

Activity F CASE STUDY

Antonia Lopez is a cousin of Alfredo Garcia; she is aged 43 years. Mrs. Lopez was recently diagnosed with cancer and the chemotherapy she will receive includes vincristine.

1. What class of traditional chemotherapy is vincristine in and what is its mechanism of action?

_____

_____

2. Following the administration of vincristine to Mrs. Lopez, what are the specific recommendations for the client to maintain good oral hygiene and reduce the symptoms associated with oral stomatitis?

_____

_____

SECTION III: PRACTICING FOR NCLEX

Activity G **NCLEX-STYLE QUESTIONS**

Answer the following questions.

1. A nurse is caring for a client who has been receiving chemotherapy for breast cancer. The client wants to know why chemotherapy is administered in a series of cycles. Which of the following should the nurse tell the client? **Select all that apply.**

   1. To allow for recovery of the normal cells

   2. To release antioxidants into the system

   3. To release polyphenols and flavonoids

   4. To destroy more of the malignant cells

   5. To minimize damage to normal cells that rapidly divide

2. A nurse is caring for a client with cancer. The client asks the nurse if drinking green tea will be beneficial. Which of the following adverse effects can occur from drinking green tea? **Select all that apply.**

   1. Nervousness

   2. Insomnia

   3. Antioxidation

   4. GI upset

   5. Restlessness

3. The nurse is caring for a client with cancer. The client is prescribed an antimetabolite drug. The client asks the nurse to explain the action of the drug. Which of the following is the action of an antimetabolite?

   1. Changes the cell to a more alkaline environment

   2. Incorporates into the cellular components at a specific phase

   3. Interferes with protein production

   4. Interferes with any phase of cell reproduction

4. A nurse is assigned to care for an older client who is receiving a traditional chemotherapy drug. Which of the following factors should be a priority for the nurse preparing a nursing care plan for the ongoing assessment of the client?

   1. Guidelines established by the health care facility

   2. The client's general condition

   3. The cancer cell type

   4. The adequacy of health insurance coverage

5. A nurse is caring for a client with diabetes who also has cancer and is to be administered an insulin injection subcutaneously. Which of the following is applicable to the subcutaneous administration of a drug?

   1. The injection should contain no more than 1 mL.

   2. Use an Angiocath for administration.

   3. Use the Z-track method for administration.

   4. The injection should contain only 3 mL.

6. A nurse is caring for a client receiving traditional chemotherapy drugs. The client's dietary requirements are not met due to loss of appetite. Which of the following nursing strategies would best help promote nutrition?

   1. Provide three large meals

   2. Provide food with less salt

   3. Provide small, frequent meals

   4. Provide food rich in fats

7. A nurse is caring for a client who is experiencing anxiety after being diagnosed with cancer. What is the nurse's role when caring for this client?

   1. Assist in making critical decisions regarding treatment

   2. Emphasize safety requirements for chemotherapy

   3. Plan and institute therapy to control the disease

   4. Offer consistent and empathetic support to the client and family

8. A nurse is caring for a client who was prescribed traditional chemotherapy drugs in oral form to take at home. Which of the following should the nurse include in the teaching plan for the client and family?
   1. Take the drug as needed.
   2. Take the drug as directed on the prescription.
   3. There is no need to inform the dentist of the therapy.
   4. Decrease the dose as the symptoms of illness decrease.

9. The part of cell growth that entails RNA and protein synthesis preparing for division is known as which of the following?
   1. G_1 phase
   2. S phase
   3. G_2 phase
   4. M phase

10. Which of the following herbal products has the benefits of overall sense of well-being, cancer prevention, dental health, and maintenance of heart and liver health as a result of being loaded with antioxidants?
    1. Licorice
    2. Kava
    3. Ma huang
    4. Green tea

11. Which of the following is an example of an traditional chemotherapy drug that interferes with amino acid production in the S phase and the formation of microtubules in the M phase?
    1. Etoposide
    2. Vinblastine
    3. Teniposide
    4. Irinotecan

12. Which of the following classes of traditional chemotherapy drugs stop cells in the S and G_2 phase, thereby causing cell division to cease?
    1. Podophyllotoxins
    2. Taxanes
    3. Vinca alkaloids
    4. Camptothecin analogs

Immune Modulating Therapies

SECTION I: ASSESSING YOUR UNDERSTANDING

Activity A FILL IN THE BLANKS

1. _____ immunity is pathogen specific and creates memory to the pathogen.

2. The ability to grow blood vessels is called _____.

3. _____ means poisonous to living cells.

4. Unique _____ on the surface of cells are called antigens.

5. The purpose of _____ system is to protect from foreign bodies and abnormal cells.

Activity B SEQUENCING

The process of adaptive immunity is outlined below, write the correct sequence of events in the boxes provided.

1. Prevents the foreign microorganism from making the body ill again

2. Presents the antigen to a B or T lymphocyte

3. Recognizes the foreign antigen

4. Produces memory cells

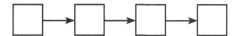

Activity C MATCHING

1. Match the types of cancer immunotherapy drug class in Column A with their corresponding descriptions in Column B.

Column A

____ **1.** Vaccines

____ **2.** Checkpoint inhibitors

____ **3.** Cytokines

____ **4.** Adoptive cell therapy

____ **5.** Monoclonal antibodies

Column B

a. Cells communicate using these proteins

b. Make tumor tissue recognizable to fight the cancer

c. These are produced with human or animal tissue

d. T cells are made to learn what cancer cells are and memorize them

e. A subgroup of monoclonal antibodies, which work inside the cell to stop activity

Activity D SHORT ANSWERS

A nurse's role in managing clients who have been administered immunotherapy drugs for the treatment of cancer involves monitoring them and implementing interventions that aid in their recovery. Answer the following questions, which involve the nurse's role in the management of such situations.

1. A client is having a scan at 10 weeks after beginning immunotherapy for a lung tumor. After seeing the oncologist, they look very sad, when asked they express sadness because the drugs are not working—reviewing the chart, you see the physician suspects pseudoprogression. How would you explain this to the client?

_____

_____

2. Another client mentions they have an "iron gut," nothing ever gives them an upset stomach. What are the concerns when a person does begin to experience gastrointestinal disturbances?

_____

_____

Activity E EXPLAIN THE DRUG NAME

Using the information in Box 51.1 of the textbook, determine the tissue used to make the following monoclonal antibodies:

1. Daratumumab

2. Pertuzumab

3. Trastuzumab

4. Nivolumab

5. Cetuximab

SECTION II: APPLYING YOUR KNOWLEDGE

Activity F CASE STUDY

Mr. Phillip recalls that his wife was started on a drug called Herceptin. During the treatments, they switched her to a drug named Enhertu. He is wondering why this happened. How can you explain the following about these drugs to him?

1. What is the difference between these two drugs?

_____

_____

2. How would you explain biosimilars to Mr. Phillip, check Chapter 49 in the text?

_____

_____

SECTION III: PRACTICING FOR NCLEX

Activity G NCLEX-STYLE QUESTIONS

Answer the following questions.

1. A client will be taking erlotinib at home as part of the immunotherapy treatment plan. What should the nurse include in client teaching?
   1. The drug may be taken at least once daily.
   2. If taken with meals, it may increase a skin rash.
   3. You must not handle the drug with bare hands.
   4. Suggest the client drink at least five glasses of water per day.

2. A nurse has administered a mouse-originated mAb to a client for the first time. Which of the following adverse reactions should the nurse monitor for in the client?
   1. Diarrhea
   2. Fungal infection
   3. Infusion reaction
   4. Acne

3. A client receiving immunotherapy for bowel cancer is complaining of loose stools. Which of the following is the best explanation of for this adverse reaction?
   1. Inflammatory response to the therapy
   2. Advancing tumor in the colon
   3. Microorganisms invading the gut tissue
   4. Reaction of drug to food being consumed

4. A client in the ambulatory clinic is schedule for a drug that is likely to cause an infusion reaction. Which of the following interventions should the nurse perform during the drug administration?
   1. Give drugs individually, not together.
   2. Provide warm blankets before starting the infusion.
   3. Be sure the client's chemo chair is not in direct sunlight.
   4. Instruct the client to eat foods high in pectin after the procedure.

5. A client has been prescribed an oral checkpoint inhibitor. Which of the following points should the nurse include in the teaching program?
   1. Monitoring for bone marrow suppression will be done weekly.
   2. Set an alarm or reminder to take the drug at the same time daily.
   3. Do not put sunscreen on if you develop a skin reaction.
   4. Flush the toilet frequently to prevent cross-contamination.

6. As the nurse is interviewing a client new to the clinic, they state "I'm too tired to get up and do anything." Which is the best statement to make at this time?
   1. "That's okay, you have plenty of time later."
   2. "Fatigue requires that you rest more."
   3. "Try a short walk, a balance of rest and activity helps."
   4. "Cold or salty foods will give you energy."

7. A drug that works by passive immunity is unable to do which of the following?
   1. Targets foreign objects
   2. Be administered repeatedly for protection
   3. Stops the growth of cancer cells
   4. Identify the antigen in the future

8. Tumor-associated antigens can help identify a tumor from a normal cell. How many cancer-specific, tumor-associated antigens have been identified?
   1. 25
   2. 150
   3. 500
   4. 1,200

9. Which of the following immunotherapy agents offer active immunity?
   1. Interferons
   2. Cytokines
   3. Monoclonal antibodies
   4. Cancer vaccines

10. Flu-like symptoms (an adverse reaction to cytokine administration) are characterized by which of the following symptoms?
    1. Chills, fever, headache
    2. Malaise, diarrhea, muscle pains
    3. Infusion pain, edema, cough
    4. Nausea, sore throat, reduced appetite

11. The reason immunotherapy adverse reactions are less than traditional chemotherapy is because:
    1. Traditional chemotherapy is stronger.
    2. Less healthy cells are harmed during therapy.
    3. Smaller doses are typically given.
    4. The drugs are newer than traditional chemotherapy.

12. Which drugs are a subclass of monoclonal antibodies?
    1. Cancer vaccines
    2. Oncoviral therapy
    3. Checkpoint inhibitors
    4. Interferons

Drugs That Affect
Other Body Systems

Skin Disorder Topical Drugs

- List the types of drugs used in the treatment of skin disorders.
- Explain the general drug actions, uses, and reactions to and any contraindications, precautions, and interactions associated with drugs used in treating skin disorders.
- Distinguish important preadministration and ongoing assessment activities the nurse should perform on clients receiving a drug used to treat skin disorders.
- List nursing diagnoses particular to a client using a drug to treat a skin disorder.
- Examine ways to promote an optimal response to therapy and important points to keep in mind when educating the client about a skin disorder.

SECTION I: ASSESSING YOUR UNDERSTANDING

Activity A FILL IN THE BLANKS

1. The prolonged use of topical antibiotic preparations may result in a superficial _____.

2. Topical _____ are drugs used to treat psoriasis.

3. Adverse reactions to topical anti-infectives may include rash, itching, urticaria (hives), or dermatitis, which may indicate a _____ reaction to the drug.

4. A(n) _____ is a drug that stops, slows, or prevents the growth of microorganisms on the skin surface.

5. A _____ drug is bactericidal and used to cleanse skin surfaces.

Activity B DOSAGE CALCULATION

1. A client has been prescribed selenium in a shampoo form for a seborrheic scalp condition. The client is concerned about cost and wants to purchase only enough for the treatment period. If the primary health care provider (PHCP) recommends use for 6 weeks and each bottle lasts 3 weeks, how many bottles should the client purchase?

_____

_____

2. A caregiver is instructed to apply acyclovir ointment to a client's lesion five times per day, for 4 days. How many total applications would the caregiver administer for the entire treatment?

_____

_____

3. A CNA has been taught to apply tolnaftate twice daily for 3 weeks to a client with tinea corporis. How many treatments would the CNA administer for the entire treatment?

_____

_____

4. A client is sent home with a preoperative skin scrub of chlorhexidine. The instructions to the client are to add three parts water to one part solution and wash their leg twice daily for 3 days. If the client uses 6 cups of water, how many cups of chlorhexidine should be added to the solution?

_____

_____

Activity C MATCHING

1. Match the antibiotic drugs in Column A with their uses in Column B.

Column A

____ **1.** Azelaic acid

____ **2.** Bacitracin

____ **3.** Gentamicin

____ **4.** Mupirocin

Column B

a. Relief of primary and secondary skin infections

b. Acne vulgaris, rosacea

c. Impetigo infections caused by *Staphylococcus aureus*

d. To help prevent infections in minor cuts and burns

2. Match the drugs in Column A with their adverse reactions in Column B.

Column A

____ **1.** Butenafine

____ **2.** Calcipotriene

____ **3.** Clotrimazole

____ **4.** Hexachlorophene

Column B

a. Hyperpigmentation

b. Burning, itching, erythema

c. Photosensitivity

d. Contact dermatitis, erythema, irritation

Activity D SHORT ANSWERS

A nurse's role in managing clients who are receiving a topical drug for a skin disorder involves assisting the clients through assessment. Answer the following questions, which involve the nurse's role in the management of clients receiving a topical drug for a skin disorder.

1. At a preadministration assessment, what are the required nursing activities?

_____

_____

_____

2. What are the tasks required as part of the ongoing assessment?

_____

_____

_____

Activity E CROSSWORD PUZZLE

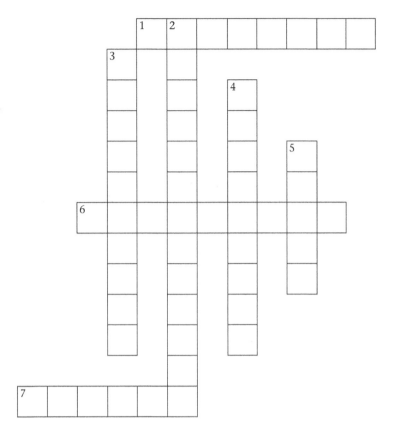

Across

1. Term for ringworm from the *Tinea* family
6. A bactericidal solution
7. Term for jock itch from the *Tinea* family

Down

2. Term for nail fungus
3. A bacteriostatic solution
4. Term for generalized trunk rash from the *Tinea* family
5. Term for athlete's foot from the *Tinea* family

SECTION II: APPLYING YOUR KNOWLEDGE

Activity F CASE STUDY

Janna Wong, a student athlete, presents to the PHCP's office seeking treatment for recurrent athlete's foot. The PHCP prescribes a topical fungal applied to affected areas BID. Janna has no known drug allergies and takes no medications.

1. What are the common adverse reactions seen with the use of an antifungal?

_____

_____

2. Janna says she is reluctant to use the ointment because another student has an infection that got worse instead of better. What might this condition be if an area is over treated with different antifungal and antibiotic preparations?

_____

_____

Now Map It Out! Use the templates provided in the appendix to add information and make client connections on a concept map.

Throughout the textbook and study guide, Janna Wong has been prescribed a number of anti-infectives. Add the above problem and intervention to Janna's concept map and analyze the map for interactions or additive reactions. Does the route of administration make a difference?

SECTION III: PRACTICING FOR NCLEX

Activity G NCLEX-STYLE QUESTIONS

Answer the following questions.

1. A nurse is caring for a client who has been diagnosed with plaque psoriasis. Which of the following topical preparations should always be used with another agent in treating infections?
    1. Antifungals
    2. Antibacterials
    3. Corticosteroids
    4. Germicides

2. A drug ointment is known to have proteolytic properties. Which of the following best describes proteolysis?
    1. Lysis of protozoa
    2. Enzyme action to remove dead tissue
    3. Formation of proteins into complex structures
    4. Bacteriocidal action on bacteria

3. The PHCP has prescribed benzocaine to be administered to a client. In which of the following should the nurse use benzocaine cautiously?
    1. In clients who are pregnant or lactating
    2. In immunocompromised clients with herpes simplex virus (HSV) infections
    3. In clients receiving class I antiarrhythmic drugs such as tocainide
    4. In clients with cutaneous candidiasis or tinea pedis

4. The PHCP has prescribed alclometasone for a client being treated for eczema. Which of the following adverse reactions should be monitored by the nurse with a client using corticosteroids?
    1. Hyperglycemia and glycosuria
    2. Mild and transient pain
    3. Numbness and dermatitis
    4. Flu-like syndrome

5. A client is undergoing treatment for debridement of a chronic dermal ulcer and the PHCP has prescribed collagenase. Which of the following adverse reactions should the nurse be monitoring for with a client administered collagenase?
    1. Flu-like syndrome
    2. Numbness and dermatitis
    3. Cushing syndrome
    4. Hyperglycemia and glycosuria

6. A nurse is caring for a client who has been prescribed salicylic acid for the treatment of a skin wart. Which of the following should the nurse consider an infrequent adverse reaction to salicylic acid?
    1. Mild and transient pains
    2. Temporary discoloration of the hair
    3. Flu-like syndrome
    4. Hyperglycemia and glycosuria

7. A nurse is caring for an infected client with isolation precautions. To avoid transmitting infections, which of the following should the nurse use to wash their own hands before and after caring for the client?
    1. Topical antipsoriatics
    2. Topical antiseptics and germicides
    3. Topical enzymes
    4. Topical antifungals

8. Which of the following might be used topically by a client with acne vulgaris?
    1. Aklief
    2. Ciclopirox
    3. Nystatin
    4. Imiquimod

9. Which of the following might a client use to treat onychomycosis?
   1. Erythromycin
   2. Acyclovir
   3. Terbinafine
   4. Vidarabine

10. Which of the following products will deactivate collagenase?
    1. Soap and water
    2. Vinegar
    3. Povidone–iodine
    4. Corticosteroid cream

11. Which of the following can a nurse recommend to a client for the treatment of HSV that is available without a prescription?
    1. Docosanol (Abreva)
    2. Penciclovir (Denavir)
    3. Acyclovir (Zovirax)
    4. Imiquimod (Aldara)

Otic and Ophthalmic Preparations

■ Explain the general actions, uses, adverse reactions, contraindications, precautions, and interactions of otic and ophthalmic preparations.

■ Distinguish important preadministration and ongoing assessment activities the nurse should perform on a client receiving otic and ophthalmic preparations.

■ List nursing diagnoses particular to a client taking an otic or ophthalmic preparation.

■ Examine ways to promote an optimal response to therapy, how to administer the preparations, and important points to keep in mind when educating clients about the use of otic or ophthalmic preparations.

SECTION I: ASSESSING YOUR UNDERSTANDING

Activity A FILL IN THE BLANKS

1. The term _____ means *auditory* in Latin.

2. The most common middle ear disorder is _____.

3. When hearing loss is suspected, the ear should be examined for excess _____.

4. _____ is a condition of the eye in which there is an increase in ocular pressure, causing progressive atrophy of the optic nerve with deterioration of vision.

5. _____ is the paralysis of the ciliary muscle, resulting in an inability to focus the eye.

Activity B DOSAGE CALCULATION

1. A child has been prescribed an otic preparation of dexamethasone for an inflamed ear. The young mother is confused regarding when to use the drug when the prescription states four times a day. How frequently would the medication be administered if the doses were spread out equally over an entire day?

2. The primary health care provider orders 0.5 mL of ciprofloxacin otic solution for a suspected ear canal infection. If the dropper used delivers 0.1 mL/drop, how many drops of solution should be instilled in the ear for each dose?

3. The primary health care provider recommends using a product to remove cerumen. The client states they already purchased the product to use 4 months ago on the same child. If the directions are to instill five drops for 3 days and the dropper delivers 0.1 mL/drop, is there enough if 5 mL is left in the container?

4. The eye care provider orders 0.5 mL of Flucaine anesthetic solution for each eye before an examination procedure. If the dropper used delivers 0.1 mL/drop, how many drops of solution should be instilled in each eye for each dose?

_____

_____

5. The ocular antibiotic gentamicin comes in a 5-mL container and each drop is 0.5 mL. How many doses are there in the container?

_____

_____

Activity C MATCHING

1. Match the ophthalmic drugs in Column A with their uses in Column B.

Column A

____ **1.** Brimonidine

____ **2.** Diclofenac

____ **3.** Dapiprazole

____ **4.** Ofloxacin

Column B

a. Reverses the diagnostic mydriasis after ophthalmic examination

b. Lowers intraocular pressure (IOP) in clients with open-angle (chronic) glaucoma

c. Treatment of bacterial eye infection

d. Postoperative anti-inflammatory

2. Match the otic drug ingredients in Column A with their uses in Column B.

Column A

____ **1.** DermOtic

____ **2.** Cerumenex

____ **3.** Cetraxal

Column B

a. Wax softening and removal

b. Otitis media

c. External ear eczema

Activity D SHORT ANSWERS

A nurse's role in managing clients who are receiving an otic preparation involves assisting the clients through assessment. Answer the following questions, which involve the nurse's role in the management of clients receiving otic preparations.

1. Before administration of an otic preparation, the primary health care provider examines the ear and external structures surrounding the ear and prescribes the drug indicated to treat the disorder. In the preadministration assessment, the nurse may be responsible for examining which areas of the ear?

_____

_____

2. How should the nurse assess the client's response to otic therapy, and what further examinations should be carried out?

_____

_____

Activity E **LABELING**

Label the different segments of the auditory structures.

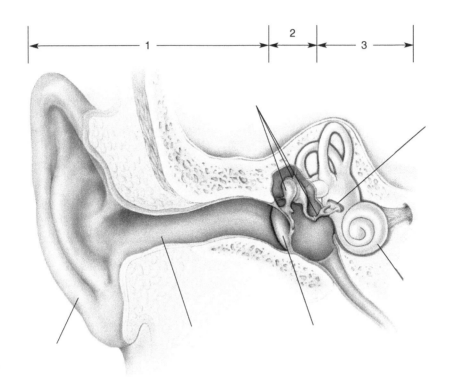

SECTION II: APPLYING YOUR KNOWLEDGE

Activity F **CASE STUDY**

Jimmy Peterson, 4 months old, is at the clinic for a well-child visit and immunizations. The infant has a runny nose and bright red ear lobes. Jimmy reacts and pulls away when the nurse attempts to take a tympanic temperature.

1. What questions should the nurse ask the mother to assess for an ear problem?

_____

_____

2. An otic solution is prescribed for Jimmy's ears. How should the nurse instruct the mother on administration of the solution?

_____

_____

Now Map It Out! Use the templates provided in the appendix to add information and make client connections on a concept map.

Janna Wong says she has been having issues with her eyes lately. She states that she is staying up late at night lately in order to study more. She asks about using the eye product Visine. Using the concept map for Janna, review the medications she is currently taking to identify any potential drug interactions.

SECTION III: PRACTICING FOR NCLEX

Activity G NCLEX-STYLE QUESTIONS

Answer the following questions.

1. A nurse is caring for a client who has been using ofloxacin for a prolonged time. Which of the following are the risks associated with the prolonged use of such otic antibiotics?
   1. Danger of superinfection in the ear
   2. Systemic effects of cholinesterase inhibitors
   3. Exacerbation of existing hypertension
   4. Additive CNS depressant effects

2. The nurse should know that ofloxacin is used with caution in which of the following?
   1. While taking monoamine oxidase inhibitors
   2. During pregnancy and lactation
   3. During activities requiring mental alertness
   4. While performing activities in dimly lit areas

3. A nurse is caring for a client who is to be administered an antibiotic ear solution. Before instilling the otic solution, what should the nurse inform the client?
   1. Local effects such as headache and visual blurring may be felt.
   2. Fatigue and drowsiness may be experienced.
   3. A feeling of fullness may be felt in the ear.
   4. Hearing in the treated ear may temporarily improve.

4. A nurse needs to administer otic drops to a client. Which of the following should the nurse do to ensure correct administration of the otic drops?
   1. Have the client lie on their side with the ear toward the ceiling.
   2. In the upright position, have the head tilted straight down toward the floor.
   3. Gently pull the cartilaginous portion of the outer ear down and forward.
   4. Insert the applicator tip or the dropper tip into the ear canal.

5. A nurse is caring for a client who is being administered Cerumenex for softening the dried ear wax inside the ear canal. When should the nurse discontinue the use of Cerumenex?
   1. After using the medication for 1 week
   2. When absolutely no cerumen remains
   3. When drainage or discharge occurs
   4. When dizziness or other sensations occur

6. A nurse is caring for a client who is being administered dipivefrin for the treatment of open-angle glaucoma. Which of the following should the nurse monitor for in the client as a transient local reaction to dipivefrin?
   1. Deposits in conjunctiva
   2. Brow ache or headache
   3. Ocular allergic reactions
   4. Foreign body sensation

7. A client has undergone an ophthalmic examination and is being administered dapiprazole to reverse the diagnostic mydriasis used in the eye examination. The nurse should know that which of the following is a local effect of dapiprazole?
   1. Abnormal corneal staining
   2. Decreased night vision
   3. Frequent urge to urinate
   4. Drooping of the upper eyelid

8. A client has been administered echothiophate iodide for the treatment of accommodative esotropia (cross-eyed). Which of the following ophthalmic adverse reactions should the nurse monitor for in the client?
   1. Eyelid muscle twitching
   2. Abdominal cramps
   3. Cardiac irregularities
   4. Urinary incontinence

9. Antipyrine is used in otic preparations as which of the following?
   1. Solvent
   2. Decongestant
   3. Analgesic
   4. Anesthetic

10. Which of the following can a nurse recommend to a client to aid in removing cerumen?
    1. Carbamide peroxide
    2. Acetic acid
    3. Phenylephrine
    4. Hydrocortisone

11. The nurse may use Cerumenex to aid in the removal of ear wax from the client's ear canal; however, Cerumenex is not allowed to stay in the ear canal for more than how long before irrigation?
    1. 5 minutes
    2. 30 minutes
    3. 10 minutes
    4. 15 minutes

12. A client should not use over-the-counter ear wax removal products for more than how long before consulting a primary health care provider?
    1. 4 days
    2. 7 days
    3. 2 days
    4. 10 days

CHAPTER 54

Fluids, Electrolytes, and Parenteral Therapy

Learning Objectives

- List the types and uses of solutions used in the parenteral management of body fluids.
- Define the types of intravenous (IV) administration of a solution or electrolyte used in the management of body fluids.
- Describe the calculations used to establish IV flow rates.
- Compare and contrast the types and uses of electrolytes used in the management of electrolyte imbalances.
- Explain the more common signs and symptoms of electrolyte imbalance.
- Distinguish preadministration and ongoing assessment activities the nurse should perform with the client administered an electrolyte or an IV solution to manage body fluids.
- List nursing diagnoses particular to a client receiving an electrolyte or a solution to manage body fluids.
- Examine ways to promote an optimal response to therapy and important points to keep in mind when educating clients about the use of an electrolyte or a solution to manage body fluids.

SECTION I: ASSESSING YOUR UNDERSTANDING

Activity A FILL IN THE BLANKS

1. An _____ is an electrically charged substance essential to the normal functioning of all cells.

2. A low pH in the blood means the body is in an acidic condition and a high blood pH indicates an _____ condition.

3. The term *fluid* _____ describes a condition when the body's fluid requirements are met and the administration of fluid occurs at a rate that is greater than the rate at which the body can use or eliminate the fluid.

4. _____ is typically the intravenous solution used for clients with burns or trauma, when significant blood loss occurs.

5. Equal analgesic conversion uses a chart to determine the amount of most opiate drugs compared to the drug _____.

Activity B DOSAGE CALCULATION

1. A client has been prescribed an IV infusion of 1000 mL lactated Ringer's to be infused every 10 hours. How many milliliters per hour should be set on the infusion pump for this infusion?

   _____

   _____

2. A client is prescribed 5 g of magnesium sulfate to be given via the IV route every 3 hours. The drug is available in the form of 1 g/2 mL. How many mL of the magnesium sulfate will be mixed into the IV secondary set for infusion?

   _____

   _____

3. A client is prescribed potassium 60 mEq/day to be taken orally. The drug is available in the form of 30 mEq. How many tablets should be administered to the client daily?

   _____

   _____

Activity C MATCHING

Match the electrolytes in Column A with their common uses in Column B.

Column A

____ 1. Potassium

____ 2. Magnesium

____ 3. Sodium

____ 4. Calcium

Column B

a. Plays an important role in the transmission of nerve impulses; is also important in the activity of many enzyme reactions such as carbohydrate metabolism

b. Necessary for the functioning of nerves and muscles, clotting of blood, building of bones and teeth, and other physiologic processes

c. Necessary for the transmission of impulses; the contraction of smooth, cardiac, and skeletal muscles; and other important physiologic processes

d. Important in maintaining acid–base balance and normal heart action and in regulating osmotic pressure in body cells

Activity D SHORT ANSWERS

A nurse's role in managing clients who are using fluids and electrolytes involves monitoring and managing interventions that aid in their recovery. Answer the following questions, which involve the nurse's role in the management of such situations.

1. A nurse has been caring for a client who has been administered intravenous replacement solutions. What factors should the nurse consider when evaluating the therapy to determine its effectiveness?

   _____

   _____

   _____

2. A nurse has been caring for a client who has been administered oral potassium supplement. What instructions should the nurse offer related to the intake of this electrolyte as part of the client teaching plan post discharge?

_____

_____

_____

Activity E Crossword Puzzle

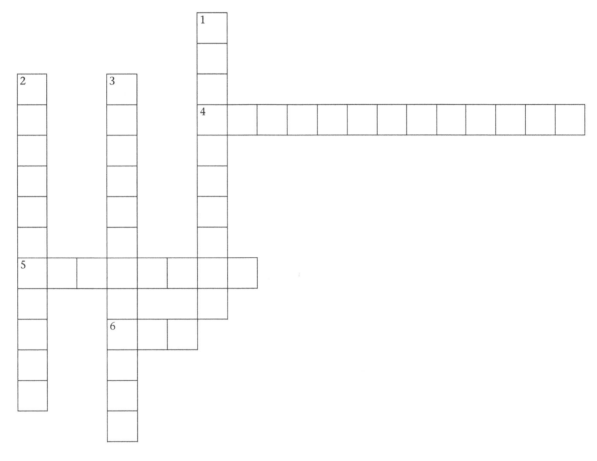

Across

4. Escape of fluid from a blood vessel into surrounding tissue
5. Condition in which the body's fluid requirements are met and the administration of fluid occurs at a rate that is greater than the rate at which the body can use or eliminate the fluid
6. Complex admixture of nutrients combined in a single container and administered to the body by an IV route (abbreviation)

Down

1. Administration of a substance, such as a drug, by any route other than through the gastrointestinal (GI) system (e.g., oral or rectal route)
2. Electrically charged substance essential to the normal functioning of all cells
3. Collection of fluid into tissue

SECTION II: APPLYING YOUR KNOWLEDGE

Activity F CASE STUDY

 Mr. Park, a 77-year-old man, is transported to the ED with symptoms of dehydration after falling and suffering a fractured leg. The ED provider has ordered dextrose in water (D_5W) IV.

1. The ED provider says to finish the infusion which came to the ED, it is not on a pump. Calculate the drip rate (drops/minute) if a 1000-mL bag of D_5W was to be infused over a period of 4 hours with a drop factor of 10.

   _____

   _____

   _____

2. Fluid overload is commonly associated with solutions administered via the parenteral route. What symptoms might Mr. Park exhibit that would indicate fluid overload?

   _____

   _____

   _____

Now Map It Out! Use the templates provided in the appendix to add information and make client connections on a concept map.

Bring out your concept map of Mr. Park and look at his various medical diagnoses. Using the information from Box 54.1 in the textbook, is dextrose in water the appropriate parenteral infusion?

SECTION III: PRACTICING FOR NCLEX

Activity G NCLEX-STYLE QUESTIONS

Answer the following questions.

1. A nurse is assigned to care for a client who needs to be administered a magnesium supplement. What piece of data should the nurse specifically look for in the client's health history section of the electronic record before administering the drug?

   1. Client does not experience fluid retention.
   2. Client does not have a heart block.
   3. Client does not have untreated Addison disease.
   4. Client is not taking digitalis.

2. A nurse is caring for a client who is being administered potassium orally. During assessment, the nurse observes that the client is experiencing GI distress after administration. What nursing interventions should the nurse perform to reduce the distress? **Select all that apply.**

   1. Offer meals in smaller quantities and more frequently.
   2. Monitor the client for any signs and symptoms of nausea.
   3. Encourage the client to take the drug with fruit juice.
   4. Ensure that the drug is taken by the client with meals.
   5. Administer antacids to the client as prescribed for nausea.

3. A nurse is caring for a client who is being administered plasma protein fractions. Which of the following adverse reactions should the nurse monitor for in this client?

   1. Urticaria
   2. Hypertension
   3. Dyspnea
   4. Diuresis

4. A nurse is caring for a client who has a peripheral IV lock device. The IV device should be flushed with a solution to prevent small clots from obstructing the cannula. Which solutions may be used for a peripheral IV lock flush? **Select all that apply.**
   1. Dilute heparin
   2. Sodium bicarbonate
   3. Normal saline
   4. Drug diluent
   5. 100 unit/mL strength heparin

5. A nurse is caring for a client who needs to be administered IV bicarbonate. In the client's health history, which finding would suggest cautious administration rather than being contraindicated in this client?
   1. Metabolic alkalosis
   2. Heart failure
   3. Hypocalcemia
   4. Severe abdominal pains

6. The student nurse is observing the surgical nurse calculate conversion of a Dilaudid infusion to oral Percocet. The nurse asks the student what drug is an equal analgesic conversion chart based upon. The correct answer is:
   1. Acetaminophen
   2. Furosemide
   3. Morphine
   4. Potassium

7. A nurse is caring for a client who is being prepared for an administration of TPN. As a general rule, how many days can an infusion of TPN be administered in a peripheral IV site?
   1. 8 hours
   2. 2 days
   3. 1 week
   4. 15 days

8. How many unsuccessful venipuncture attempts on the same client warrants having a more skilled individual attempt the procedure?
   1. 1
   2. 2
   3. 3
   4. 4

9. Which of the following is a major intracellular fluid electrolyte?
   1. Potassium
   2. Sodium
   3. Calcium
   4. Phosphate

10. Which of the following is a major extracellular fluid electrolyte?
    1. Potassium
    2. Magnesium
    3. Phosphate
    4. Sodium

11. Which of the following electrolytes is necessary for the contraction of smooth, cardiac, and skeletal muscles?
    1. Calcium
    2. Potassium
    3. Sodium
    4. Magnesium

12. How frequently should an IV site be inspected when normal saline is infusing into a critical client?
    1. Every 4 hours
    2. Every 1–2 hours
    3. Hourly
    4. Every 5–15 minutes

Answers

CHAPTER 1

SECTION I: ASSESSING YOUR UNDERSTANDING

Activity A FILL IN THE BLANKS

1. living organisms
2. natural sources
3. potentially harmful
4. Nonprescription
5. abuse

Activity B LABELING

1. Pharmaceutic
2. Pharmacokinetic
3. Pharmacodynamic

Activity E CROSSWORD PUZZLE

Activity C MATCHING SHORT ANSWERS

1. **1.** b   **2.** c   **3.** a
2. **1.** c   **2.** d   **3.** a   **4.** b

Activity D SHORT ANSWERS

1. **Drug tolerance** is a decreased response to a drug, requiring an increase in dosage to achieve the desired effect. **Physical dependency** is the habitual use of a drug, and physical withdrawal symptoms result from abrupt discontinuation. **Psychological dependency** is a compulsion or craving to use a drug for a pleasurable experience.
2. The U.S. Food and Drug Administration (FDA) is responsible for approving new drugs and monitoring drugs currently in use for adverse or toxic reactions. The process of drug development takes about 7–12 years and sometimes even more.

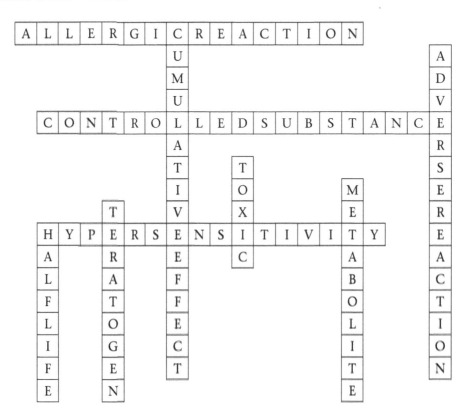

SECTION II: APPLYING YOUR KNOWLEDGE
Activity F CASE STUDY

1. As you discuss the use of comfrey for digestive purposes, remember many of these natural substances have strong pharmacologic activity, and some may interact with prescription drugs or be toxic in the body. For example, *comfrey,* an herb that was once widely used to promote digestion, can cause liver damage. Although it may still be available in some areas, it is a dangerous herb and is not recommended for use as a supplement.
2. Specific teaching points:
   - Herbal preparations are not necessarily safe because they are natural.
   - If you have health problems, there may be an increased danger in taking herbal preparations.
   - If you are going to have surgery, be sure to tell your doctor if you use herbal products.
   - Herbal products can change the way prescription and over-the-counter drugs work.
   - Herbal products can cause other problems.

SECTION III: PRACTICING FOR NCLEX
Activity G NCLEX-STYLE QUESTIONS

1. **Answer: 4**
   RATIONALE: The nurse should refer to a drug by its generic name to avoid confusion. A generic name is the name given to a drug before it becomes official and can be used in many countries by all manufacturers. The scientific name, also called the *chemical name,* gives the molecular structure of that particular drug. The trade or brand name is the name registered by the manufacturer and is followed by the trademark symbol. This name can be used only by the manufacturer holding the trademark.
2. **Answers: 2, 3, 4**
   RATIONALE: The purpose of the Controlled Substances Act of 1970 is to regulate the manufacture, distribution, and dispensing of drugs that have abuse potential.
3. **Answer: 3**
   RATIONALE: The nurse should administer the fluid intravenously, as it is rapidly absorbed by the system. Absorption occurs slowly when a drug is administered orally, intramuscularly, or subcutaneously. Because of the complex membranes of the gastrointestinal mucosal layers, muscle and skin delay the drug passage.

4. **Answers: 1, 3, 5**
   RATIONALE: Most drugs act on the body by altering cellular function. A drug that alters cellular function can increase or decrease certain physiologic functions, such as increasing heart rate, decreasing blood pressure, or increasing urine output.
5. **Answer: 1**
   RATIONALE: Weakening the cell membrane is working from the outside environment of the cell. Cancer drugs act on the cell membrane and the cell processes, eventually causing starvation and death of the cancer cells.
6. **Answers: 1, 2, 3**
   RATIONALE: The client's age and weight are important in determining the drug dosage to be administered for effective action of the drug. If the client has some disease, it could interfere with the drug action, so the dosage has to be adjusted accordingly. Client's appetite and income do not influence the drug response.
7. **Answer: 3**
   RATIONALE: Clients with impaired liver function need to be monitored frequently during the drug administration, as impaired liver function influences the drug response. Impaired vision, speech, or hearing does not affect the drug response.
8. **Answer: 1**
   RATIONALE: Administration of a drug is primarily the responsibility of the nurse.
9. **Answer: 2**
   RATIONALE: Pharmacology is the study of drugs and their action on living organisms.
10. **Answer: 1**
    RATIONALE: The Food and Drug Administration (FDA) is responsible for the approval of new drugs in the United States.
11. **Answer: 3**
    RATIONALE: Prescription drugs are also called *legend drugs.*
12. **Answer: 1**
    RATIONALE: The generic name of a drug is the name found in the *National Formulary* or the *U.S. Pharmacopeia.*
13. **Answer: 1**
    RATIONALE: Physical dependence is the habitual use of a drug, in which negative physical withdrawal symptoms result from abrupt discontinuation.

CHAPTER 2

SECTION I: ASSESSING YOUR UNDERSTANDING

Activity A FILL IN THE BLANKS

1. insulin, heparin
2. subcutaneous
3. unit
4. sublingual
5. allergies
6. Workplace

Activity B SEQUENCING

1. 4   3   1   2

Activity C MATCHING

1. 1. c   2. d   3. f   4. b   5. a   6. e

Activity D SHORT ANSWERS

1. At least two of the methods listed are used to ensure that the right client is administered the medication:
   - Check the client's wristband containing the client's name. If there is no written identification verifying the client's name, the nurse can obtain a wristband or other form of identification before administering the drug.
   - Ask the client to identify themselves and state their date of birth prior to administering the drug.
   - Some long-term care or rehabilitation care facilities have pictures of the client available, which allows the nurse to verify the correct client. If pictures are used, it is critical that they are recent and bear a good likeness of the individual.
2. The term *Just Culture* means focusing on finding the system problem, not punishing the person who made an error. Therefore, it is even more important for you and other nurses to report errors and omissions so problems can be discovered and changed.

Activity E CROSSWORD PUZZLE

			B				P	
	S	T	A	N	D	A	R	D
	T		R				N	
	A		C					
J	O	I	N	T				
	S		O					
	M		R					
	P		D					
	E							
	P	A	R	E	N	T	E	R	A	L

SECTION II: APPLYING YOUR KNOWLEDGE

Activity F CASE STUDY

1. The nurse should compare the medication, container label, and medication record to ensure that the right drug is administered to the right client.
2. Immediate documentation is particularly important when drugs are given on an as-needed (PRN) basis. Immediate documentation prevents accidental administration of a drug by another individual. Proper documentation is essential to the process of administering drugs correctly.

SECTION III: PRACTICING FOR NCLEX

Activity G NCLEX-STYLE QUESTIONS

1. **Answer: 4**
   RATIONALE: The nurse should remove the old patch when the next dose is applied to a new site. Removing all old patches prevents added dosing of the drug. The rotation of sites for transdermal patches prevents skin irritation. The nurse should not shave the area to apply the patch; shaving may cause skin irritation. The area where the transdermal patch is to be applied should be dry, not moist.

2. **Answer: 2**
   RATIONALE: The nurse should obtain instructions for application of the drug from the primary health care provider. The instructions may include whether to apply the drug in a thin or even layer or whether or not to cover the area after application of the drug to the skin. It is not essential to obtain information about the cause of the skin infection, reasons for selecting the drug, and composition of the drug before administering the prescribed drug.

3. **Answer: 3**
   RATIONALE: The inner part of the forearm is ideal for administering an intradermal injection. The nurse should not administer the drug near moles, areas with hair cover, or pigmented skin. The thigh and the upper arm are ideal sites for intramuscular injections, but not for intradermal injections.

4. **Answer: 3**
   RATIONALE: Most hospitals use needles designed to prevent needle-stick injuries. This needle has a plastic guard that slips over the needle and locks in place as it is withdrawn from the injection site. Do not recap syringes. Discard needles and syringes into clearly marked, appropriate containers to prevent needle-stick injuries.

5. **Answer: 1**
   RATIONALE: If an intramuscular injection volume is more than 3 mL, the nurse should divide the drug and give it as two separate injections, as volumes larger than 3 mL will not be absorbed properly. The nurse should use a 1½-in. needle for the injection, not ½ in. The upper back is not an ideal site for intramuscular injections. When giving a drug by the intramuscular route, the nurse should insert the needle at a 90-degree angle.

6. **Answers: 1, 3, 4, 5**

   RATIONALE: The nurse should crush the tablets and ensure that they are completely dissolved before administering to the client. The nurse should check the tube for placement and flush the tube with water to clear it. The nurse should not put the tablets in water without crushing them, as the drug may not dissolve properly. The tube should be flushed after the drug has been administered.

7. **Answer: 2**

   RATIONALE: A nurse should use two methods to identify the client before administering the medication.

8. **Answer: 3**

   RATIONALE: This order represents a PRN order, an order to administer the drug as needed.

9. **Answer: 3**

   RATIONALE: The abbreviation mL may be used for milliliter; all others are on the "do not use" list.

10. **Answer: 2**

    RATIONALE: The Joint Commission updates the NPSG on a yearly basis.

11. **Answers: 1, 4**

    RATIONALE: The Institute for Safe Medication Practices is responsible for the Medication Errors Reporting Program. MedWatch is the program run by the U.S. Food and Drug Administration (FDA).

12. **Answer: 4**

    RATIONALE: The nurse is responsible for the administration part of the drug distribution process. Primary and specialty providers are responsible for ordering and pharmacists are responsible for dispensing.

CHAPTER 3

SECTION I: ASSESSING YOUR UNDERSTANDING

Activity A FILL IN THE BLANKS

1. calculating
2. accuracy
3. metric
4. formulas
5. zeros, mL
6. vials, ampules

Activity B LABELING

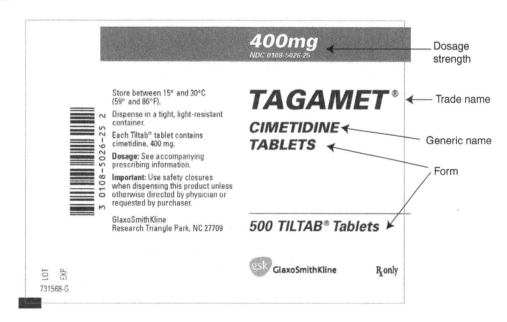

Activity C MATCHING

1. 1. b **2.** d **3.** a **4.** c

Activity D SHORT ANSWERS

Think about the rationale for the redundancy system. Is that removed by the computer system? This is a system in which each person in the process of medication prescription and delivery checks the drug dosage for accuracy.

Activity E SUDOKU PUZZLE

mL	kg	mg	g	lb	C	m	F	mcg
g	lb	m	mcg	F	mg	kg	C	mL
mcg	C	F	mL	kg	m	g	lb	mg
C	m	g	mg	mcg	kg	lb	mL	F
kg	mcg	lb	m	mL	F	C	mg	g
mg	F	mL	C	g	lb	mcg	kg	m
lb	g	C	F	mg	mcg	mL	m	kg
m	mg	mcg	kg	C	mL	F	g	lb
F	mL	kg	lb	m	g	mg	mcg	C

SECTION II: APPLYING YOUR KNOWLEDGE

Activity F CASE STUDY

1. Mr. Garcia weighs 97.7 kg (215 lb × 1 kg/2.2 lb = 97.7 kg)
2. 37 °C is 98.6 °F (9/5 × 37 = 66.6; 66.6 + 32 = 98.6)

SECTION III: PRACTICING FOR NCLEX

Activity G NCLEX-STYLE QUESTIONS

1. **Answer: 1**
   RATIONALE: The best method of error detection is the manual redundancy system.
2. **Answer: 3**
   RATIONALE: Problems can arise if a client recognizes the brand name of the drug but does not recognize the generic name and refuses the medication. The nurse should know both the generic and trade names of each drug by reviewing the label and drug information carefully.
3. **Answer: 1**
   RATIONALE: There are three systems of measurement associated with drug dosing: the metric system, the apothecary system, and household measurements. The metric system is the most commonly used system of measurement in medicine. The apothecary system at one time was used for weight measurement. In 1994, recommendations were made by the Institute for Safe Medication Practices (ISMP) to eliminate this system due to the high rate of medication errors it produced. The household system is rarely used in a hospital setting but may be used to measure drug dosages in the home.

4. **Answer: 1**
   RATIONALE: When there is no number to the left of the decimal, a zero is written; for example, 0.75 shows correct placement of the zero in a decimal.
5. **Answer: 3**
   RATIONALE: There are 2.2 lb in 1 kg.
6. **Answers: 2, 3, 1**
   RATIONALE: 1000 milliliters = 1 liter, 10 liters = 1 deciliter
7. **Answer: 4**
   RATIONALE: 1 milligram (mg) = 1000 micrograms (mcg)
8. **Answer: 4**
   RATIONALE: There are 3 teaspoons in 1 tablespoon.
9. **Answer: 3**
   RATIONALE: A tablet is the compressed form of a powdered substance. Ampules, vials, and syringes may all involve a solvent used to make a drug solution when the drug is added.
10. **Answer: 3**
    RATIONALE: There are 1000 milligrams in 1 gram.
11. **Answer: 3**
    RATIONALE: When using dimensional analysis to calculate dosage problems, the identified unit of measure to be calculated is written followed by an equal sign. Then the dosage strength is written with the numerator always expressed in the same unit that was identified before the equal sign. Expressing the dosage strength as a fraction with the numerator having the same unit, writing the next fraction with the numerator having the same unit of measure as the denominator, and expanding the equation by filling in the missing numbers using the appropriate equivalent are the steps associated with performing metric conversion using dimensional analysis.
12. **Answers: 2, 4**
    RATIONALE: The body surface area is the square meter of measurement according to the client's height and weight.
13. **Answers: 1, 2, 4, 5**
    RATIONALE: Drug labels may contain two names: the trade (brand) name and the generic name. On the label, the form will be listed; in other words, it will list the drug as a capsule, tablet, or other form of the drug. The dosage strength is also given on the container. Drugs may have more than one use, so the use of the drug is not always listed. One exception is over-the-counter drugs.
14. **Answer: 4**
    RATIONALE: The generic name is written in smaller print and is usually located under the trade name. The trade name is capitalized, written first on the label, and identified by the trademark or registration symbol.

15. Answer: 3

RATIONALE: A gram represents a unit of weight; a liter represents a unit of volume; a meter represents a unit of length; and a deciliter represents one-tenth of a liter (unit of volume).

CHAPTER 4

SECTION I: ASSESSING YOUR UNDERSTANDING

Activity A FILL IN THE BLANKS

1. Objective
2. ongoing
3. diagnosis
4. implementation
5. individual

Activity B SEQUENCING

1.	5	3	1	4	2

Activity C MATCHING

1. 1. c   2. e   3. a   4. b   5. d
2. 1. b   2. a   3. c   4. d   5. d

Activity D SHORT ANSWERS

1. a. The nursing process is a framework for nursing action consisting of problem-solving steps that help members of the health care team provide effective client care. It is both a specific and an orderly plan used to gather data, identify client problems from the data, develop and implement a plan of action, and then evaluate the results of nursing activities, including the administration of drugs.

    b. The five phases of the nursing process are:
       - Assessment
       - Analysis
       - Planning
       - Implementation
       - Evaluation

2. An initial assessment is made based on objective and subjective data collected when the client is first seen in a hospital, outpatient clinic, health care provider's office, or other type of health care facility. The initial assessment is usually more thorough and provides a database from which later data can be compared and decisions made. An ongoing assessment is one that is made at the time of each client contact and may include the collection of objective data, subjective data, or both. The scope of an ongoing assessment depends on many factors, such as the client's diagnosis, the severity of illness, the response to treatment, and the prescribed medical or surgical treatment.

Activity E WORD FIND PUZZLE

O	N	G	O	I	N	G			I
			U					E	N
			T				V		D
P	R	O	C	E	S	S	I		E
			O			T	N		P
			M		C		I		E
			E	E			T		N
S	U	B	J	E	C	T	I	V	E	D
		B					A		E
	O						L		N
									T

SECTION II: APPLYING YOUR KNOWLEDGE

Activity F CASE STUDY

Check Box 4.1 in the text for some reasons that clients have problems staying on medications. Which of these factors does the client have control or no control over when taking medications? What does the nurse need to know about client habits to be sure the client takes the prescribed medications?

SECTION III: PRACTICING FOR NCLEX

Activity G NCLEX-STYLE QUESTIONS

1. **Answer: 1**

    RATIONALE: To obtain subjective data from the client, the nurse should inquire about the number of cigarettes smoked in a day. Subjective data include facts that are supplied to the nurse and other health care professionals by the client and the client's family. Monitoring the client's body temperature, blood pressure, and pulse rate and rhythm are objective data that the nurse should obtain. Objective data include facts that the nurse obtains through physical assessment or physical examination.

2. **Answer: 2**

    RATIONALE: When developing an expected outcome, the nurse should focus on the client's ability to carry out a plan. Expected outcome describes the maximum level of wellness that is reasonably attainable for the client. The expected outcome defines the expected behavior of the client or family that indicates the problem is being resolved or that progress toward resolution is occurring. When developing an expected outcome, the nurse need not focus on the type of drug administered, its dosage pattern, or the client's ability to recuperate, since these will not determine if the client has the ability to achieve the maximum level of wellness.

3. Answer: 1
RATIONALE: In selecting a nursing diagnosis, a nurse should include problems that can be solved by independent nursing actions (i.e., actions that do not require a physician's order and may be legally performed by a nurse). The nurse should not include problems that have a definite cure or problems that cannot be prevented by nursing actions. Nursing diagnosis also does not include identification of the client's condition or criticality.

4. Answers: 1, 3, 5
RATIONALE: Planning for nursing actions specific for the drug to be administered promotes a greater accuracy in drug administration, client understanding of the drug regimen, and improved client adherence with the prescribed drug therapy after hospital discharge. The planning for nursing actions does not bring about prevention of a relapse. Planning and implementing nursing actions do promote an optimal response to drug therapy, but they do not always promote an optimal response in minimum time.

5. Answers: 3, 1, 4, 2, 5
RATIONALE: The nursing process steps described are assessment, analysis, and planning. Assessment involves collecting objective and subjective data. The data collected during assessment are analyzed, the client's needs (problems) are identified, and one or more nursing diagnoses are formulated. After the nursing diagnoses are formulated, a client-oriented goal and expected outcomes are developed for each nursing diagnosis.

6. Answer: 1
RATIONALE: Facts obtained by means of a physical assessment or physical examination are considered objective data.

7. Answer: 3
RATIONALE: Facts supplied by the client or the client's family are considered subjective data.

8. Answer: 3
RATIONALE: Assessment is the first step of the nursing process because none of the other steps can be accomplished without assessment.

9. Answer: 3
RATIONALE: Assessment involves collecting objective and subjective data.

10. Answer: 1
RATIONALE: A nursing diagnosis identifies problems that can be solved or prevented by independent nursing actions that do not require a physician's order.

11. Answer: 4
RATIONALE: NANDA-I was formed to standardize the terminology used for nursing diagnoses and continues to define, explain, classify, and research summary statements about health problems related to nursing.

12. Answer: 1
RATIONALE: Planning is the next step of the nursing process after the formulation of nursing diagnoses.

13. Answer: 2
RATIONALE: When related to the administration of drugs, implementation refers to the preparation and administration of one or more drugs to a specific client.

CHAPTER 5

SECTION I: ASSESSING YOUR UNDERSTANDING

Activity A FILL IN THE BLANKS
1. teaching
2. trust, respect
3. limited health
4. Motivation
5. affective

Activity B SEQUENCING
1. 2   3   1   4

Activity C MATCHING
1. 1. b   2. c   3. a
2. 1. c   2. a   3. b

Activity D SHORT ANSWERS
1. a. To ensure that the client perfectly remembers all the exercises taught, the nurse should observe while the client demonstrates the exercises.
   b. To ensure that the client's relative has understood the procedure of measuring the client's temperature using an ear thermometer, the nurse should:
   ■ Ask the relative to perform a return demonstration of the procedure.
   ■ Refrain from using questions such as "Do you understand? or "Is there anything you

don't understand?" because the relative may be uncomfortable in admitting a lack of understanding.

2. **a.** Since the client is deficient in cognitive knowledge and psychomotor skills, the nursing diagnosis *Deficient Knowledge* should be used to teach the client about diabetes type 2 and administration of the insulin injection.

   b. Kinesthetic learners—they learn by moving, touching, and doing.

   c. The affective domain of learning comes into the picture when the client expresses her feelings about what she knows.

Activity E CROSSWORD PUZZLE

```
                                  D           B
           P  A  T  R  I  A  R  C  H  A  L
           A              I           D
 C  U  L  T  U  R  A  L               L
              T              Y
 D            N              C
 W  E  L  L  N  E  S  S      A  D  U  L  T  S
    C  I        R            L
    I  M        S            E
    S  I                     N
    I  T                     D
    O  E  X  P  E  R  T       A
    N  D                     R
```

SECTION II: APPLYING YOUR KNOWLEDGE

Activity F CASE STUDY

1. The factor making Mr. Garcia at risk for limited health literacy is speaking limited English; ask the couple what they know about the disease and how long they have been in the United States.

2. Limit the amount of information at each interaction with the client. Make it relevant to his current needs or situation. Focus communication on the use of the glucometer because this was identified as the most important thing the client needs to know at this time.

SECTION III: PRACTICING FOR NCLEX

Activity G NCLEX-STYLE QUESTIONS

1. **Answers: 1, 2, 3**

   RATIONALE: Ineffective Health Management helps in discharge teaching, in managing a complicated medication regimen, and in providing positive results to clients. It also describes clients who successfully manage Readiness for Enhanced Health Management, which is used when the client has mastered basic information and is learning more about drug reactions and management of adverse reactions.

2. **Answers: 2, 3, 4**

   RATIONALE: Plans for teaching should begin when a client comes to the facility, and sessions can be held at a time when the client is alone, alert, and free of distractions. If the client has a learning impairment (such as sedation), a family member or friend should be included in the teaching process. For example, do not perform client teaching when there are visitors (unless they are to be involved in the administration of the client's drugs) or if the client is sedated or in pain.

3. **Answers: 1, 4, 5**

   RATIONALE: Carrying out a client assessment before formulating a teaching plan helps a nurse to identify barriers and obstacles in the learning process, to choose teaching methods that fit learning styles, and to identify effective teaching tools. Client motivation and participation will be improved by the correct implementation, not the assessment.

4. **Answer: 2**

   RATIONALE: The psychomotor domain involves the learning of physical skills. The affective domain involves the client's or the caregiver's attitudes, feelings, beliefs, and opinions. The cognitive domain involves intellectual activities such as thought, recall, decision making, and drawing conclusions.

5. **Answer: 2**

   RATIONALE: Health literacy is the ability to understand information about health and disease, then use the information to make decisions about health care. Diabetics measure carbohydrates in dietary education. All the other statements are false.

6. **Answer: 3**

   RATIONALE: Written instructions are translated into different languages. During conversations, interpreters are used to explain the foreign words.

7. **Answer: 3**

   RATIONALE: There are three basic types of learners: auditory, learn by listening; visual, learn by seeing or watching; and kinesthetic, learn by moving, touching, and doing. Although only a small percentage of people learn best by listening, they can do other tasks (knitting) while learning.

8. **Answer: 1**

   RATIONALE: Client teaching is an ongoing process.

9. **Answer: 3**

   RATIONALE: When individualized written material is developed for limited English proficiency clients, be sure the material includes the basic information that a client would receive in English. The nurses and doctors on the hospital staff would know if the medical information in the materials is the same as the English versions provided by the facility.

10. **Answers: 1, 2, 3, 4**

    RATIONALE: Making sure the client is not distracted by physical conditions, such as pain, rapid heartbeat, hyperglycemia, or hypotension, is vital to the teaching/learning process.

11. **Answer: 4**

    RATIONALE: Limited health literacy is higher in individuals who do not speak English and can be identified in behaviors such as frequently missed appointments.

12. **Answer: 2**

    RATIONALE: Most adults are visual learners, others learn hands on, while only a few learn best by listening. The DVD provides the best visual learning opportunity.

13. **Answer: 1**

    RATIONALE: When you take the time to develop a therapeutic relationship, the client/family has confidence in the nurse and more confidence in the information conveyed by the nurse.

CHAPTER 6

SECTION I: ASSESSING YOUR UNDERSTANDING

Activity A FILL IN THE BLANKS

1. 2
2. bacteriostatic
3. photosensitivity
4. Cranberry
5. thrombocytopenia

Activity B DOSAGE CALCULATION

1. 3 tablets
2. 1 tablet
3. 1 gram or 1000 mg, 20 mL
4. 3 tablets
5. 5 tablets

Activity C MATCHING

1. **1.** c   **2.** d   **3.** a   **4.** b
2. **1.** d   **2.** a   **3.** b   **4.** c

Activity D SHORT ANSWERS

1. As part of the preadministration assessment, a nurse would perform the following:
   - Assess the client's general appearance, general health history (surgeries, medical conditions, and medications), and allergies.

- Take and record vital signs.
- Obtain a description of the signs and symptoms of infection from the client or family.
- Review any results of tests previously done.

2. A nurse's teaching plan should include the following:
   - Take the drug as prescribed.
   - Drink at least six to eight 8-ounce glasses of fluid every day.

- Complete the full course of therapy.
- Take the drug on an empty stomach either 1 hour before or 2 hours after a meal if indicated.
- Exposure to sunlight may result in skin reactions similar to severe sunburn.
- Keep all follow-up appointments to ensure the infection is treated correctly.

Activity E CROSSWORD PUZZLE

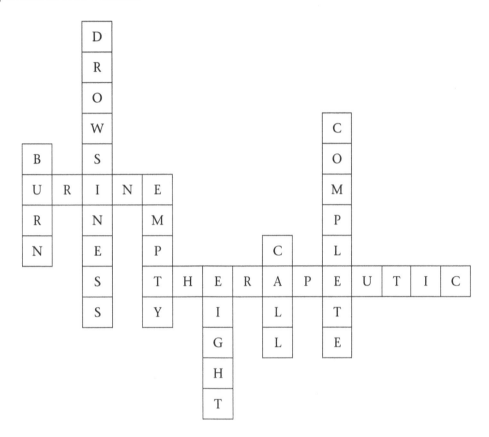

SECTION II: APPLYING YOUR KNOWLEDGE

Activity F CASE STUDY

1. When triaging a client who may have an infection, the nurse should assess the client's general appearance; take and record vital signs; obtain information regarding symptoms experienced by the client and the length of the symptoms; ask the client about self-remedies used; and review the results of labs and tests. The nurse should also obtain a list of current medications and medical conditions and ask the client about allergies to food, drugs, or environmental factors.

2. The nurse should discuss the possible side effects of sulfonamides with Mrs. Moore (nausea, vomiting, anorexia, stomatitis, chills, fever, crystalluria, and photosensitivity). The client should be advised to take the medication with a full glass of water and to increase daily fluid intake. The client should be instructed to call the physician's office if an allergic reaction occurs, if she experiences any unusual bruising, or if worsening of her condition occurs. Mrs. Moore should be instructed to take the Bactrim DS until it is gone even if she is feeling better and to keep all follow-up appointments with the physician.

SECTION III: PRACTICING FOR NCLEX

Activity G NCLEX-STYLE QUESTIONS

1. **Answer: 1**
   RATIONALE: The nurse should clean and remove the debris present on the surface of the client's burnt skin before the application of cream. The nurse should not apply a thick layer of cream on the burned area. The drug is normally applied

1/16-in. thick; thicker application is not recommended. Applying drugs with a bare hand involves a risk of passing infection. It is advisable to use gloves while applying cream. The nurse should remove debris present on the surface of the skin before each application of the drug.

2. **Answer: 4**
   RATIONALE: The nurse should inspect the client's skin daily to assess the extent of bruising and evidence of exacerbation of existing ecchymotic areas. The client can be shifted if required, but care should be taken to prevent bruising. There is no need to avoid brushing teeth as long as a soft-bristled toothbrush is used. While it is necessary to examine the client's skin for trauma, palpating the client's body can create unnecessary pain and may trigger bleeding.

3. **Answers: 2, 4**
   RATIONALE: Sunscreen should be applied on exposed body parts, but this is not enough to protect from photosensitivity and the client should wear protective clothing even after applying sunscreen. Sulfasalazine, not sulfadiazine, causes a yellow stain on contact lenses. There is no need to avoid indoor lights as the effects of photosensitivity are caused by sunlight.

4. **Answer: 3**
   RATIONALE: Facial edema may indicate a possible allergic reaction that may occur due to the application of mafenide, and the nurse should monitor the client for edema. Urine turning orange-yellow is one of the symptoms of sulfasalazine, not mafenide. Crystalluria does not occur during mafenide therapy. A burning sensation while applying the drug to the skin is unpleasant, yet it is an anticipated, normal reaction.

5. **Answer: 3**
   RATIONALE: The nurse should inform the client that using soft contact lenses during the sulfonamide therapy may result in a permanent yellow stain on the lenses. Wearing lenses will not, however, cause a burning sensation in the eyes, headache and dizziness, or impaired vision.

6. **Answers: 1, 2, 5**
   RATIONALE: While caring for clients with ulcerative colitis, the nurse should inspect the stool samples, record their appearance, and monitor for evidence of the relief or intensification of the symptoms. The nurse should also ensure that sulfasalazine is administered during meals or immediately afterward. There is no need to measure urine output as the client does not have impaired urinary elimination as the diagnosis resulting in prescription of the sulfa drug.

Loss of appetite is a mild adverse effect of sulfonamides.

7. **Answer: 1**
   RATIONALE: The nurse should inform the client that using cranberries with antibiotics prevents bacteria from attaching to the walls of the urinary tract. Crystalluria or the formation of crystals in urine can be prevented by increasing fluid intake. Specifically consuming cranberry juice will not have any significant effect in preventing crystalluria. The effects of photosensitivity can be reduced by wearing protective clothing or sunscreen when traveling outside and consumption of cranberry juice will not have any effect. Clots can be prevented by using oral anticoagulants with sulfonamides.

8. **Answer: 1**
   RATIONALE: The nurse should inform the client that sulfonamide is used in the treatment of urinary tract infection because it is easily absorbed by the gastrointestinal system. Sulfonamides do not kill bacterial cells directly. They inhibit the activity of folic acid in bacterial cell metabolism, which are then subsequently destroyed by the body's defense mechanisms. A decrease in the number of white blood cells is caused by leukopenia, which is also an adverse effect of sulfonamides. Sulfonamides may have life-threatening complications such as Stevens–Johnson syndrome (SJS).

9. **Answer: 2**
   RATIONALE: The nurse should assess for lesions on the mucous membranes to determine whether the client is showing signs of SJS. Inflammation of the mouth (stomatitis), crystals in the urine (crystalluria), and diarrhea are some of the common adverse reactions of sulfonamides and do not necessarily indicate that the client has SJS.

10. **Answers: 1, 2, 3, 4**
    RATIONALE: The body is equipped with a natural defense system that includes our skin and bodily secretions.

11. **Answers: 1, 2, 3, 4**
    RATIONALE: Microbes enter the body in different ways, such as through a break in the skin or by ingestion, breathing, or contact with the mucous membranes of the body.

12. **Answer: 1**
    RATIONALE: Sulfonamides treat bacterial infection and are considered antibacterial.

13. **Answer: 2**
    RATIONALE: Drugs that slow or retard the multiplication of bacteria are known as bacteriostatic.

14. **Answer: 1**
    RATIONALE: Drugs that destroy bacteria are known as bactericidal.

CHAPTER 7

SECTION I: ASSESSING YOUR UNDERSTANDING

Activity A FILL IN THE BLANKS

1. wall
2. penicillin
3. kidneys
4. beta-lactam (β-lactam) ring
5. penicillinase

Activity B DOSAGE CALCULATION

1. 2 tablets
2. 3 mL
3. 1 mL
4. 1 capsule
5. 2 capsules
6. 100 mL

Activity C OUT IN THE COMMUNITY

Class discussion: Keeping antibacterial drugs past expiration makes the drug less effective and later taking the drugs will contribute to resistance. Are they disposed of safely?

Activity D SHORT ANSWERS

1. Before administering penicillin for the first time, a nurse should perform the following assessments:

- Obtain client's general health history including medical and surgical treatments, drug history, history of drug allergies to penicillin or cephalosporin, and present symptoms of infection.
- Take and record vital signs.
- Obtain description of signs and symptoms of infection from the client or family.
- Assess infected area and record findings on the client's chart.
- Describe signs and symptoms relating to the client's infection accurately, such as color and type of drainage from a wound, pain, redness and inflammation, color of sputum, and presence of odor.
- Note client's general appearance.
- Obtain results of the culture and sensitivity test if possible before giving the first dose.

2. When a client is to be administered cephalosporin IV, the following interventions are important:

- Check for history of drug allergies to penicillin or cephalosporin.
- Inspect the needle insertion site for signs of extravasation or infiltration.
- Inspect the needle insertion site and the area above the site several times a day for phlebitis or thrombophlebitis.
- If problems occur, contact the primary health care provider, and discontinue the IV line and restart it in another vein.

Activity E CROSSWORD PUZZLE

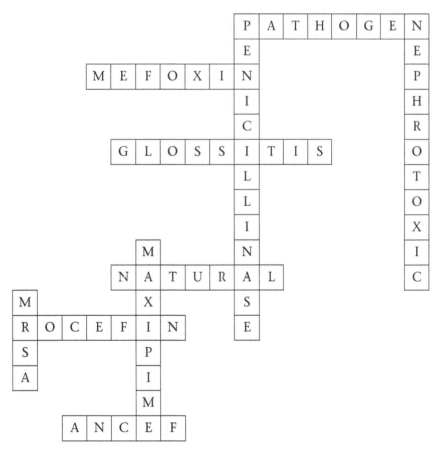

SECTION II: APPLYING YOUR KNOWLEDGE

Activity F CASE STUDY

1. The nurse should reassure Janna's mother that the bee allergy is not related to a penicillin allergy. It is good to know the signs and symptoms of a hypersensitivity reaction. The nurse should advise Janna's mother to watch for skin rash; hives; sneezing; wheezing; itching; difficulty breathing; swelling of the skin and mucous membranes, especially around and in the mouth and throat; and signs resembling serum sickness (chills, fever, edema, joint and muscle pain, and malaise). If any of these are present in Janna during treatment, her mother should stop the medication immediately and seek medical attention.

2. The nurse should advise Janna's mother to keep the container refrigerated, shake the drug well before pouring, and return the drug to the refrigerator immediately after pouring the dose. Drugs that are kept refrigerated like amoxicillin lose their potency when kept at room temperature. A small amount of the drug may be left after the last dose is taken. Any remaining amoxicillin should be discarded because the drug begins to lose its potency after a few weeks. Janna's mother should use a medicine spoon or an oral syringe to measure the dose accurately, as not all spoons are created equal.

SECTION III: PRACTICING FOR NCLEX

Activity G NCLEX-STYLE QUESTIONS

1. **Answer: 1**
   RATIONALE: When cephalosporin is given intravenously, the nurse should monitor the needle insertion site and the area above the site several times a day for signs of redness, which may indicate phlebitis or thrombophlebitis. The nurse should inspect the site for tenderness when the drug is administered to the client intramuscularly. Administration of cephalosporin intravenously does not cause fever or angina.

2. **Answer: 3**
   RATIONALE: Anemia is the result of a low red blood cell count.

3. **Answers: 3, 4, 5**
   RATIONALE: As part of the ongoing assessment, the nurse evaluates the client's response to the therapy, such as a decrease in temperature, relief from pain or discomfort, an increase in appetite, and a change in the appearance or in the amount of drainage. These evaluations are then recorded on the client's chart to monitor progress. Additional culture and sensitivity tests may be performed to check if the microorganisms have become penicillin resistant or if a superinfection has occurred. The client's general health history is obtained *before*

the appropriate penicillin therapy is determined, not in the ongoing assessment, and the client's stools are saved *only* if they show signs of diarrhea and there are signs of blood and mucus in the stools.

4. **Answers: 3, 2, 4, 1**
   RATIONALE: In situations where diarrhea is suspected, the nurse first inspects all stools. The primary health care provider has to be notified immediately if diarrhea occurs because it may be necessary to stop the drug. If there are signs of blood and mucus in the stool, it is important to save a sample to test it for occult blood to confirm presence of blood. If the stool tests positive for blood, the nurse saves another sample for possible further laboratory analysis.

5. **Answers: 1, 3, 4**
   RATIONALE: Some of the signs of anaphylactic shock are severe hypotension, loss of consciousness, and acute respiratory distress. Pain at the injection site is normal for penicillins administered intramuscularly. Nausea and vomiting are signs of gastrointestinal disturbances that may or may not be serious.

6. **Answers: 2, 3, 5**
   RATIONALE: In cases of impaired comfort or increased fever, the nurse should take vital signs every 4 hours or more. The nurse should report any rise in temperature to the primary health care provider, who may take additional treatment measures, such as administering an antipyretic drug or changing the drug or dosage to bring down the temperature. The nurse should not discontinue the dosage unless specifically instructed by the primary health provider. Changing the client's diet to a soft, nonirritating diet is not necessary unless the client shows signs of impaired oral mucous membranes.

7. **Answers: 1, 2**
   RATIONALE: Fourth-generation cephalosporins have a broader spectrum of action and a longer duration of resistance to beta-lactamase (β-lactamase); however, they have no ability to treat viral infections.

8. **Answer: 1**
   RATIONALE: Natural penicillins exert a bactericidal effect on bacteria.

9. **Answer: 1**
   RATIONALE: Penicillinase is an enzyme produced by certain bacteria that inactivates the penicillin.

10. **Answers: 1, 3**
    RATIONALE: Chemical modification to slow excretion of penicillins from the kidney and addition of a chemical compound to inhibit β-lactamase inhibitors are ways the penicillins can be modified to broaden their spectrum of action.

11. **Answer: 4**
    RATIONALE: Aztreonam is contraindicated in clients who are allergic to cephalosporins and penicillins.

12. **Answer: 1**
    RATIONALE: Administer each IV dose of vancomycin over 60 minutes. Too rapid an infusion may result in a sudden and profound fall in blood pressure and shock.

CHAPTER 8

SECTION I: ASSESSING YOUR UNDERSTANDING

Activity A FILL IN THE BLANKS

1. bacteriostatic
2. bactericidal
3. positive, negative
4. tetracyclines
5. Ototoxicity
6. hepatic

Activity B DOSAGE CALCULATION

1. 1 tablet
2. 34.09 or rounded to 34 kg
3. 4 mL
4. 2 tablets
5. 2 tablets
6. 2 mL

Activity C MATCHING

1. 1. c   **2.** a   **3.** d   **4.** b
2. 1. b   **2.** c   **3.** a

Activity D SHORT ANSWERS

1. Roles of a nurse in monitoring and managing clients' needs are as follows:
   - Observe the client at frequent intervals, especially during the first 48 hours of therapy.
   - Report to the primary health care provider the occurrence of any adverse reaction before the next dose of the drug is due.
   - Report serious adverse reactions, such as a severe hypersensitivity reaction, respiratory difficulty, severe diarrhea, or a decided drop in blood pressure, to the primary health care provider immediately, because a serious adverse reaction may require emergency intervention.
2. In the teaching plan, the nurse should include the following information:
   - Take the correct dose of the drug as prescribed.
   - Complete the entire course of treatment.
   - Take each dose on an empty stomach with a full glass of water.
   - Avoid dairy products, antacids, laxatives, or products containing iron during the course of treatment.
   - Notify the primary health care provider of any adverse reactions.
   - Avoid the use of alcoholic beverages during therapy unless use has been approved by the primary health care provider.

Activity E WORD FIND PUZZLE

C									
C	O	N	F	U	S	I	O	N	
		M						O	
			F					I	
	D			O				S	
	I	N	J	U	R	Y		U	
	A					T		F	
	R							R	
	R							E	
	H							P	
	E								
	A								

SECTION II: APPLYING YOUR KNOWLEDGE

Activity F CASE STUDY

1. Tetracyclines such as doxycycline can decrease the effectiveness of oral contraceptives, leading to breakthrough bleeding or pregnancy. The nurse should advise Ms. Chase to use a backup method of contraception while taking the tetracycline.
2. The nurse should advise Ms. Chase that doxycycline can cause nausea, vomiting, dizziness, photosensitivity reaction (wear sunscreen and avoid tanning beds), pseudomembranous colitis (report diarrhea to the physician immediately), and hematologic changes (which the physician will monitor with periodic blood work).

SECTION III: PRACTICING FOR NCLEX

Activity G NCLEX-STYLE QUESTIONS

1. **Answer: 1**

   RATIONALE: Lincosamides as well as other antibacterials are contraindicated for clients with viral infections. Use is contraindicated in clients younger than 1 year. Clients with cardiac disease are not contraindicated.

2. **Answer: 2**

   RATIONALE: Increased action of a neuromuscular blocking drug may lead to severe and profound respiratory depression. Increased risk for bleeding is caused by the interaction of oral anticoagulants with tetracyclines. Decreased absorption of the lincosamide is caused by the interaction of kaolin- or aluminum-based antacids with lincosamides. Increased risk for digitalis toxicity is caused by the interaction of digoxin with tetracyclines.

3. **Answers: 1, 4, 5**

   RATIONALE: General malaise, chills, fever, and redness are signs and symptoms of an infection. Diabetes is not a cause of any infection. Blood dyscrasia is an abnormality of the blood cell structure or function, which is an adverse effect of lincosamides.

4. **Answers: 2, 4, 5**

   RATIONALE: Tests that are done before the first dose of a drug is administered are culture and sensitivity tests to see if the bacteria are sensitive to doxycycline. Because this is a tetracycline, which is harmful to the kidney, a renal function test and urinalysis should be done to evaluate the kidney. A stress test is done to monitor heart conditions. A glucose tolerance test is done to check for diabetes.

5. **Answer: 4**

   RATIONALE: Tetracyclines are not given to children younger than 9 years unless their use is absolutely necessary because these drugs may cause permanent yellow-gray-brown discoloration of the teeth.

6. **Answer: 4**

   RATIONALE: Because a GI disorder is suspected, the appropriate nursing intervention should be to save a sample of the stool for a *Clostridium difficile* test. Taking urine samples, measuring and recording vital signs, and checking blood pressure are not immediately required; these may follow at a later stage and as required.

7. **Answer: 2**

   RATIONALE: The client should take nothing by mouth (except water) for 1–2 hours before and after taking lincomycin because food impairs its absorption. The client can have food 1–2 hours before the administration; they should not be administered the drug on an empty stomach. The drug is to be administered only with water.

8. **Answer: 2**

   RATIONALE: Signs and symptoms of nephrotoxicity may include proteinuria (protein in the urine), hematuria (blood in the urine), an increase in the blood urea nitrogen (BUN) level, a decrease in urine output, and an increase in the serum creatinine concentration. Ototoxicity includes tinnitus (ringing in the ears), dizziness, roaring in the ears, vertigo, and a mild to severe loss of hearing. Neuromuscular blockade includes acute muscular paralysis and apnea. Cardiac issues do not occur with aminoglycosides.

9. **Answers: 1, 4, 5**

   RATIONALE: As part of the preadministration assessment, the nurse should obtain a swab for the culture. The nurse should also ensure that the client's hepatic and renal function tests are conducted, and that urine is obtained for testing. Monitoring the client's vital signs every 4 hours and recording observations in the client's chart are interventions related to the client's ongoing assessment, not preadministration assessment.

10. **Answer: 3**

    RATIONALE: Neuromuscular blockade or respiratory paralysis may occur after administration of the aminoglycosides. The best vital sign measurement of respiration would be the respiratory rate. Temperature measures fever and the pulse, and blood pressure indicates the workings of the heart and circulatory system.

CHAPTER 9

SECTION I: ASSESSING YOUR UNDERSTANDING

Activity A FILL IN THE BLANKS

1. Fluoroquinolones
2. IV or intravenously
3. Metronidazole or Flagyl
4. superinfection
5. tendon rupture

Activity B DOSAGE CALCULATION

1. 1 tablet
2. 325 mL
3. 1 tablet
4. 12 mL

Activity C MATCHING

1. **1.** c   **2.** d   **3.** a   **4.** b
2. **1.** a   **2.** c   **3.** d   **4.** b

Activity D SHORT ANSWERS

1. A nurse should perform the following assessments for a client who is being administered fluoroquinolones via the IV route:
   - Inspect needle site and area around the needle every hour.
   - Perform the assessment frequently if the client is found restless or uncooperative.
   - Check the rate of infusion every 15 minutes.
   - Inspect the vein used for IV infusion every 4 hours for signs of tenderness, pain, and redness.
   - In apparent situations, restart IV in another vein and notify the primary health care provider.
2. To determine the effectiveness of the treatment plan, the nurse should ensure the following:
   - Pain or discomfort following IM or IV administration is relieved or eliminated.
   - Anxiety is reduced.
   - The client and family demonstrate understanding of the drug regimen.

Activity E CHART THE FINDING

1. *The bacteria are not sensitive to the antibacterial drug ordered.*

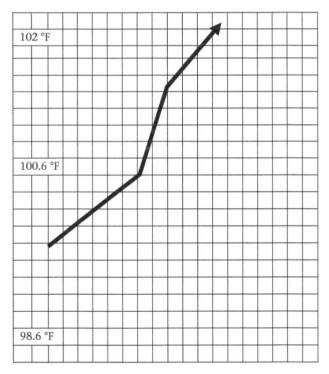

2. *The bacteria are sensitive to the antibacterial drug ordered.*

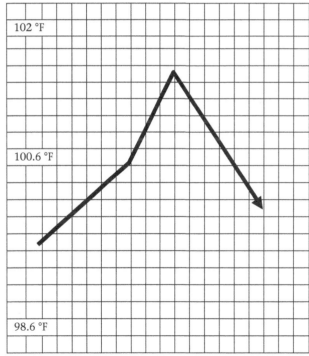

SECTION II: APPLYING YOUR KNOWLEDGE

Activity F CASE STUDY

1. Before administering a fluoroquinolone like Cipro, the nurse identifies and records the signs and symptoms of the infections, takes a thorough allergy history, takes and records vital signs, and obtains a urine specimen for urinalysis, if ordered.
2. The syringe pump should have 40 mL of solution for one 400-mg dose of Cipro to be administered to Mrs. Peterson.

SECTION III: PRACTICING FOR NCLEX

Activity G NCLEX-STYLE QUESTIONS

1. **Answer: 3**
   RATIONALE: Common adverse effects from the administration of ciprofloxacin (a fluoroquinolone) include nausea, diarrhea, headache, abdominal pain or discomfort, dizziness, and photosensitivity. These are primarily gastrointestinal.

2. **Answer: 1**
   RATIONALE: To maintain continuity in care, the nurse should instruct the client and client's family to complete the full course of treatment. All drugs need not be taken with food. The nurse should instruct the client to administer the drug with or without food in the stomach, depending on what has been prescribed by the physician. Although it is a good idea to avoid drinking alcoholic beverages, these particular drugs do not adversely interact with alcohol, except Flagyl. The nurse should instruct the client and client's family to monitor for adverse symptoms for 5–7 days or longer depending on how long the drug is taken.

3. **Answer: 1**
   RATIONALE: The nurse should prepare and administer a dose of 2 mL of ciprofloxacin to the client IV. The available strength of the drug dose is 2 g/5 mL. The prescribed dose is 800 mg, so the nurse should prepare a dose of 2 mL. The nurse should not prepare a dose of 15 mL, 1 mL, or 4 mL.

4. **Answer: 2**
   RATIONALE: Photosensitivity (exaggerated skin reaction to sun exposure) is a more serious adverse reaction seen with the administration of the fluoroquinolones, especially ofloxacin.

5. **Answers: 1, 2, 4**
   RATIONALE: Some drugs are made so that they release the drug over time in the body; these formulations are known as extended-release (XR), sustained-release (SR), or controlled-release (CR) drugs. Immediate release indicates that all of the drug is released immediately.

6. **Answers: 2, 3, 4**
   RATIONALE: When conducting an ongoing assessment, the nurse should monitor vital signs of the client, observe for an increase in temperature in the client indicating the antibacterial is not effective, and ask the client about ongoing urinary tract symptoms such as pain or urgency. Determining initial signs of infection in the client is part of the nurse's preadministration assessment before the administration of the drug, not during ongoing assessment. The nurse should monitor for an increase and not a decrease in the pulse and respiratory rate.

7. **Answer: 4**
   RATIONALE: Pseudomembranous colitis is one type of bacterial superinfection. This potentially life-threatening problem develops because of an overgrowth of the microorganism *Clostridium difficile* in the bowel.

8. **Answers: 2, 3, 5**
   RATIONALE: When caring for a client receiving an intramuscular anti-infective, the nurse should rotate and monitor the injection sites if more than one injection is to be given. Ensure that any IM injection contains no more than 3 mL. If an injection is more than 3 mL, divide the drug and give it as two separate injections. Volumes larger than 3 mL will not be absorbed properly. The following items are done when the route is IV: assess the vein used for infusion for any signs of irritation and check the infusion site more frequently.

9. **Answer: 1**
   RATIONALE: The nurse should know that fluoroquinolones have to be administered cautiously in clients with a history of seizures. Aminoglycosides and not fluoroquinolones are administered cautiously to elderly clients, clients who have neuromuscular disorders, and clients who have renal failure.

10. **Answers: 1, 3, 5**
    RATIONALE: Symptoms of bacterial superinfection of the bowel include diarrhea or bloody diarrhea, rectal bleeding, and abdominal cramping. Vomiting is a common adverse reaction to a number of antibacterials, and lesions may occur due to a hypersensitivity reaction.

11. **Answer: 2**
    RATIONALE: When caring for a client receiving fluoroquinolones, the nurse should inspect the vein used for infusion frequently. The nurse should check the rate of infusion every 15 minutes and not every 2 hours. The nurse should change the vein used for infusion only in case of thrombophlebitis or phlebitis seen in the client and not otherwise. Raising the arm does not reduce vein inflammation.

12. **Answer: 1**
    RATIONALE: The nurse should ensure that the client is not younger than 18 years to be certain that fluoroquinolone is not contraindicated. The nurse checks that the client does not have preexisting hearing loss, myasthenia gravis, or Parkinson disease when aminoglycoside is considered.

13. Answers: 1, 2, 4
> **RATIONALE:** The nurse should instruct the client to wear long-sleeve clothing, sunscreen, and brimmed hats to assist in preventing photosensitive reactions. Wearing light makeup will not help the client avoid a skin reaction. Venturing out on hazy and cloudy days cannot be considered safe. The nurse should inform the client that the glare during hazy or cloudy days can cause skin reactions as much as when the sky is clear.

CHAPTER 10

SECTION I: ASSESSING YOUR UNDERSTANDING

Activity A FILL IN THE BLANKS

1. isoniazid
2. immunodeficiency
3. Extrapulmonary
4. tyramine
5. 2

Activity B DOSAGE CALCULATION

1. 1.5 tablets
2. 2 tablets
3. 4 tablets

Activity C MATCHING

1. **1.** d **2.** c **3.** a **4.** b

Activity D SHORT ANSWERS

1. When caring for a client with tuberculosis, many laboratory and diagnostic tests may be necessary before starting antitubercular therapy, including skin or blood testing for disease, radiographic studies, sputum culture and sensitivity tests, and various types of laboratory tests, such as a complete blood count. The nurse should see that results of these tests are on the chart for the primary health care provider to use in the determination of therapy. It also is important to assess the family history and a history of contacts if the client has active TB.
2. To decrease the chance of nonadherence with the drug regimen, the nurse emphasizes the following points when any of these drugs are prescribed on an outpatient basis:
   - Ask the client what they think causes the symptoms, and promote health literacy by integrating the client's beliefs and fears into how the bacteria invade the body and how the drugs work to kill it.
   - Discuss tuberculosis, its causes and communicability, and the need for long-term therapy for disease control using simple, nonmedical terms.
   - Use visual props or educational materials to help emphasize that short-term treatment is ineffective.
   - Review the drug therapy regimen, including the prescribed drugs, doses, and frequency of administration.
   - Reassure the client that various combinations of drugs are effective in treating tuberculosis.
   - Urge the client to take the drugs exactly as prescribed and not to omit, increase, or decrease the dosage unless directed to do so by the health care provider.
   - Instruct the client about possible adverse reactions and the need to notify the primary health care provider should any occur.
   - Arrange for direct observation therapy with the client and family.
   - Instruct the client in measures to minimize gastrointestinal upset.
   - Advise the client to avoid alcohol and the use of nonprescription drugs, especially those containing aspirin, unless use is approved by the health care provider.
   - Reassure the client and family that the results of therapy will be monitored by periodic laboratory and diagnostic tests and follow-up visits with the health care provider.
3. The nurse should keep the following things in mind when evaluating the treatment plan:
   - The therapeutic drug effect is achieved and the infection is controlled.
   - Adverse reactions are identified, reported to the primary health care provider, and managed successfully.
   - No evidence of injury.
   - Adequate nutritional status is maintained.
   - The client manages the drug routine.

Activity E WORD FIND PUZZLE

Q	U	I	E	S	C	E	N	T
C								
H								
R	O							
O		U			H			
N	P	O	S	I	T	I	V	E
I			E		V			
C				H				
			A	N	Y	O	N	E
							L	
								D

SECTION II: APPLYING YOUR KNOWLEDGE

Activity F CASE STUDY

1. Additional assessment before antitubercular drugs are started should include sputum culture and sensitivity testing, complete blood count, radiographic studies, medication history, and a family and contacts history for those with active TB.
2. Ongoing assessment of clients taking antitubercular drug therapy should include monitoring for adverse reactions and vital signs, as well as adherence to taking the scheduled medications.

SECTION III: PRACTICING FOR NCLEX

Activity G NCLEX-STYLE QUESTIONS

1. **Answer: 3**
   RATIONALE: When caring for a client who has been administered rifampin, the nurse should monitor for reddish-orange discoloration of the bodily fluids as one of the drug's generalized adverse reactions. Myalgia is an adverse reaction of pyrazinamide and not rifampin. Jaundice is an adverse reaction of isoniazid. Dermatitis and pruritus are adverse reactions of ethambutol and not rifampin.
2. **Answers: 1, 2, 3**
   RATIONALE: The nurse should ensure that the client is not younger than 13 years, does not have cataracts, and does not have a hypersensitivity to the drug. Any of these conditions in the client contraindicate the use of ethambutol. The nurse should ensure that the client does not have diabetes mellitus or gout only if the client has to be administered pyrazinamide and not ethambutol.
3. **Answer: 1**
   RATIONALE: The nurse knows that an alternative regimen of twice-weekly dosing promotes nutrition and decreases the incidence of gastric upset in the client. It also promotes client compliance to the drug regimen on an outpatient basis. An alternative dosing regimen of twice weekly does not promote fluid balance in the body or reduce the incidence of liver dysfunction. Taking vitamin B_6 or pyridoxine prevents the occurrence of neuropathy, not following an alternative regimen of twice-weekly dosing.
4. **Answers: 1, 2, 3**
   RATIONALE: The nurse should know if the client is taking digoxin, oral anticoagulants, or oral contraceptives along with prescribed rifampin. Rifampin when taken along with digoxin decreases the serum level. Rifampin when taken along with oral anticoagulants leads to decreased anticoagulant effectiveness and when taken with oral contraceptives leads to decreased contraceptive effectiveness. Colchicine and allopurinol more commonly interact with pyrazinamide, leading to decreased effectiveness.
5. **Answer: 1**
   RATIONALE: The nurse should monitor for jaundice in the form of skin discoloration as a manifestation of a severe hepatotoxic reaction to pyrazinamide. Epigastric distress and hematologic changes are some of the reactions of isoniazid but may indicate other issues than liver involvement. Yellow-colored sclera indicates jaundice, but discolored body fluids (tears) are not from jaundice; instead, they are an expected reaction of the medications.
6. **Answer: 2**
   RATIONALE: Rifampin is contraindicated in clients with hepatic or renal impairment. Pyrazinamide is contraindicated in clients with diabetes mellitus and those who have tested positive for HIV. Ethambutol is contraindicated in clients with diabetic retinopathy.
7. **Answers: 1, 2, 5**
   RATIONALE: Individuals living in crowded conditions, those with compromised immune systems (like those with HIV), and individuals with debilitative conditions are especially susceptible to tuberculosis.
8. **Answer: 3**
   RATIONALE: Tuberculosis is transmitted from one person to another by droplets dispersed in the air when an infected person coughs or sneezes.

9. **Answers: 1, 2, 3, 4, 5**
   RATIONALE: Tuberculosis primarily affects the lungs, but it can affect other organs including the liver, kidneys, spleen, and uterus. Tuberculosis found to affect organs outside the lungs is known as *extrapulmonary* tuberculosis.
10. **Answers: 1, 2, 3, 4**
    RATIONALE: Antitubercular drugs treat active tuberculosis infection and are used as prophylactic therapy to prevent the activation of tuberculosis, which may be dormant in the lungs. They render the client noninfectious to others.
11. **Answers: 1, 3, 5**
    RATIONALE: X-ray studies, sputum analyses, and physical examinations can be used to determine if a client with HIV and a negative skin test has active TB.
12. **Answer: 1**
    RATIONALE: Optic neuritis is a dose-related adverse reaction that can occur during treatment with ethambutol. The symptoms of optic neuritis are a decrease in visual acuity and change in color perception.

CHAPTER 11

SECTION I: ASSESSING YOUR UNDERSTANDING

Activity A FILL IN THE BLANKS

1. living cell
2. 200
3. Ritonavir
4. Antibiotics
5. Antiretroviral

Activity B DOSAGE CALCULATION

1. 325 mL
2. 5 mL
3. 2 tablets
4. 4 mL
5. 250 mg

Activity C MATCHING

1. 1. a   2. d   3. b   4. c
2. 1. c   2. a   3. d   4. b

Activity D SHORT ANSWERS

1. Before administering an antiviral drug, the preadministration assessment of the client

receiving an antiviral drug depends on the client's symptoms or diagnosis. HSV is divided into HSV-1, which causes oral, ocular, or facial infections, and HSV-2, which causes genital infection. However, either type can cause disease at either body site. The client may appear irritable, lethargic, and jaundiced and may have difficulty breathing or experience seizures. The nurse assesses the site of the lesion (e.g., the mouth, face, eyes, or genitalia) as a baseline for comparison during therapy. The client's general state of health and resistance to infection is also assessed. The nurse then records the client's symptoms and complaints. In addition, the nurse takes and records the client's vital signs.

2. During the administration of an antiviral drug, a nurse should perform the following ongoing assessments, which will depend on the reason for giving the antiviral drug. The nurse monitors for and reports any adverse reactions from the antiviral drug. Additionally, the nurse inspects the client with hepatitis B (an inflammation of the liver) for symptoms of increasing liver involvement such as nausea, vomiting, and abdominal pain; changes in color of urine or stool; and jaundice. Liver function studies are also indicated.

Activity E VIRAL SUDOKU PUZZLE

FLU	HZV	HIV	HPV	HCV	HSV	RSV	CMV	HBV
HPV	HCV	HBV	CMV	RSV	FLU	HZV	HIV	HSV
CMV	RSV	HSV	HZV	HIV	HBV	FLU	HPV	HCV
HSV	FLU	RSV	HCV	HPV	CMV	HIV	HBV	HZV
HIV	HBV	HPV	HSV	FLU	HZV	HCV	RSV	CMV
HCV	CMV	HZV	RSV	HBV	HIV	HSV	FLU	HPV
RSV	HPV	CMV	FLU	HZV	HCV	HBV	HSV	HIV
HBV	HSV	HCV	HIV	CMV	RSV	HPV	HZV	FLU
HZV	HIV	FLU	HBV	HSV	HPV	CMV	HCV	RSV

SECTION II: APPLYING YOUR KNOWLEDGE

Activity F CASE STUDY

1. The nurse needs to obtain Mr. Atain's vital signs, a medication history (prescription and nonprescription), and his symptoms and complaints and assess his general state of health.
2. The nurse should caution Mr. Atain regarding St. John's wort because it can reduce the effectiveness of his antiretroviral therapy. The nurse should encourage Mr. Atain to disclose the use of all over-the-counter medications and supplements to his primary health care provider and not to begin taking any over-the-counter medications or supplements without consulting the primary health care provider first. The nurse can suggest the client talk to the primary health care provider about combination medications that include multiple antiretrovirals. The nurse should also encourage Mr. Atain to discuss his depressive mood with the primary health care provider.

SECTION III: PRACTICING FOR NCLEX

Activity G NCLEX-STYLE QUESTIONS

1. **Answers: 1, 2, 4**
   RATIONALE: While administering ribavirin, the nurse should use a small-particle aerosol generator and discard and replace the solution every 24 hours. Ribavirin can worsen the respiratory status and the nurse should monitor the client's respiratory system for any signs of deterioration. Ribavirin does not induce anorexia or nephrotoxicity in the client.

2. **Answer: 2**
   RATIONALE: When clarithromycin is taken along with an antiretroviral drug, it results in an increased serum level of both drugs. An increased serum level of the antiretroviral is the effect of the interaction of antifungals and antiretroviral drugs. There is no risk of toxicity associated with combining the two drugs. Combining the two drugs also does not significantly decrease the effectiveness of either of the drugs.

3. **Answer: 3**
   RATIONALE: Before beginning treatment of the client with HSV-1 (HSV-1 causes painful vesicular lesions), the nurse should inspect the areas of the body affected with the lesions as a baseline for comparison during therapy. Recording a client's temperature and blood pressure are routine interventions that the nurse should follow and are not specific to the treatment of HSV-1. There

is no need to save a sample of the client's urine unless specifically instructed to do so by the health care provider.

4. **Answer: 3**
   RATIONALE: Phlebitis refers to the inflammation of the veins of the client. It commonly occurs when drugs are administered intravenously. Phlebitis does not occur in clients who are being administered drugs orally, intramuscularly, or transdermally.

5. **Answer: 4**
   RATIONALE: The nurse should exercise caution while caring for clients who have been administered indinavir and have a history of bladder stone formation. Indinavir does not react significantly to exacerbate the condition of clients with cardiac disorders or renal impairment. The drugs fosamprenavir and amprenavir, and not indinavir, should be used cautiously in clients with sulfonamide allergy.

6. **Answer: 3**
   RATIONALE: Avoid generating dust while preparing to administer didanosine to the client. Didanosine should be given on an empty stomach and not with meals. The drug should be dissolved in 4 ounces of water and not 2 ounces. The solution should be given immediately to the client after preparation and not refrigerated.

7. **Answer: 3**
   RATIONALE: Required dosage is 800 mg. Available drug is 200 mg. Number of tablets required is 4 (800/200) per dosage.

8. **Answers: 1, 3, 4, 5**
   RATIONALE: A virus can enter the body through various routes including being swallowed, inhaled, injected with a contaminated needle or transmitted through the bite of an insect. Intact skin is a protective barrier for both viral and bacterial invasion.

9. **Answers: 1, 3, 4, 5**
   RATIONALE: Viruses can cause infections of the skin, eye, nose, throat, and respiratory system such as warts, the common cold, or influenza. Viruses can also cause systemic infections including West Nile, hepatitis B and C, and HIV.

10. **Answer: 1**
    RATIONALE: HAART is multidrug therapy that is used to treat HIV.

11. **Answers: 1, 2, 3**
    RATIONALE: Retroviruses contain an enzyme called reverse transcriptase, which is used to turn the primary component RNA into DNA. Human immunodeficiency virus is an example of a retrovirus.

CHAPTER 12

SECTION I: ASSESSING YOUR UNDERSTANDING

Activity A FILL IN THE BLANKS

1. Systemic
2. Superficial
3. Paromomycin
4. Renal
5. prophylactically

Activity B DOSAGE CALCULATION

1. 125.25 mg = 5 mL
2. 28 capsules
3. 16 tablets

Activity C SEQUENCING AND MATCHING

1. **3**   **1**   **4**   **2**
2. **1.** b   **2.** d   **3.** a   **4.** e   **5.** c
3. **1.** b   **2.** c   **3.** d   **4.** a

Activity D SHORT ANSWERS

1. The nurse should perform the following preadministration assessments before administering an antifungal drug for a vaginal yeast infection:
   - Assess client for signs of infection before first dose of an antifungal drug.
   - Assess whether the woman is pregnant or lactating. Most antifungals are contraindicated.
   - Ask about pain; describe white plaques or sore areas on mucous membranes or oral or perineal areas, and inquire about any vaginal discharge or odor.
   - Take and record vital signs.
2. The client should teach the following items to prevent the spread of pinworms to others:
   - Wash all bedding and bed clothes once treatment has started.
   - Daily bathing (showering is best) is recommended.
   - Disinfect toilet facilities daily, and disinfect the bathtub or shower stall immediately after bathing.
   - Keep towels and facecloths for bathing separate from those of other family members.
   - Wash hands thoroughly after urinating or defecating and before preparing and eating food.
   - Clean under the fingernails daily and avoid putting fingers in the mouth or biting the nails.
   - Food handlers should not resume work until a full course of treatment is completed and stools do not contain the parasite.
   - Child care workers should be especially careful of diaper disposal and proper hand washing to prevent the spread of infections.

Activity E CROSSWORD PUZZLE

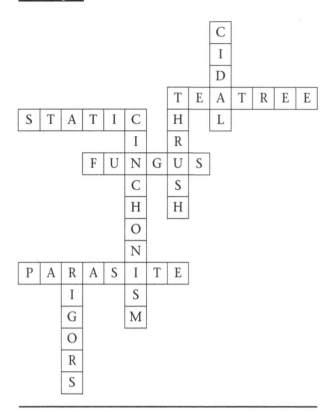

SECTION II: APPLYING YOUR KNOWLEDGE

Activity F CASE STUDY

1. Yeast infections, such as those caused by *Candida albicans,* are known as candidiasis. Infection of the mouth by the microorganism *C. albicans* is commonly called thrush. Candidiasis affects women in the vulvovaginal area and immunocompromised clients with chronic conditions such as diabetes or who are pregnant. Johnnie is HIV positive and is immunocompromised. The HAART therapy does not put him at risk, but it will not prevent an opportunistic infection either.
2. Each dose will contain 5 mL of the nystatin suspension. The nurse should instruct Johnnie to swish and hold the solution in the mouth for several seconds (or as long as possible), gargle, and then swallow the solution.

SECTION III: PRACTICING FOR NCLEX

Activity G NCLEX-STYLE QUESTIONS

1. **Answer: 3**
   RATIONALE: The client needs to observe for any redness or stinging reaction in a client who is treated with topical administration of an antifungal drug. Topical administration is unlikely to cause nausea and diarrhea; these are adverse reactions that can be caused by systemic administration of an antifungal drug.

2. Answer: 3
RATIONALE: History of heart failure is a contraindication the nurse must consider when assessing a client for itraconazole therapy. The drug is not contraindicated in clients with bone marrow suppression, severe liver disease, or history of asthma.

3. Answer: 1
RATIONALE: When administering an IV solution of amphotericin B, the nurse should ensure that the IV solution is protected from light since it is light sensitive. The nurse should ensure that the solution is used within 8 hours after the drug is reconstituted, not 48, to prevent loss of drug activity. The nurse should not freeze the unused solution; it should be discarded. The solution should not be stored.

4. Answers: 1, 3, 4
RATIONALE: When administering amphotericin B by IV infusion, be aware that immediate adverse reactions can occur. Nausea, vomiting, hypotension, tachypnea, fever, and chills may occur within 15–20 minutes of beginning the IV infusion. Hypertension is not an adverse reaction.

5. Answer: 2
RATIONALE: The nurse should encourage the client to verbalize feelings since it will help reduce the client's anxiety regarding the situation. The nurse need not check the client's blood pressure, provide the client with a blanket, or keep the client away from light, since her highest need is assistance in problem solving her situation.

6. Answer: 4
RATIONALE: In the teaching plan, the nurse should include informing the client about keeping towels and facecloths separate from those of other family members to avoid the spread of the infection.

7. Answer: 3
RATIONALE: The nurse should instruct the client that the following adverse reactions can occur when taking ketoconazole: headache, dizziness, and drowsiness. The client is unlikely to experience unusual fatigue, yellow skin, darkened urine, fever, sore throat, skin rash, nausea, vomiting, or diarrhea, since these are not the adverse reactions caused by ketoconazole. Unusual fatigue, yellow skin, and darkened urine are reactions caused by itraconazole, while fever, sore throat, or skin rash are reactions caused by griseofulvin. Nausea, vomiting, or diarrhea is caused by flucytosine.

8. Answer: 4
RATIONALE: As the client is acutely ill, the nurse should carefully measure and record the fluid intake and output. The nurse should record the vital signs of the client every 4 hours, not 12 hours, and observe the client every 2 hours, not 4 hours, for malaria symptoms. There is no need to collect urine samples of the client for testing.

9. Answer: 1
RATIONALE: Quinine is contraindicated in clients with myasthenia gravis as it may cause respiratory distress and dysphagia. Quinine, however, is not contraindicated in clients with thyroid disease, blood dyscrasias, or diabetes.

10. Answer: 2
RATIONALE: The nurse should follow hospital procedure for transporting the stool sample to the laboratory. Unless ordered otherwise, the nurse should save all stools that are passed after the drug is given. The nurse should visually inspect all stools and not just when the client reports something unusual. Specimens should be taken by swabbing the perianal area with a cellophane tape–covered swab to get a good sample.

11. Answer: 3
RATIONALE: The nurse should educate the client to use chlorine bleach to disinfect toilet facilities or the shower stall after bathing. The barrier method and not birth control pills for contraception is the proper recommendation. The entire dose for treatment should be adhered to even if the symptoms of the condition have disappeared. The drug should be taken with water and not milk.

12. Answer: 2
RATIONALE: Nephrotoxicity and ototoxicity are adverse reactions associated with paromomycin. Peripheral neuropathy may occur with metronidazole use but not paromomycin. Thrombocytopenia is associated with anthelmintic medications, and vertigo and hypotension are the adverse effects of chloroquine.

13. Answer: 1
RATIONALE: The nurse should instruct the client to take metronidazole with meals or immediately afterward. Alcohol should be avoided for the duration of the treatment and not just for the first week. Cimetidine should not be taken as it decreases the metabolism of metronidazole. Metronidazole does not cause photosensitivity, so there is no need to wear additional clothing to protect the skin from the sun.

CHAPTER 13

SECTION I: ASSESSING YOUR UNDERSTANDING

Activity A FILL IN THE BLANKS

1. prostaglandins
2. platelets
3. Pancytopenia
4. Reye
5. Tinnitus

Activity B DOSAGE CALCULATION

1. 2 tablets
2. 2 tablets
3. No, it is 1950 mg
4. 150 mg, 0.5 or ½ tablet
5. 4 tablets
6. 2 tablets

Activity C MATCHING

1. **1.** b   **2.** d   **3.** a   **4.** c
2. **1.** c   **2.** a   **3.** d   **4.** b

Activity D SHORT ANSWERS

1. The difference between acute and chronic pain are as follows:
   - Acute pain is brief and lasts less than 3–6 months. Causes range from a sunburn to post-operative, procedural, or traumatic pain. Acute pain usually subsides when the injury heals.
   - Chronic pain lasts more than 6 months and is often associated with specific diseases, such as cancer, sickle cell anemia, and end-stage organ or system failure. Various neuropathic and musculoskeletal disorders, such as headaches, fibromyalgia, rheumatoid arthritis, and osteoar-thritis, are also causes of chronic pain.
2. The nurse can monitor and manage the discomfort of the client receiving a salicylate or a nonsalicylate in the following ways:
   - Notify primary health care provider if there has been no relief from pain or discomfort.
   - Assess for bleeding or inflammation.
   - To minimize GI distress, administer drug with food or milk or give antacids.
   - Check color of stools (bright red or black indicating bleeding) and report.

Activity E CROSSWORD PUZZLE

(Crossword puzzle grid with answers: PAIN, ASTRICIDIS/GASTRITIS column, INFLAMMATION column, CHRONIC, TINNITUS, ACUTE)

SECTION II: APPLYING YOUR KNOWLEDGE

Activity F CASE STUDY

1. Many people use acetaminophen for pain relief because it does not cause GI distress. Because acetaminophen is contained in many cold preparations, the 3250 mg daily maximum can be unintentionally surpassed when combining cold and pain relievers. You should instruct parents to be aware of the different drug preparations being used, especially when teens and adolescents may self-administer these drugs for cold or flu symptoms. Examples of nonpain relievers containing acetaminophen include Actifed, Benadryl, Cepacol, DayQuil, Formula 44, NyQuil, Robitussin, Sudafed, and Theraflu.
2. In a 24-hour period, what is the potential acetaminophen intake you have when ill with a cold or flu? How close are you to the 3250 mg daily maximum?

SECTION III: PRACTICING FOR NCLEX

Activity G NCLEX-STYLE QUESTIONS

1. **Answer: 2**
   RATIONALE: The nurse needs to monitor the client for GI bleeding, as it is an adverse reaction caused by the administration of salicylates. Skin eruptions, jaundice, and neurologic disorders are not adverse reactions of the administration of salicylates. Skin eruptions and jaundice are the adverse reactions of administration of acetaminophen.

2. **Answers: 1, 3, 4**
   RATIONALE: For clients with influenza, viral illness, or bleeding disorders, salicylate use is contraindicated. Salicylates are also contraindicated for clients with a known history of hypersensitivity to the salicylates. Salicylates are not known to be contraindicated in clients with heart disease. Salicylates are administered with caution in clients with hepatic or renal disorders, but incidence of these conditions does not contraindicate the administration of salicylates.

3. **Answer: 1**
   RATIONALE: Nausea is one of the symptoms that can be observed in a client with salicylate levels between 150 and 250 mcg/mL. Respiratory alkalosis, hemorrhage, and asterixis are associated with salicylate levels in excess of 400 mcg/mL.

4. **Answer: 4**
   RATIONALE: Combining loop diuretics with acetaminophen may result in decreased effectiveness of the diuretic. Combining loop diuretics with acetaminophen does not increase the possibility of toxicity or bleeding, nor does it decrease the effectiveness of acetaminophen.

5. **Answers: 1, 4, 5**
   RATIONALE: The nurse should instruct the client to avoid OTC drugs that may contain aspirin on the label. The client should purchase the drug in small quantities when used on an occasional basis to prevent deterioration. If a surgery or a dental procedure is anticipated, the client should notify the primary health care provider or dentist. The client should avoid eating foods such as paprika, licorice, prunes, and raisins as they are rich in salicylates. Salicylates should be stored in tightly closed containers and not in ventilated locations.

6. **Answer: 1**
   RATIONALE: One of the adverse reactions that the nurse should monitor for in a client who has been administered salicylates is GI bleeding. Hypoglycemia, pancytopenia, and hemolytic anemia are symptoms associated with acetaminophen and not salicylates.

7. **Answer: 2**
   RATIONALE: Aspirin can be used to treat inflammatory conditions such as rheumatoid arthritis. Since aspirin increases bleeding tendencies, it is contraindicated in clients with hemophilia, clients who have just undergone surgical operations, or clients taking anticoagulants.

8. **Answer: 1**
   RATIONALE: Malaise is one of the symptoms associated with acetaminophen toxicity when a client has been prescribed acetaminophen. Increased anxiety, hyperglycemia, and bradycardia are not symptoms generally associated with acetaminophen toxicity.

9. **Answers: 1, 3**
   RATIONALE: Terms used to describe pain duration are acute (less than 3–6 months) pain and chronic (more than 6 months) pain.

10. **Answers: 1, 2**
    RATIONALE: Acute pain is brief and lasts less than 3–6 months. Postoperative pain and procedural pain represent acute pain.

11. **Answer: 4**
    RATIONALE: Chronic pain lasts more than 6 months.

12. **Answers: 1, 4, 5**
    RATIONALE: Chronic pain lasts more than 6 months and is often associated with specific diseases, such as fibromyalgia, rheumatoid arthritis, and osteoarthritis.

CHAPTER 14

SECTION I: ASSESSING YOUR UNDERSTANDING

Activity A FILL IN THE BLANKS

1. location, intensity
2. cyclooxygenase
3. Celecoxib
4. NSAIDs
5. Reye
6. inflammation

Activity B DOSAGE CALCULATION

1. 3 tablets
2. 2 tablets
3. 1 tablet
4. 1 tablet
5. 1 tablet

Activity C MATCHING

1. 1. c   **2.** a   **3.** b

2. 1. d   **2.** c   **3.** a   **4.** b

Activity D SHORT ANSWERS

1. NSAIDS are used to treat the following:
   - Pain and inflammation associated with osteoarthritis, rheumatoid arthritis, and other musculoskeletal disorders
   - Mild to moderate pain
   - Primary dysmenorrhea (menstrual cramps)
   - Fever reduction
2. Pain is often considered the "fifth vital sign" in nursing assessment; it is important to appropriately assess pain in order to provide effective pain management. Failure to assess pain adequately is a major factor in the under treatment of pain.
3. The nurse should monitor the client for the following adverse reactions of NSAIDs on the sensory organs:
   - Visual disturbances, blurred or diminished vision, diplopia (double vision), swollen or irritated eyes, photophobia (sensitivity to light), reversible loss of color vision
   - Tinnitus (ringing in the ears)
   - Taste change
   - Rhinitis (runny nose)

Activity E CROSSWORD PUZZLE

```
L           P           M
O           R           I       I
C  Y  C  L  O  O  X  Y  G  E  N  A  S  E  -  1
A     A     S           R       T
T     R     T           A       E
I     D     A           I       N
O     I     G           N       S
N     O     L           E       I
      V     A                   T
      A     N                   Y
      S     D
      C     I
      U     N
      L     S
      A
      R
```

SECTION II: APPLYING YOUR KNOWLEDGE

Activity F CASE STUDY

1. The nurse should tell Mr. Park that ibuprofen works in a way similar to his aspirin (inhibition of prostaglandin synthesis), and he may experience easy bruising and bleeding with the combination. He should notify other health care providers, including the dentist, that he is taking ibuprofen. The nurse should relay that prolonged use of ibuprofen can increase blood pressure and that home monitoring is recommended to ensure the dosage of his antihypertensive continues to be appropriate.

2. The nurse should educate Mr. Park about the following key aspects of the administration of his medication:
   - Take the medication every 8 hours as needed for pain.
   - Do not increase the dose without discussing it with the physician first.
   - Take the medication with food or milk and a full glass of water.

SECTION III: PRACTICING FOR NCLEX

Activity G NCLEX-STYLE QUESTIONS

1. **Answers: 1, 3, 5**
   RATIONALE: The nurse should inform the client that epigastric pain, abdominal distress, and intestinal ulceration are GI system adverse reactions of NSAIDs. Appendicitis and indigestion are not adverse reactions of NSAIDs.

2. **Answer: 1**
   RATIONALE: The nurse should identify the client using sulfonamides as the only client not at risk for using ibuprofen. Clients with peptic ulceration, cardiac disease, or stroke are contraindicated for treatment with ibuprofen.

3. **Answer: 4**
   RATIONALE: Before administering an NSAID to the client, the nurse should assess the client for bleeding disorders. Visual disturbances, allergic skin reactions, and dizziness are monitored during ongoing assessments.

4. **Answer: 3**
   RATIONALE: The nurse should suggest that the client take medication with food. This will promote an optimal response to therapy. Avoiding exercise, restricting to a liquid diet, or restricting mobility will not promote an optimal response to therapy. Exercise and mobility are essential in maintaining free movement of the joints. Clients taking NSAIDs may be affected by acid production in the stomach, hence the need for a complete, nutritious diet.

5. **Answer: 4**
   RATIONALE: The nurse should monitor the client for GI bleeding, which is an adverse reaction of indomethacin administration.

6. **Answer: 4**
   RATIONALE: NSAID treatment for clients older than 65 years should begin with a reduced dosage, which is increased slowly due to escalated risk of serious ulcer diseases. Older clients are not at an increased risk for inflammation, erythema, or an increase in the number of RBCs due to NSAIDs.

7. **Answers: 2, 4, 5**
   RATIONALE: The nurse should instruct the client not to use the drugs on a regular basis unless notifying the primary health care provider, to avoid use of aspirin, and to take the drug with a full glass of water or with food in the client's teaching plan. Avoiding physical activities during drug therapy and keeping towels separate from those of other family members are not points that the nurse should include in the plan.

8. **Answer: 2**
   RATIONALE: Blocking cyclooxygenase-2 is responsible for the pain-relieving effects of NSAIDs. Cyclooxygenase-1 is responsible for maintenance of the stomach lining, not pain and inflammatory regulation.

9. **Answer: 1**
   RATIONALE: The most common side effects caused by the NSAIDs involve the GI tract, including the stomach.

10. **Answer: 3**
    RATIONALE: A hypersensitivity to aspirin is a contraindication for all NSAIDs.

11. **Answer: 1**
    RATIONALE: Celecoxib (Celebrex) is the NSAID that appears to work by specifically inhibiting cyclooxygenase-2, without inhibiting cyclooxygenase-1.

12. **Answer: 3**
    RATIONALE: Cyclooxygenase-1 is responsible for maintenance of the stomach lining, not pain and inflammatory regulation.

CHAPTER 15

SECTION I: ASSESSING YOUR UNDERSTANDING

Activity A FILL IN THE BLANKS

1. morphine
2. antagonist
3. opium
4. Heroin
5. cachectic

Activity B DOSAGE CALCULATION

1. ½ tablet
2. 2 tablets
3. 2 tablets
4. 1 mL
5. 12.5 mL

Activity C OUT IN THE COMMUNITY

Class discussion: Review Chapter 15 and the discussion of the use of the term *opioid*. Can you identify the relationship between the term *narcotic* and the fear of opiates for pain relief?

Activity D SHORT ANSWERS

1. When a client is receiving drugs through a PCA infusion pump, the nurse should educate the client on the following points:
   - The location of the control button that activates the administration of the drug.
   - The difference between the control button and the button to call the nurse (when both are similar in appearance and feel).
   - The machine regulates the dose of the drug as well as the time interval between doses.
   - If the control button is used too soon after the last dose, the machine will not deliver the drug until the correct time.
   - Pain relief should occur shortly after pushing the button.
   - Call the nurse if pain relief does not occur after two successive doses.
2. The nurse should evaluate the following factors to confirm the success of an opioid treatment plan:
   - The breathing pattern is maintained.
   - No evidence of injury is seen.
   - Bowel movements are normal for the client.
   - Body weight is maintained.
   - Diet is adequate.
3. Pain intensity is used to determine what type of drug is necessary to achieve proper pain management. Opioid analgesics are used primarily for the treatment of moderate to severe acute and chronic pain. If the intensity of the client's pain is mild, then nonopioid analgesics can be used. The WHO pain ladder is an effective tool that can be utilized to determine what type of drug is necessary according to a client's reported pain intensity.

Activity E CROSSWORD PUZZLE

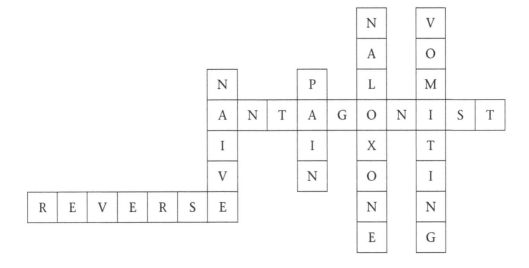

SECTION II: APPLYING YOUR KNOWLEDGE

Activity F CASE STUDY

1. The nurse should tell Mr. Garcia that clients who are relaxed and sedated when an anesthetic agent is given are easier to anesthetize (requiring a smaller dose of an induction anesthetic). This will make the procedure easier to do in a quicker manner. Clients receiving opioid analgesics for short-term acute pain do not develop physical dependence.
2. Decreased GI motility due to the opioids, in addition to lower food and water intake and decreased mobility, cause the constipation. If the client is constipated, try the use of a stool softener or laxative.

SECTION III: PRACTICING FOR NCLEX

Activity G NCLEX-STYLE QUESTIONS

1. **Answer: 2**
   RATIONALE: The most critical preadministration assessment conducted by the nurse before the administration of an opioid analgesic involves assessing and documenting the type, onset, intensity, and location of the pain. Other preadministration assessments include reviewing the client's health history, allergy history, and past and current drug therapies. The nurse obtains the blood pressure, pulse and respiratory rate, and pain rating in 5–10 minutes if the drug is given

intravenously (IV), 20–30 minutes after the drug is taken intramuscularly or subcutaneously, and 30 or more minutes if the drug is given orally, but these interventions are part of the ongoing assessment conducted while the client is on the drug therapy and not before the administration of the drug.

2. **Answer: 1**

   RATIONALE: The nurse should confirm that the client is not taking anticoagulants (blood thinners, NSAIDS, or aspirin), which interact with marijuana and may cause an increased risk of bleeding. Acetaminophen does not interact with marijuana. Medical marijuana is approved in some states for treatment of GI and seizure disorders when they are unrelieved by standard treatments or medications. Providers (MD, DO, naturopath, or nurse practitioner) may *recommend* use for a qualified condition that is unrelieved by standard treatments or medications. Medical marijuana is not *prescribed* to date because this would be a violation of federal laws.

3. **Answer: 2**

   RATIONALE: The nurse should assess food intake after each meal when caring for a client with imbalanced nutrition as a result of anorexia. It is important for the nurse to notify the primary health care provider of continued weight loss and anorexia. The intake summary will help the nurse determine if the client's meal requires additional protein supplements. The client's bowel movements are recorded if the client has constipation, which can affect appetite, but food intake is a better measurement for nutritional imbalance. Ensuring an increase in the client's fluid intake specifically is not a necessary intervention, since it will not help improve the client's nutrition.

4. **Answer: 2**

   RATIONALE: Opioid-naïve clients are most at risk for respiratory depression after opioid administration.

5. **Answer: 1**

   RATIONALE: A nurse should administer naloxone with great caution to a client who is prescribed an opioid for treatment for a decrease in respiratory rate. Naloxone removes all the pain-relieving effects of the opioid and leads to withdrawal symptoms or return of intense pain. Naloxone is not known to cause vomiting, dizziness, or headache.

6. **Answers: 1, 2, 3**

   RATIONALE: The primary health care provider should be contacted immediately if the nurse observes a significant decrease in the respiratory rate or a respiratory rate of 10 breaths/minute or below, a significant increase or decrease in the pulse rate or a change in the pulse quality, a significant decrease in blood pressure (systolic or diastolic), or a systolic pressure below 100 mm Hg. Opioid analgesics do not lead to an increase in body weight or an increase in body temperature; therefore, the nurse is not likely to make these observations when caring for the client.

7. **Answers: 1, 3, 4**

   RATIONALE: The nurse should know that opioid analgesics are administered with caution in clients with undiagnosed abdominal pain, hepatic or renal impairment, and hypoxia. Other conditions that require cautious use of opioid analgesics include supraventricular tachycardia, prostatic hypertrophy, lactating clients, clients of an advanced age, opioid-naïve clients, and clients undergoing biliary surgery. The drug need not be used cautiously with clients who are aged 13 years or in clients with fungal infections.

8. **Answer: 3**

   RATIONALE: Administration of barbiturates when the client is on opioid therapy leads to respiratory depression, hypotension, and sedation. Barbiturates interacting with opioid analgesics are not known to cause bacterial infections, hypertension, or hypothyroidism.

9. **Answer: 2**

   RATIONALE: The nurse should instruct the client to avoid alcohol after being treated with opioid analgesics. Alcohol may intensify the action of the drug and cause extreme drowsiness or dizziness. In some instances, the use of alcohol and an opioid can have extremely serious and even life-threatening consequences that may require emergency medical treatment. The nurse need not instruct the client to avoid traveling, avoid exercising, and avoid eating starchy food since they will not have a negative effect on the client's health when the client is on an opioid.

10. **Answer: 1**

    RATIONALE: Morphine sulfate is considered the gold standard in pain management and is considered the prototype opioid. Charts called equal-analgesic conversions compare other opioid doses with the doses of morphine sulfate that would be used for the same level of pain control.

11. **Answer: 1**

    RATIONALE: The one bodily system that does not adapt and compensate for the secondary effects of opioids is the GI system. Slow GI motility and the resulting constipation are always a problem in opioid therapy.

12. **Answer: 2**

    RATIONALE: A lactating female should wait at least 4–6 hours after taking an opioid analgesic to breastfeed the infant.

13. Answers: 1, 3, 4

> **RATIONALE:** PCA allows postsurgical clients to administer their own analgesic by means of an IV pump system. The medication can be delivered, for example, when the client begins to feel pain or when the client wishes to ambulate but wants some medication to prevent pain on getting out of bed. The client does not have to wait for the nurse to administer the medicine. As a result, clients medicate before they cannot tolerate the pain, use less medication, and resume activity faster. When clients take less opioid, they also experience fewer unpleasant adverse reactions, such as nausea and constipation.

CHAPTER 16

SECTION I: ASSESSING YOUR UNDERSTANDING

Activity A FILL IN THE BLANKS

1. conduction
2. General
3. Anesthesia
4. anesthetist
5. anesthesiologist
6. cholinergic

Activity B SEQUENCING

1. 4   3   1   2

Activity C MATCHING

1. 1. c   2. d   3. a   4. b
2. 1. d   2. c   3. b   4. a

Activity D SHORT ANSWERS

1. The nurse must ensure that the surgeon and the anesthesiologist are made aware of the abnormality. The nurse must attach a note to the front of the chart and also try to contact the surgeon or anesthesiologist via telephone or in person.
2. After surgery, the nurse has the following unique responsibilities, when a client has been given a regional anesthetic. With regional anesthesia, check limbs and body for proper position to prevent injury.
3. The administration of general anesthesia requires the use of one or more drugs. The choice of anesthetic drug depends on many factors, including:

- The general physical condition of the client
- The area, organ, or system being operated on
- The anticipated length of the surgical procedure.

Activity E CROSSWORD PUZZLE

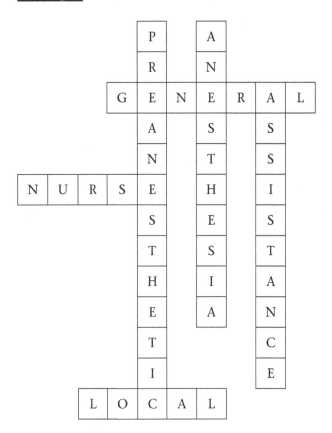

SECTION II: APPLYING YOUR KNOWLEDGE

Activity F CASE STUDY

1. The preoperative nurse is responsible for describing the preparation for surgery ordered by the physician, assessing the physical status of the client, describing postoperative care, demonstrating postoperative client activities, and demonstrating the use of a PCA pump. If this is an outpatient procedure, the nurse needs to ensure a responsible person will take him home after.
2. The nurse should administer 5 mL to the client (5 mg × 1 mL/1 mg = 5 mL). When caring for a client receiving a preanesthetic drug, the nurse assesses the client's physical status and gives an explanation of the anesthesia. If this is to be given IM, the nurse must draw up two syringes with no more than 3 mL in each.

SECTION III: PRACTICING FOR NCLEX

Activity G NCLEX-STYLE QUESTIONS

1. **Answer: 1**

   RATIONALE: Stage I of anesthesia, known as the *induction* or analgesic stage of general anesthesia, begins with a loss of consciousness. Delirium, along with excitement, is marked in the second stage of anesthesia. Surgical analgesia and respiratory paralysis are noted in the third and fourth stages, respectively.

2. **Answer: 2**

   RATIONALE: Topical anesthesia leads to desensitization of the skin and mucous membranes. Topical anesthesia does not bring about a decrease in anxiety and apprehension, cardiovascular stimulation, or a loss of feeling in the lower extremities.

3. **Answer: 3**

   RATIONALE: As part of the postoperative interventions after the administration of anesthesia, the nurse should position the client to prevent aspiration of vomitus and secretions. The nurse should review the client's laboratory test records before the administration of anesthesia and not after. The nurse should also monitor the blood pressure, pulse, and respiratory rate every 5–15 minutes until the client is discharged from the area, not every 12 hours. As part of the postoperative interventions done after the administration of anesthesia, the nurse should review the client's surgical and anesthesia records. This will show if a hypnotic agent was administered to the client before the administration of anesthesia and not after.

4. **Answer: 2**

   RATIONALE: If a client shows an increase in his respiratory secretions in the operating room, the nurse should understand that the preanesthetic drug was not given to the client on time. Preanesthetic drugs must be administered on time to produce their intended effects. Failure to give the preanesthetic drug on time may result in such events as increased respiratory secretions caused by the irritating effect of anesthetic gases and the need for an increased dose of the induction drug because the preanesthetic drug has not had time to affect the client. Not assessing the client's IV lines well, not assessing the client's respiratory status, and not reviewing the client's anesthesia records do not cause an increase in the client's respiratory secretions.

5. **Answers: 1, 2, 3**

   RATIONALE: When caring for a client receiving local anesthesia, the nurse should apply dressing to surgical areas and observe for any bleeding or oozing in the client. Assessing the client's pulse rate every 5–15 minutes and exercising caution when administering opioids to the client are postoperative interventions, which are not appropriate when caring for a client who has undergone local anesthesia.

6. **Answer: 1**

   RATIONALE: The nurse should confirm that the client is not older than 60 years. Preanesthetic drugs may be omitted in clients aged 60 years or older because many of the medical disorders for which these drugs are contraindicated are seen in older individuals. Preanesthetic drugs are not contraindicated in cases of the application of anesthesia to the extremities. Preanesthetic drugs are not known to be contraindicated in clients who are younger than 13 years or who have a low body weight.

7. **Answer: 2**

   RATIONALE: The nurse should know that the transsacral block is a conduction block. It is a type of regional anesthesia produced by injection of a local anesthetic drug into or near a nerve trunk. A transsacral (caudal) block (injection of a local anesthetic into the epidural space at the level of the sacrococcygeal notch) is often used in obstetrics.

8. **Answer: 4**

   RATIONALE: The nurse should confirm that the client does not require anesthesia to be administered on the extremities to ensure that the use of epinephrine along with local anesthesia is not contraindicated in the client. The anesthetic stays in the tissue longer when epinephrine is used. This is contraindicated, however, when the local anesthetic is used on an extremity. Epinephrine used with local anesthesia is not known to be contraindicated in clients who are anemic, clients who have low blood pressure, or clients who are older than 60 years.

9. **Answer: 1**

   RATIONALE: Regional anesthesia is a type of local anesthesia and includes spinal anesthesia and conduction block.

10. **Answer: 3**

    RATIONALE: Topical anesthesia may be applied by the nurse with a cotton swab or sprayed on the area to be desensitized.

11. **Answer: 1**

    RATIONALE: Local infiltration anesthesia is commonly used for dental procedures, for the suturing of small wounds, or for making an incision into a small area.

12. **Answer: 1**

    RATIONALE: A nurse may be asked to administer an antianxiety drug, such as midazolam, prior to a colonoscopy to help the client relax.

CHAPTER 17

SECTION I: ASSESSING YOUR UNDERSTANDING

Activity A FILL IN THE BLANKS

1. carotid
2. narcolepsy
3. sympathomimetic
4. medulla
5. arrhythmias

Activity B DOSAGE CALCULATION

1. 2 tablets
2. 2 mL
3. 2 tablets
4. 1.5 tablets
5. 1 tablet

Activity C MATCHING

1. 1. b   2. c   3. a

Activity D SHORT ANSWERS

1. The nursing interventions while caring for a client with an ineffective breathing pattern who is being administered CNS stimulants are as follows:
   - Record blood pressure, pulse, and respiratory rate.
   - Before administering drug, ensure patent airway, and provide oxygen as needed.
   - Monitor respirations closely after administration.
   - Record the effects of therapy.
2. The instructions for a client starting CNS stimulants for ADHD are as follows:
   - Give the drug in the morning 30–45 minutes before breakfast and before lunch.
   - Do not give the drug in the late afternoon.
   - Monitor the eating patterns of the child while they are taking CNS stimulants.
   - Provide nutritious meals and snacks; a good breakfast is important to provide because the drug will cause the child to possibly not feel hungry at lunchtime in school where the parent cannot monitor nutritional intake.
   - The child should be checked frequently with height and weight measurements to monitor growth.
   - Keep a journal of the child's behavior, including the general patterns, socialization with others, and attention span.
   - Bring this record to each primary health care provider or clinic visit because this record may help the primary health care provider determine future drug dose adjustments or additional treatment modalities.
   - The primary health care provider may prescribe drug therapy only on school days, when high levels of attention and performance are necessary.

Activity E WORD FIND PUZZLE

A							
N							N
A			A	P	N	E	A
L			D				R
E	U	P	H	O	R	I	C
P	A		D	B			O
T		C		E			L
I			T	S			E
C				I			P
				T	V		S
				Y		E	Y

SECTION II: APPLYING YOUR KNOWLEDGE

Activity F CASE STUDY

1. Yes, he is a candidate for weight loss anorexiant drugs. A weight of 215 lb and 5′6″ equals a BMI of 33.7 kg/m². These drugs may be used for obesity (BMI kg/m² of 30 or greater) or overweight (BMI of 27 kg/m²) when comorbid conditions exist, such as hypertension.
2. Amphetamines and anorexiants should not be taken concurrently or within 14 days of antidepressant medications.

SECTION III: PRACTICING FOR NCLEX

Activity G NCLEX-STYLE QUESTIONS

1. **Answer: 2**
   RATIONALE: Hyperactivity is one of the adverse reactions of CNS stimulants that a nurse should monitor for. Bradycardia, not tachycardia, is a reaction of CNS stimulants. Fever or high BP are not adverse effects generally associated with CNS stimulants.
2. **Answer: 3**
   RATIONALE: The CNS stimulants are contraindicated in clients with ventilation disorders (such as COPD). The drug is not contraindicated in clients

with bone marrow suppression, severe liver disease, or ulcerative colitis.

3. **Answer: 3**

RATIONALE: The conscious level should be monitored in 5–15-minute intervals, and the respirations monitored until a return of the respiratory rate to normal.

4. **Answer: 3**

RATIONALE: Amphetamines work by blocking the reuptake of norepinephrine and dopamine. This lessens the action of other neurotransmitters, thus helping to focus concentration and attention.

5. **Answers: 1, 2, 5**

RATIONALE: The nurse should instruct the parents to monitor the eating patterns of the child and check height and weight measurements to monitor growth. The nurse should also stress the importance of preparing nutritious meals and snacks. The child should be encouraged to have a substantial breakfast, as they may be in school during lunchtime and may not feel hungry. Sleeping pills should be avoided.

6. **Answer: 3**

RATIONALE: When an anorexiant is used as part of obesity treatment, the nurse obtains and records the client's weight before therapy is started. Weight reduction is used to determine the extent of therapy. There is no need to observe the urinary output or measure blood glucose.

7. **Answers: 1, 2**

RATIONALE: The CNS is composed of the brain and spinal cord.

8. **Answers: 1, 4**

RATIONALE: Analeptics are CNS stimulant drugs that stimulate the respiratory center of the brain and dilate vessels of the cardiovascular system.

9. **Answer: 2**

RATIONALE: Anorexiants are drugs used to suppress the appetite.

10. **Answer: 1**

RATIONALE: Provigil is used to treat narcolepsy and does not cause cardiac and other systemic stimulatory effects like other CNS stimulants.

11. **Answer: 4**

RATIONALE: Most anorexiants are pregnancy category X and should not be used during pregnancy.

12. **Answer: 1**

RATIONALE: Pediatric clients given atomoxetine (Strattera) should be monitored closely for suicidal ideation.

CHAPTER 18

SECTION I: ASSESSING YOUR UNDERSTANDING

Activity A FILL IN THE BLANKS

1. Alzheimer
2. parasympathetic or cholinergic
3. dementia
4. brain
5. delirium

Activity B DOSAGE CALCULATION

1. 1.5 tablets
2. 20 tablets
3. 2 capsules/dose or 3 mg
4. Patch 2: the dose is 18 mg and the patch is kept on for 3 days. This is lower than the "daily" dose (9.5 mg) because patches lose potency over time, and therefore, the dose is not consistent each of the 3 days.

Activity C MATCHING

1. **1.** d **2.** c **3.** b **4.** a
2. **1.** b **2.** c **3.** a

Activity D SHORT ANSWERS

1. The nurse should assess the following in clients who are prescribed antidementia drugs:
   - Cognitive ability, such as orientation, calculation, recall, and language, and functional ability such as performance of daily activities and self-care
   - Agitation and impulsive behavior
   - Mental health and medical history, including history of Alzheimer symptoms
   - Physical assessments such as blood pressure measurements (on both arms with client in a sitting position), pulse, respiratory rate, and weight

2. The nurse should perform the following interventions when caring for a client with loss of appetite partly due to drug therapy:
   - Mealtime should be simple and calm.
   - Offer the client a well-balanced diet with foods that are easy to chew and digest.
   - Frequent, small meals may be tolerated better than three regular meals.
   - Offering foods of different consistency and flavor is important in case the client can handle one form better than another.
   - Fluid intake of six to eight glasses of water daily is encouraged to prevent dehydration.

Activity E CROSSWORD PUZZLE

							D	E	L	I	R	I	U	M
										N				
								P		H		T		
								A		I		R		
								R		B		A		
								A		I		N		
								S		T		S		
					A	M	Y	L	O	I	D			
					C		M		R		E			
		M	M	S	E		P		S		R			
					T		A				M			
					Y		T				A			
					L		H				L			
					C		E							
					H		T							
	G	I	N	K	G	O		I						
					L		C							
D	E	M	E	N	T	I	A							
					N									
				M	E	M	A	N	T	I	N	E		

SECTION II: APPLYING YOUR KNOWLEDGE

Activity F CASE STUDY

1. **Stage I: Preclinical AD (may occur 20 years before clinical symptoms)**
   - *Focus on research*
   - Measureable changes are seen in the brain on MRI
   - Biomarkers may be present in blood or cerebrospinal fluid
   - No changes in cognitive or functional ability

   Stage II: Mild Cognitive Impairment (MCI) due to AD
   - *Focus on limiting progression with medications*
   - Changes in thinking ability noticeable to client and family members
   - Thinking or memory changes due to other causes ruled out
   - Functional ability remains intact
   - Mild to moderate anxiety noted by person

   Stages III–V: Dementia due to AD
   - *Focus on supporting function*
   - Memory, thinking, and behavior limit ability to function
   - Variable degrees of assistance needed for activities of daily living
   - Reasoning and judgment impaired

2. The most common adverse effects with the use of donepezil (Aricept) include headache, nausea, diarrhea, insomnia, and muscle cramps.

SECTION III: PRACTICING FOR NCLEX

Activity G NCLEX-STYLE QUESTIONS

1. **Answer: 1**
   RATIONALE: The nurse should monitor for diarrhea in the client as an adverse reaction of antidementia drugs. High blood pressure, seizure disorders, and renal dysfunction are not adverse reactions of antidementia drugs.

2. **Answer: 1**
   RATIONALE: The cholinesterase inhibitors act to increase the level of acetylcholine in the central nervous system (CNS) by inhibiting its breakdown and slowing neural destruction.

3. **Answer: 4**
   RATIONALE: Some of the most common adverse reactions of these drugs include dry mouth, nausea, and vomiting. Nutrition becomes a primary issue in treatment because clients with AD also may have difficulty with appetite and eating.

4. **Answer: 3**
   RATIONALE: Increased risk of GI bleeding is the effect of the interaction of nonsteroidal anti-inflammatory drugs with cholinesterase inhibitors. Asthma, sick sinus syndrome, and increased risk of theophylline toxicity are not effects of the interaction of nonsteroidal anti-inflammatory drugs with cholinesterase inhibitors. Increased risk of theophylline toxicity is the effect of the interaction of theophylline with cholinesterase inhibitors.

5. **Answer: 1**
   RATIONALE: In individuals with a history of ulcer disease, bleeding may recur.

6. **Answers: 3, 5**
   RATIONALE: When caring for a client receiving antidementia drugs, the nurse should keep the bed in a low position or use night lights in order to reduce the risk of injury in the client. The nurse should monitor the client frequently to reduce the risk of injury, instead of monitoring every 12 hours. The nurse need not use soft bedding, as it may not help reduce the risk of injury in the client, and clients should not be restrained.

7. **Answer: 1**
   RATIONALE: Ginkgo is contraindicated in clients receiving monoamine oxidase inhibitors (MAOIs) because of the risk of a toxic reaction. Ginkgo is not contraindicated in clients receiving sedatives and hypnotics, opioid analgesics, or anticholinergic drugs.

8. **Answer: 1**
   RATIONALE: It is important for the nurse to pay proper attention to the dosing of medication as it helps to decrease the adverse GI reactions. Paying proper attention to the dosing of medication is not related to the client's faster recovery, maintenance of the client's normal body temperature, or decreased variations in the client's pulse rate.

9. **Answer: 2**
   RATIONALE: NMDA receptor antagonists are utilized for the treatment of Alzheimer disease.

10. **Answer: 2**
    RATIONALE: Rivastigmine (Exelon) is available in a transdermal form of the drug.

11. **Answer: 1**
    RATIONALE: Ginkgo is a herbal product that has been used to improve mental performance.

12. **Answer: 2**
    RATIONALE: Thinking or memory changes due to other causes are ruled out, changes in thinking are noticeable to people close to the individual, functional ability remains intact, and anxiety does play a part in the decline.

CHAPTER 19

SECTION I: ASSESSING YOUR UNDERSTANDING

Activity A FILL IN THE BLANKS

1. anxiolytics
2. normal
3. antidepressants
4. Parenteral
5. Withdrawal

Activity B DOSAGE CALCULATION

1. 0.5 tablet or ½ tablet
2. Every 6 hours
3. 3 tablets
4. 2.5 tablets
5. 30 mg

Activity C MATCHING

1. 1. b   2. c   3. d   4. a
2. 1. c   2. a   3. b

Activity D SHORT ANSWERS

1. Before administering alprazolam for the first time, the nurse should perform the following assessments:
   - Obtain the client's complete medical history, including mental status.
   - Have the client rate their level of anxiety similar to rating pain.
   - If the client is moderately anxious, obtain the history from a family member or friend.
   - Observe the client for behavioral signs indicating anxiety.
   - Assess the blood pressure, pulse, respiratory rate, and weight.
   - Obtain a history of any past drug or alcohol use.

2. When caring for a client receiving alprazolam who has developed constipation, the nurse should perform the following interventions:
   - Encourage more water to provide adequate hydration.
   - Meals should include fiber, fruits, and vegetables to prevent constipation.

Activity E CROSSWORD PUZZLE

Across/Down answers:
- GABA
- BENZODIAZEPINES
- ANXIETY
- TOLERANCE
- PHYSICAL
- DEPENDENCE
- ATAXIA
- PTSD
- ANXIOLYTICS

SECTION II: APPLYING YOUR KNOWLEDGE

Activity F CASE STUDY

1. Due to Mrs. Moore's age, the lorazepam will be excreted more slowly, leading to prolonged drug effects and an increase in adverse reactions. Therefore, the drug should be initiated at a low dose and titrated slowly. Mrs. Moore should also be monitored closely for side effects and falls.
2. The nurse's ongoing assessment of Mrs. Moore should include blood pressure check, mental status, anxiety level, and any side effects that may occur.

SECTION III: PRACTICING FOR NCLEX

Activity G NCLEX-STYLE QUESTIONS

1. **Answer: 2**
   RATIONALE: Diarrhea is an adverse reaction to antianxiety drugs in the client, which is a cause of concern. Seizures are not caused by antianxiety drugs. On the contrary, antianxiety drugs are used to control seizures or convulsions in clients. Abdominal cramps and bradycardia are not known to be adverse reactions to antianxiety drugs.

2. **Answer: 4**
   RATIONALE: The nurse should monitor the client for increased risk of digitalis toxicity due to the interaction of digoxin with diazepam. Increased risk for central nervous system depression is caused by the interaction of alcohol with diazepam. Increased risk for respiratory depression and sedation are caused by the interaction of tricyclic antidepressants or antipsychotics with diazepam.

3. **Answer: 2**
   RATIONALE: Acute panic is an alcohol withdrawal symptom. Diarrhea, dry mouth, and lightheadedness are not known to be alcohol withdrawal symptoms. These are adverse reactions to chlordiazepoxide therapy, which is administered for acute alcohol withdrawal.

4. **Answer: 2**
   RATIONALE: The nurse should ensure that the client is not breastfeeding.

5. **Answer: 2**
   RATIONALE: The nurse should inform the client to avoid alcohol.

6. **Answer: 1**
   RATIONALE: The nurse should administer the drug intramuscularly in the gluteus muscle, which is a large muscle mass, and not on the arm, which has less muscle mass.

7. **Answer: 3**
   RATIONALE: The nurse should monitor the client for a metallic taste in the mouth, which is a withdrawal symptom of alprazolam. Diarrhea, dizziness, and dry mouth are adverse effects of the treatment.
8. **Answer: 1**
   RATIONALE: Antianxiety drugs are also referred to as anxiolytics.
9. **Answer: 3**
   RATIONALE: The type of questions asked depends on the client and the diagnosis and may include open-ended questions such as "How are you feeling?", "Do you feel less nervous?", or "Would you like to tell me how everything is going?" Sometimes you may need to rephrase questions or direct the conversation toward other subjects until the client feels comfortable enough to discuss their therapy.
10. **Answer: 1**
    RATIONALE: Buspirone (Buspar) exerts its anxiolytic effect by acting on the brain's serotonin receptors.
11. **Answer: 3**
    RATIONALE: Hydroxyzine (Vistaril) exerts its anxiolytic effect by acting on the hypothalamus and brainstem reticular formation.
12. **Answer: 4**
    RATIONALE: Typically, benzodiazepine withdrawal symptoms occur when the drug is stopped after 4–6 months (when used daily as a sedative) or 2–3 months when high doses are used daily.

CHAPTER 20

SECTION I: ASSESSING YOUR UNDERSTANDING

Activity A FILL IN THE BLANKS

1. healing
2. insomnia
3. hypnotic
4. wakefulness
5. Melatonin
6. sedative

Activity B DOSAGE CALCULATION

1. 1 tablet
2. 3 tablets
3. 2 tablets
4. 2 tablets
5. 1 tablet

Activity C MATCHING

1. **1.** c   **2.** a   **3.** d   **4.** e   **5.** b
2. **1.** b   **2.** c   **3.** a

Activity D SHORT ANSWERS

1. Before administering a sedative, the nurse takes and records the client's blood pressure, pulse, and respiratory rate. The nurse also assesses the following client needs by asking:
   - Is the client female, if so is she pregnant?
   - Does the client receive an opioid analgesic every 4–6 hours? Is the issue pain related?
   - If the sedative is for a surgical procedure, then is its administration correctly timed?
   - Has a consent form been signed for the procedure before the drug is administered?
2. Nursing diagnoses particular to a client taking a sedative or hypnotic are as follows:
   - Injury risk related to drowsiness or impaired memory
   - Altered breathing pattern related to respiratory depression
   - Coping impairment related to excessive use of medication

Activity E WORD FIND PUZZLE

	I						
	N	E	W	J	O	B	
	S						H
	O	T					E
	M		R	J			A
A	N	X	I	E	T	Y	D
	I			T	S		A
P	A	I	N	L		S	C
				A			H
C	H	A	N	G	E	S	E

SECTION II: APPLYING YOUR KNOWLEDGE

Activity F CASE STUDY

1. Temazepam (Restoril) is a hypnotic drug.
2. A hypnotic is a drug that induces drowsiness or sleep, which allows the client to fall asleep and stay asleep. A sedative is a drug that produces a relaxing, calming effect.

SECTION III: PRACTICING FOR NCLEX
Activity G NCLEX-STYLE QUESTIONS

1. **Answer: 3**
   RATIONALE: The nurse can evaluate the effectiveness of the treatment being given to the client from an improvement in the client's sleep pattern. An improvement in the client's consciousness level, a normalcy in the client's respiration rate, and a decrease in the client's restlessness do not indicate the effectiveness of the treatment.

2. **Answer: 2**
   RATIONALE: The nurse should record the client's blood pressure before administering the sedative. Platelet count, hematocrit, and blood sugar are not altered by the sedative; hence, these factors are not necessarily recorded before administration of the sedative.

3. **Answer: 1**
   RATIONALE: The nurse should monitor the client for nausea, which is an adverse reaction of sedatives. Headache, restlessness, and anxiety are causes of insomnia for which a sedative may be prescribed.

4. **Answer: 4**
   RATIONALE: Sedatives must be administered cautiously to clients with renal impairment. Clients with hearing impairment, hyperglycemia, or glucose intolerance are not high-risk candidates for sedative administration.

5. **Answer: 2**
   RATIONALE: The nonbenzodiazepine effects diminish after approximately 2 weeks.

6. **Answer: 3**
   RATIONALE: According to the National Sleep Foundation, sleep/wake problems affect nearly 40 million people in the United States.

7. **Answers: 2, 3, 4**
   RATIONALE: A high-fat meal or snack can interfere with the absorption of the following drugs: eszopiclone, ramelteon, and zaleplon.

8. **Answers: 1, 3, 5**
   RATIONALE: Relaxation, calming, and drowsiness are beneficial effects of sedatives. Nausea and dizziness are the adverse reactions of sedatives and hypnotics.

9. **Answer: 1**
   RATIONALE: Sedatives and hypnotics are used primarily to treat insomnia.

10. **Answers: 1, 3**
    RATIONALE: Due to a specific enzyme reaction, grapefruit or its juice should not be given to clients who are on triazolam or zaleplon.

11. **Answer: 4**
    RATIONALE: Older adult clients may require a smaller hypnotic dose, and in some instances, a sedative dose may act like a hypnotic and produce sleep.

12. **Answer: 2**
    RATIONALE: Benzodiazepines are classified in pregnancy category X and their use is contraindicated in pregnancy.

CHAPTER 21

SECTION I: ASSESSING YOUR UNDERSTANDING
Activity A FILL IN THE BLANKS

1. Psychotherapy
2. Coming out
3. 2 weeks
4. tricyclic
5. 2, 4

Activity B DOSAGE CALCULATION

1. 3 tablets
2. 2 tablets
3. 2 capsules
4. 1 tablet
5. 10 mL
6. 3 tablets

Activity C OUT IN THE COMMUNITY

Class discussion: To measure geriatric depression risk, the tool should be relatively simple with not too many questions. Did you find people at risk? If not, check to see if they are taking antidepressants already.

Activity D SHORT ANSWERS

1. Clinical depression may be treated with antidepressant drugs. Psychotherapy is used with antidepressants in treating clinical depression, too.
2. There are four classes of antidepressants: selective serotonin reuptake inhibitors (SSRIs), serotonin/norepinephrine or dopamine/norepinephrine reuptake inhibitors (SNRIs or DNRIs), tricyclic antidepressants (TCAs), and monoamine oxidase inhibitors (MAOIs). Discovery of the role of dopamine in depression and the ability to be more selective in reuptake make the TCA and MAOI classes of drugs less frequently prescribed than the SSRI and SNRI/DNRI classes.
3. Treatment with antidepressants increases the sensitivity of postsynaptic alpha-adrenergic and serotonin receptors and decreases the sensitivity of the presynaptic receptor sites. This enhances recovery from the depressive episode by making neurotransmission activity more effective.

Activity E SUDOKU PUZZLE

EPI	MAOI	TCA	CNS	DNRI	SNRI	DOPA	SSRI	SERO
DNRI	SSRI	SERO	DOPA	MAOI	EPI	SNRI	TCA	CNS
DOPA	SNRI	CNS	SERO	SSRI	TCA	MAOI	EPI	DNRI
SERO	DNRI	EPI	SNRI	DOPA	SSRI	TCA	CNS	MAOI
SNRI	TCA	SSRI	DNRI	CNS	MAOI	EPI	SERO	DOPA
CNS	DOPA	MAOI	EPI	TCA	SERO	DNRI	SNRI	SSRI
TCA	SERO	DNRI	SSRI	EPI	DOPA	CNS	MAOI	SNRI
MAOI	CNS	SNRI	TCA	SERO	DNRI	SSRI	DOPA	EPI
SSRI	EPI	DOPA	MAOI	SNRI	CNS	SERO	DNRI	TCA

SECTION II: APPLYING YOUR KNOWLEDGE

Activity F CASE STUDY

1. The following is a list of symptoms that may be present in clients who are depressed:
   - Feelings of hopelessness or helplessness
   - Diminished interest in activities of life
   - Significant weight loss or gain (without dieting)
   - Insomnia or hypersomnia
   - Agitation, restlessness, or irritability
   - Fatigue or loss of energy
   - Feelings of worthlessness
   - Excessive or inappropriate guilt
   - Diminished ability to think or concentrate, or indecisiveness
   - Recurrent thoughts of death or suicide (or suicide attempt)
2. The nurse should tell Mrs. Smith to take the escitalopram (Lexapro) in the morning, as this will lessen the likelihood of insomnia, and that it can take 2–4 weeks to see a difference in mood.

SECTION III: PRACTICING FOR NCLEX

Activity G NCLEX-STYLE QUESTIONS

1. **Answer: 1**
   RATIONALE: Photosensitivity is one of the adverse reactions to tricyclic antidepressant drugs.

Hypertensive episodes and severe convulsions are the effects observed when tricyclic antidepressants are administered along with MAOIs. Nervous system depression is the effect of the interaction of tricyclic antidepressants with sedatives, hypnotics, and analgesics.

2. **Answer: 2**
   RATIONALE: Due to a specific enzyme reaction, grapefruit or its juice should not be taken if on sertraline (Zoloft).

3. **Answer: 1**
   RATIONALE: The nurse should monitor the client for an increased risk of bleeding. Increased risk for hypotension is observed when antihypertensive drugs interact with antidepressants. Increased anticholinergic symptoms are observed when cimetidine used for GI upset interacts with antidepressants. Increased risk for nervous system depression is observed in clients when an analgesic interacts with antidepressants.

4. **Answer: 3**
   RATIONALE: The nurse should monitor the client for somnolence, a possible reaction of SSRIs. Vertigo and blurred vision are adverse reactions observed when MAOIs are administered. Tremor is an adverse reaction indicating a greater issue such as serotonin syndrome.

5. Answer: 1
RATIONALE: Extremely high blood pressure results in hypertensive crisis. The medical intervention involves lowering of the blood pressure. Blood sugar, temperature, and respiration rate are not causes of hypertensive crisis.

6. Answers: 1, 2, 5
RATIONALE: The nurse should obtain a complete medical history, blood pressure measurements, pulse, and respiratory rate as part of the preadministration assessment. Complete blood count and blood sugar levels are not adversely affected before antidepressant drugs.

7. Answer: 2
RATIONALE: The nurse should closely monitor the client for hypertensive crisis, a life-threatening adverse effect of tyramine interacting with MAOI antidepressants. Orthostatic hypotension and blurred vision are adverse effects of MAOIs. Photosensitivity is an adverse reaction of tricyclic antidepressants.

8. Answer: 1
RATIONALE: The nurse should instruct the client to change positions slowly and assist the client if required. Instructing the client to drink plenty of fluids, monitoring changes in vital signs, or monitoring for hyperglycemia will not help the client overcome orthostatic hypotension due to antidepressants.

9. Answer: 3
RATIONALE: The nurse should administer fluoxetine in the morning because it is an SSRI, which is the best time for its administration. Most antidepressant drugs, except SSRIs, are best administered at night before bedtime, rather than with lunch or dinner, so that the sedative effects promote sleep and the adverse reactions appear less troublesome.

10. Answer: 1
RATIONALE: Anticholinergic side effects commonly occur with the use of the tricyclic class of antidepressants.

11. Answer: 4
RATIONALE: MAOIs such as phenelzine (Nardil) exert their effects by inhibiting the activity of monoamine oxidase.

12. Answer: 1
RATIONALE: The smoking cessation product Zyban is a form of the antidepressant drug bupropion.

Smokers should not use Zyban if they are currently taking bupropion for management of depression because of the possibility of bupropion overdose.

CHAPTER 22

SECTION I: ASSESSING YOUR UNDERSTANDING
Activity A FILL IN THE BLANKS
1. psychosis
2. dopamine
3. serotonin
4. Flattened
5. extrapyramidal

Activity B DOSAGE CALCULATION
1. 1 tablet
2. 1.28 or 1.3 mL
3. 1 capsule
4. 15 mL
5. 1 capsule

Activity C MATCHING
1. 1. b   2. d   3. a   4. c
2. 1. c   2. a   3. d   4. b

Activity D SHORT ANSWERS
1. Before administering antipsychotics for the first time, the nurse should perform the following assessments:
   - Obtain a complete mental health, social, and medical history.
   - Obtain a medical history and a history of the symptoms of the mental disorder from the client, a family member, or the client's hospital documents.
   - Observe the client for any behavior patterns that appear to be deviations from normal.
2. When caring for a client who is being administered parenteral medication, the nurse should perform the following interventions:
   - Repeat parenteral administration every 1–4 hours until the desired effect is obtained.
   - Monitor the client closely for cardiac arrhythmias, rhythm changes, or hypotension.

Activity E CROSSWORD PUZZLE

Crossword answers (as filled in the grid): AKATHISIA, PSYCHOSIS, DELUSIONS, ALOGIA, DOPAMINE, CONVOLUTION, RECIDIVISM, TARDIVE, ANHEDONIA

SECTION II: APPLYING YOUR KNOWLEDGE

Activity F CASE STUDY

1. The nurse should relay the following to Mr. Chase regarding his new medication:
   - The administration of atypical antipsychotic (SGA) drugs with the adverse reaction of weight gain can put the client at higher risk of acquiring type 2 diabetes (clozapine and olanzapine users gain the most weight).
   - Before starting treatment with an SGA, the client should be weighed and a family history documented to indicate the risk of type 2 diabetes.
2. Laboratory work for fasting blood sugar, total and LDL cholesterol, and triglycerides should be taken and compared at periodic intervals.

SECTION III: PRACTICING FOR NCLEX

Activity G NCLEX-STYLE QUESTIONS

1. **Answer: 2**
   RATIONALE: The nurse should ask the client to avoid sunlight, as photosensitivity can result in severe sunburn. Tanning beds should also be avoided. Minimizing alcohol use or drinking five glasses of water a day will not have a significant impact on photosensitivity.

2. **Answer: 4**
   RATIONALE: The use of the drug clozapine has been associated with severe agranulocytosis, or decreased white blood cell (WBC) count; neutropenia is the reduction in the WBC neutrophil.

3. **Answer: 4**
   RATIONALE: The nurse should ensure that assistance is available for securing the client as the client is displaying markedly violent behavior patterns. The drug should be given intramuscularly, not intravenously, and preferably in a large muscle mass. The nurse should keep the client lying down, not upright, for about 30 minutes after administering the drug.

4. **Answer: 3**
   RATIONALE: The nurse can mix the oral drugs in liquids such as fruit juices, tomato juice, or milk. The nurse can administer the drugs together; they do not need to be given individually. To confirm whether the client has swallowed the drug, the nurse should inspect the client's mouth, since the client may lie when questioned. The nurse should not compel the client to swallow the drug and should instead report this to the primary health care provider.

5. **Answer: 4**
   RATIONALE: The nurse should monitor the client for bone marrow suppression and other adverse reactions. The client should be informed that only a 1-week supply of this drug is dispensed at a

time. WBC count tests should be scheduled every week, not every 2 weeks, and the testing should continue for 4 weeks, not 1 week, after therapy is discontinued.

6. **Answer: 2**
   RATIONALE: Frequently, clients in a psychotic episode do not perceive reality and moving forward or touching may be thought of as a violent act against themselves instead of a therapeutic gesture as with other client populations. The client may strike out due to fear caused by the psychosis; therefore, touching can be perceived by the client as a threatening gesture and should be avoided.

7. **Answer: 4**
   RATIONALE: The nurse should administer the drug at bedtime so the client is in bed during the effects to minimize risk of injury to the client. Providing the drug with food or a calcium supplement or administering the drug every 8 hours will not help in minimizing the risk of injury to the client.

8. **Answers: 1, 2, 5**
   RATIONALE: The nurse should include the following points in an education plan: report any unusual changes or physical effects, inform the client about the risks of EPS and TD, and avoid exposure to the sun. Altering dosage if the symptoms increase and taking the drug on an empty stomach are not the instructions provided in the nurse's education plan for clients undergoing antipsychotic drug therapy.

9. **Answer: 1**
   RATIONALE: Anhedonia is a symptom of psychosis that is defined as finding no pleasure in activities that are normally pleasurable.

10. **Answer: 2**
    RATIONALE: Antipsychotic medications are thought to act by inhibiting the release of dopamine in the brain and possibly increasing the firing of nerve cells in certain areas of the brain.

11. **Answer: 1**
    RATIONALE: Chlorpromazine may be administered rectally to clients with nausea and vomiting.

12. **Answer: 3**
    RATIONALE: The name of the tool used to monitor clients for involuntary movements is AIMS, or the Abnormal Involuntary Movement Scale screening tool.

CHAPTER 23

SECTION I: ASSESSING YOUR UNDERSTANDING

Activity A FILL IN THE BLANKS

1. myocardial
2. sympathetic
3. hypertension
4. C
5. Vasopressors

Activity B SEQUENCING
1. 2   1   4   3

Activity C MATCHING
1. **1.** b   **2.** c   **3.** d   **4.** a
2. **1.** c   **2.** a   **3.** d   **4.** b

Activity D SHORT ANSWERS

1. Before administering an adrenergic drug for shock, the nurse should perform the following assessments:
   - Assess the client's symptoms, problems, or needs before administering the drug and document any subjective or objective data on the client's record.
   - Obtain blood pressure, pulse rate and quality, and respiratory rate and rhythm.
   - A general survey of the client is done to look for additional symptoms of shock, such as cool skin, cyanosis, diaphoresis, and a change in the level of consciousness.

2. The following nursing interventions are involved during the ongoing administration of metaraminol:
   - Observe the client for the drug's effect.
   - Evaluate and document the drug's effect.
   - Obtain and document vital signs.
   - Compare assessments made before and after administration.
   - Report adverse drug reactions to the primary health care provider.

Activity E CHART THE FINDING

⟶ The client is in hypovolemic shock.
┄┄➤ The client is administered an adrenergic drug.

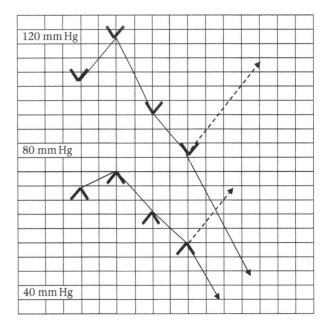

SECTION II: APPLYING YOUR KNOWLEDGE
Activity F CASE STUDY

1. Ms. Chase was most likely suffering from neurogenic shock, a type of distributive shock, as a result of the head trauma and spinal cord injury from the motor vehicle accident.
2. Other symptoms of shock the nurse may observe in Ms. Chase are decreased cardiac output, cool and clammy skin, pallor, cyanosis, sweating, decrease in urinary output, hypoxia, increased concentration of intravascular fluid, tachypnea, pulmonary edema, tachycardia, arrhythmias, wide pulse pressure, gallop rhythm, confusion, agitation, disorientation, and coma.

SECTION III: PRACTICING FOR NCLEX
Activity G NCLEX-STYLE QUESTIONS

1. **Answer: 3**
   RATIONALE: When caring for a client who has been administered metaraminol and is taking digoxin, the nurse should monitor for cardiac arrhythmias. Epigastric distress or a decrease in blood pressure is not known to be caused by the interaction of digoxin and metaraminol, although an increase in blood pressure is an adverse reaction caused by the action of adrenergic drugs. Dopamine, which is an adrenergic drug, is contraindicated in those with pheochromocytoma. Pheochromocytoma is not an adverse reaction caused by the interaction between digoxin and metaraminol.

2. **Answer: 2**
   RATIONALE: Isoproterenol is contraindicated in clients with tachyarrhythmias, tachycardia, or heart block caused by digitalis toxicity; ventricular arrhythmias; and angina pectoris. It is not contraindicated in clients with narrow-angle glaucoma, hypotension, or pheochromocytoma. Dopamine is contraindicated in those with pheochromocytoma (adrenal gland tumor). Epinephrine is contraindicated in clients with narrow-angle glaucoma. Norepinephrine is contraindicated in clients who are hypotensive from blood volume deficits.

3. **Answer: 2**
   RATIONALE: The nurse should immediately report any changes in the pulse rate or rhythm, as older adults are more likely to have preexisting cardiovascular disease that predisposes them to potentially serious cardiac arrhythmias. Nausea, headache, and urinary urgency are not known to occur in older clients due to the administration of adrenergic drugs.

4. **Answer: 1**
   RATIONALE: The nurse should monitor for supine hypertension while caring for a client who is being administered midodrine. Midodrine causes bradycardia, not tachycardia. Orthostatic hypotension is not an adverse effect of midodrine; instead, the drug is taken to reduce orthostatic hypotension. Midodrine is not known to cause respiratory distress.

5. **Answer: 1**
   RATIONALE: The nurse should immediately report a consistent fall in the client's blood pressure, especially if the systolic blood pressure is below 100 mm Hg. A decrease in gastric motility and an increase in the heart rate are desirable outcomes of administering metaraminol. Blood glucose levels are not known to increase with the administration of metaraminol.

6. **Answers: 1, 2, 3**
   RATIONALE: The nurse should identify circumstances that disturb sleep and work toward minimizing their effect. Curtains can be drawn over windows to filter light. The nurse can also provide comfort measures such as a back rub to the client. Caffeinated beverages such as tea and coffee should be avoided. Administering drugs only during daytime will disrupt the blood level of the medication.

7. **Answer: 1**
   RATIONALE: The nurse should immediately discontinue the old IV line and establish another IV line before calling the primary health care provider. Moving the head of the bed to an elevated position will not help minimize the effect of tissue perfusion. Norepinephrine should not be diluted with alkaline solutions.

8. **Answer: 2**
   RATIONALE: The sympathetic nervous system is also known as the adrenergic branch.

9. **Answer: 1**
   RATIONALE: The sympathetic branch of the autonomic nervous system is stimulated during the body's fight, flight, or freeze response to a stressful condition.

10. **Answer: 1**
    RATIONALE: Norepinephrine is the primary neurotransmitter of the sympathetic nervous system.

11. **Answer: 1**
    RATIONALE: Vasoconstriction of peripheral blood vessels occurs as the result of stimulation of $alpha_1$ receptors.

12. **Answer: 1**
    RATIONALE: Decreased tone, motility, and secretions of the GI tract are the result of stimulation of $alpha_2$ receptors.

CHAPTER 24

SECTION I: ASSESSING YOUR UNDERSTANDING

Activity A FILL IN THE BLANKS

1. Norepinephrine
2. Sympatholytic
3. inhibit
4. blockers
5. Glaucoma
6. slower

Activity B DOSAGE CALCULATION

1. 2 tablets
2. 20 tablets
3. 1 tablet
4. 1.5 tablets
5. 2 tablets

Activity C MATCHING

1. **1.** b   **2.** d   **3.** a   **4.** c
2. **1.** c   **2.** d   **3.** b   **4.** a

Activity D SHORT ANSWERS

1. The nurse will perform the following during a teaching session to be certain the client is able to monitor blood pressure in the home:
   - Assess the client's and a family member's ability to see numbers on equipment and handle the apparatus as you help the client determine the best equipment to be used in the home.
   - Be sure the proper size cuff is purchased for the client to minimize inaccurate readings. Remind the client to deflate the cuff completely before putting on or taking off the device.
   - Teach the client and a family member how to inflate and deflate the device and have them demonstrate use before doing the procedure independently. Be sure the arm used is stretched out and at the level of the heart.
   - Teach the client and a family member to use the same extremity for taking the blood pressure.
   - Instruct the client to continue taking the medication regardless of the readings of the blood pressure. Give the parameters of when to call the primary health care provider or emergency services if needed.
   - Explain how to document the blood pressure readings so both the client and primary health care provider can see the trends of the readings.

Activity E CROSSWORD PUZZLE

C								
O								
N						D		
S						I		
T						L		
R						A		
I	N	H	I	B	I	T	S	
C				L		E		
T		S	L	O	W	S		
S				C				
				K				

R	E	L	A	X	E	S
E						
D						
U						
C						
E						
S						

SECTION II: APPLYING YOUR KNOWLEDGE

Activity F CASE STUDY

1. The nurse should include the following in the preadministration assessment of metoprolol to Mrs. Garcia: blood pressure on both arms, pulse rate and rhythm, general appearance, complaints or description of symptoms, and an electrocardiogram.
2. Referring back to Chapter 5 and LEP strategies, find and use written instructions that have been translated into the familiar language. Contact a service of professional interpreters to relay oral instructions or find a fellow employee who speaks Spanish. Avoid using family and friends for interpretation.

SECTION III: PRACTICING FOR NCLEX
Activity G NCLEX-STYLE QUESTIONS

1. **Answer: 2**
   RATIONALE: The nurse needs to monitor for orthostatic hypotension in a client who is treated with phentolamine.

2. **Answer: 3**
   RATIONALE: Coronary artery disease is a contradiction that the nurse must consider when assessing a client for alpha-adrenergic (α-adrenergic blocking) blocking drug therapy. The drug is used to treat pheochromocytoma and is not contraindicated in clients with kidney disease or emphysema.

3. **Answer: 1**
   RATIONALE: The nurse should monitor for vascular insufficiency in the elderly client when administering a beta-adrenergic (β-adrenergic) blocking drug. The nurse need not monitor occipital headache, dizziness, and CNS depression in the elderly client when administering a beta-adrenergic blocking drug, since these conditions are not known to occur in older clients on the administration of beta-adrenergic blocking drugs.

4. **Answer: 4**
   RATIONALE: The nurse should monitor for lightheadedness as the adverse reaction in a client who is administered peripherally acting antiadrenergic drugs.

5. **Answer: 1**
   RATIONALE: The nurse should measure the apical pulse rate when the client is administered a sympatholytic drug. If pulse is below 60 bpm, if there is any irregularity in the client's heart rate or rhythm, or if systolic blood pressure is less than 90 mm Hg, the nurse should withhold the drug and contact the primary health care provider. The nurse need not measure the body temperature, weight, or respiratory rate in the client who is to be administered the sympatholytic drug, since these are not likely to be affected with the administration of a sympatholytic drug.

6. **Answer: 3**
   RATIONALE: The nurse should include contacting the primary health care provider in the teaching plan of the client who is prescribed adrenergic blocking drugs for glaucoma if changes in vision occur.

7. **Answer: 2**
   RATIONALE: The nurse should assess the client for increased risk of psychotic behavior due to the interaction of the antiadrenergic drug with haloperidol. Interaction of an antiadrenergic drug with lithium causes increased risk of lithium toxicity. Increased risk of hypertension is the result of interaction between antiadrenergic drugs and beta blockers. Increased effect of anesthetic is a result of the interaction between antiadrenergic drugs and anesthetic agents.

8. **Answer: 2**
   RATIONALE: Alpha blockers result in vasodilation when administered to clients.

9. **Answer: 1**
   RATIONALE: Phentolamine is an alpha-adrenergic blocker.

10. **Answer: 1**
    RATIONALE: The majority of the beta-adrenergic receptors are found in the heart.

11. **Answer: 4**
    RATIONALE: Peripherally acting (i.e., acting on peripheral structures) antiadrenergic drugs are used to treat benign prostatic hypertrophy (BPH).

12. **Answer: 4**
    RATIONALE: Carvedilol (Coreg) is an example of an alpha/beta-adrenergic drug.

CHAPTER 25

SECTION I: ASSESSING YOUR UNDERSTANDING

Activity A FILL IN THE BLANKS

1. Muscarinic
2. parasympathetic
3. Acetylcholine
4. anticholinesterases
5. Nicotinic

Activity B DOSAGE CALCULATION

1. 8 tablets
2. 2 tablets
3. 3 doses per day

Activity C MATCHING

1. **1.** b **2.** c **3.** a

Activity D SHORT ANSWERS

1. Before administering pyridostigmine for the first time, a nurse should perform the following assessments:
   - Perform a complete neurologic assessment.
   - Assess for signs of muscle weakness, such as drooling, inability to chew and swallow, drooping of the eyelids, double vision, inability to perform repetitive movements, difficulty breathing, and extreme fatigue.

2. The nurse should explain that myasthenia gravis is a disease that involves rapid fatigue of skeletal muscles because of the lack of acetylcholine released at the nerve endings of the parasympathetic nerves. Cholinergic drugs are used primarily to treat symptoms of the disease. Ocular symptoms such as double vision or drooping eyelids are not impacted much with this drug.

Activity E WORD FIND

P		A							
A		C							
R		E							
A		T							
S	N	Y							
Y		I	L						
M	U	S	C	A	R	I	N	I	C
P		H	O						
A		O		T					
T		L			I				
H		I				N			
E		N					I		
T		E						C	
I									
C	H	O	L	I	N	E	R	G	I	C

SECTION II: APPLYING YOUR KNOWLEDGE

Activity F CASE STUDY

1. Before the nurse gives a medication for urinary retention, the nurse should palpate the abdomen in the pelvic area and scan the bladder to determine if urine retention is present. A rounded swelling over the pelvis usually indicates retention and a distended bladder. The client may also complain of discomfort in the lower abdomen. In addition, take and document the client's blood pressure and pulse rate.
2. The nurse should advise Mr. Park that voiding usually occurs in 5–15 minutes after subcutaneous drug administration and 30–90 minutes after oral administration.

SECTION III: PRACTICING FOR NCLEX

Activity G NCLEX-STYLE QUESTIONS

1. **Answer: 1**
   RATIONALE: The nurse should observe for temporary reduction of visual acuity and headache as adverse reactions of the topical administration of cholinergic drugs. Increased ocular tension, decreased sweat production, and anaphylactic shock are not related adverse reactions. They are adverse reactions of cholinergic blocking drugs.

2. **Answer: 3**
   RATIONALE: When developing a teaching plan for the client and family, emphasize the importance of uninterrupted drug therapy.

3. **Answer: 2**
   RATIONALE: The nurse should anticipate the decreased effect of the cholinergic as the effect of the interaction between pyridostigmine and corticosteroids. Increased neuromuscular blocking effect, increased absorption of the cholinergic, and decreased serum levels of corticosteroids are not related effects of the interactions between pyridostigmine and corticosteroids.

4. **Answers: 2, 4, 5**
   RATIONALE: Stimulation of this pathway results in the opposite reactions to those triggered by the adrenergic system: blood vessels dilate, sending blood to the gastrointestinal (GI) tract; secretions and peristalsis are activated and salivary glands increase production; the heart slows and pulmonary bronchioles constrict; the smooth muscle of the bladder contracts; and the pupils of the eyes constrict.

5. **Answer: 3**
   RATIONALE: The nurse caring for a client who is being administered a cholinergic drug should ensure that aminoglycoside antibiotics are administered cautiously, as they increase the risk of neuromuscular blocking effects.

6. **Answers: 3, 4, 5**
   RATIONALE: The nurse should observe for salivation, clenching of the jaw, and muscle rigidity and spasm as symptoms of drug overdose in the client to make frequent dosage adjustments. Drooping of the eyelids and rapid fatigability of the muscles are symptoms of drug underdosing.

7. **Answer: 3**
   RATIONALE: The nurse should place the call light and items that the client might need within easy reach while managing the care of client-administered cholinergic therapy for urinary retention.

8. **Answers: 1, 3, 5**
   RATIONALE: The nurse should ensure that a bedpan or bathroom is readily available, encourage the client to ambulate to assist the passing of flatus, and keep a record of the number, consistency, and frequency of stools if the client develops diarrhea after administering the urecholine drug orally.

9. **Answer: 1**
   RATIONALE: The stimulation of muscarinic receptors in the parasympathetic nervous system stimulates smooth muscle.

10. **Answer: 2**
    RATIONALE: The stimulation of nicotinic receptors in the parasympathetic nervous system stimulates skeletal muscle.

11. Answer: 1

RATIONALE: Acetylcholinesterase is the enzyme responsible for deactivating acetylcholine, the primary neurotransmitter in the parasympathetic nervous system.

12. Answer: 1

RATIONALE: Bethanechol is an example of a direct-acting cholinergic that acts like the neurotransmitter acetylcholine.

CHAPTER 26

SECTION I: ASSESSING YOUR UNDERSTANDING

Activity A FILL IN THE BLANKS

1. Acetylcholine
2. parasympathetic
3. Cycloplegia
4. atropine
5. idiosyncrasy

Activity B DOSAGE CALCULATION

1. 1 tablet
2. 1 tablet
3. No, 6 doses × 2 puffs = 12 inhalations
4. Total dose is 10 tablets; 12 pack is sufficient

Activity C MATCHING

1. **1.** c **2.** b **3.** a
2. **1.** c **2.** a **3.** d **4.** b

Activity D SHORT ANSWERS

1. The nurse should include the following when evaluating the client's treatment plan:
   - Therapeutic effect is achieved.
   - Oral mucous membranes remain moist.
   - Client reports adequate bowel movements.
   - No evidence of injury is seen.
2. The nurse should offer the following instructions to an older client's family when caring for the client receiving cholinergic blocking drugs for treatment:
   - The nurse should inform the family of possible visual and mental impairments (blurred vision, confusion, agitation) that may occur during therapy with these drugs. Objects or situations that may cause falls, such as throw rugs, footstools, and wet or newly waxed floors, should be removed or remedied whenever possible.
   - The nurse should instruct the family to place against the walls any items of furniture (e.g., footstools, chairs, stands) that obstruct walkways.
   - The nurse should alert the family to the dangers of heat prostration and explain the steps to take to avoid this problem.
   - The client must be closely observed during the first few days of therapy, and the primary health care provider should be notified if mental changes occur.

Activity E CROSSWORD PUZZLE

SECTION II: APPLYING YOUR KNOWLEDGE

Activity F CASE STUDY

1. The following is a list of adverse reactions that should be included in the nurse's teaching plan for Mrs. Moore: photophobia, dry mouth, constipation, heat prostration, and drowsiness.
2. The nurse should instruct the daughter to observe for the following in an older client receiving a cholinergic drug such as tolterodine (Detrol LA): excitement, agitation, mental confusion, drowsiness, urinary retention, or other adverse effects. These effects may be seen even with small doses in the older adult. If any of these adverse effects occur, it is important to withhold the next dose and contact the primary health care provider.

SECTION III: PRACTICING FOR NCLEX

Activity G NCLEX-STYLE QUESTIONS

1. **Answer: 4**

RATIONALE: A nurse should use atropine cautiously in clients with asthma.

2. Answer: 2
RATIONALE: When caring for a client on cholinergic drugs complaining of constipation, the nurse should instruct the client to increase fluid intake up to 2000 mL daily (if health conditions permit). Depending on the type of antacids, they can cause constipation, since antacids will not help relieve the client's condition. The nurse need not instruct the client to increase the consumption of citrus juices because this will not offer the fiber content as well as the fruit to relieve the client's constipation.

3. Answers: 1, 2, 3, 4
RATIONALE: The nurse should instruct the client to do the following: avoid going outside on hot, sunny days; garden early in the day; use fans to cool the body if the day is extremely warm; sponge the skin with cool water if other cooling measures are not available; and wear loose-fitting clothes in warm weather. Wearing sunglasses will shade the eyes, yet will not change the heat or warmth of the client.

4. Answers: 1, 2
RATIONALE: Unintended adverse reactions include nausea and altered taste perceptions. Tachycardia, dry mouth, and mydriasis are generalized responses to blocking the parasympathetic nervous system.

5. Answer: 1
RATIONALE: The nurse should ensure that the cholinergic drug is to be administered preoperatively for this 65-year-old client because cholinergic blocking drugs are usually not included in the preoperative drugs of clients older than 60 years due to their effects on the eyes and central nervous system.

6. Answer: 3
RATIONALE: The nurse should administer the drug at the exact time prescribed by the physician in order to allow the drug to produce the greatest effect before the administration of the anesthetic.

7. Answer: 2
RATIONALE: Mouth dryness after the oxybutynin is administered to the client will be a daily ongoing issue.

8. Answer: 4
RATIONALE: The nurse should identify drowsiness as part of the desired response for the client who has been administered atropine preoperatively. Vomiting, elevated temperature, and low pulse rate are not known to be the desired responses to the administration of atropine when it is administered preoperatively.

9. Answer: 1
RATIONALE: Oxybutynin is an example of a parasympatholytic drug.

10. Answer: 2
RATIONALE: The Parkinson drug is used to decrease skeletal muscle spasms by inhibiting the nicotinic receptors in skeletal muscles.

11. Answer: 4
RATIONALE: The cholinergic blocking drug glycopyrrolate (Robinul) is used in conjunction with anesthesia to reduce oral and bronchial secretions.

12. Answer: 3
RATIONALE: The nurse should observe clients receiving a cholinergic blocking drug during the hot summer months because these clients are at increased risk of heat prostration.

CHAPTER 27

SECTION I: ASSESSING YOUR UNDERSTANDING

Activity A FILL IN THE BLANKS
1. Parkinson disease
2. tremors, rigidity, bradykinesia
3. shuffled
4. extrapyramidal symptoms
5. irresistible

Activity B DOSAGE CALCULATION
1. 1 capsule (100 mg/dose)
2. 75 mg
3. 0.5 mL

Activity C MATCHING
1. 1. b 2. d 3. a 4. c
2. 1. c 2. a 3. d 4. b

Activity D SHORT ANSWERS
1. The nurse should observe for the following as part of the neuromuscular assessment of the client:
- Tremors of the hands or head while the client is at rest
- A masklike facial expression
- Changes (from the normal) in walking
- Type of speech pattern (halting, monotone)
- Postural deformities
- Muscular rigidity
- Drooling, difficulty in chewing or swallowing
- Changes in thought processes
- Client's ability to carry out any or all of the activities of daily living (e.g., bathing, ambulating, dressing).

2. Lack of balance is an issue for those with Parkinson disease. Research indicates a reduction in injury when clients participate in activities to improve balance, such as Tai Chi. You can refer clients to occupational or activity directors who may have listings of exercise programs that cater to individuals with balance issues.

Activity E WORD FIND

							P				
B		A	C	H	A	L	A	S	I	A	
	R	K					R				
		A					K				
		T	D				I			A	
		H		Y			N		I		
		I			K		S	N			
		S				I	O				
		I				T	N				
		A			S		I	E	P	S	
				Y			S		S		
			D				M			I	
											A

SECTION II: APPLYING YOUR KNOWLEDGE

Activity F CASE STUDY

1. It is hard to supplement dopamine because of the blood–brain barrier, the meshwork of tightly packed cells in the walls of the brain's capillaries that screen out certain substances. Dopamine is a large molecule that is prohibited from crossing the blood–brain barrier.
2. The language on the National Parkinson Foundation website can turn into Spanish with the click of a mouse. What other resources did students find?

SECTION III: PRACTICING FOR NCLEX

Activity G NCLEX-STYLE QUESTIONS

1. **Answer: 2**
   RATIONALE: When caring for a client exhibiting choreiform and dystonic movements, the nurse should withhold the next dose of the drug and notify the primary health care provider because it may be necessary to reduce the dosage of levodopa or discontinue use of the drug.
2. **Answers: 1, 2, 3**
   RATIONALE: The nurse should carefully monitor for muscular rigidity, elevated body temperature, and mental changes in the client with neuroleptic malignant-like syndrome, which occurs when the antiparkinson drugs are discontinued or the dosage of levodopa is reduced abruptly.

3. **Answer: 3**
   RATIONALE: The nurse should anticipate the increased effect of levodopa as the effect of the interaction between levodopa and antacids.
4. **Answer: 1**
   RATIONALE: The nurse should know that catechol-O-methyltransferase (COMT) inhibitors should be used with caution in clients with decreased renal function.
5. **Answers: 1, 2, 3**
   RATIONALE: When preparing a discharge care plan for a client who has had antiparkinson drugs, the nurse should instruct the client to avoid taking vitamin B_6 with levodopa. The nurse should also instruct the client to avoid consuming alcohol and to contact the PHCP in case the client experiences any symptoms of dry mouth, chewing, urination, depression, dizziness, or unusual muscle movement.
6. **Answer: 1**
   RATIONALE: When caring for a client on antiparkinson drugs experiencing GI disturbances like nausea and vomiting, the nurse should discontinue the antiparkinson drug or change it. Severe nausea or vomiting may necessitate discontinuing the drug and changing to a different antiparkinson drug. Administering the drug before meals, administering antacids after meals, and refraining from giving liquids after meals are not very appropriate interventions when caring for a client who is vomiting or experiencing other GI disturbances.
7. **Answer: 3**
   RATIONALE: When caring for a client on antiparkinson drugs who is responding to therapy, the nurse would closely monitor the client's behavior at frequent intervals.
8. **Answer: 1**
   RATIONALE: The nurse should observe for changes in facial expression that may indicate abdominal pain in the client. The nurse observes the client with Parkinson-like symptoms for outward changes that may indicate one or more adverse reactions, like a sudden change in the facial expression or changes in posture that may indicate abdominal pain or discomfort, which may be caused by urinary retention, paralytic ileus, or constipation.
9. **Answer: 1**
   RATIONALE: *Parkinsonism* is the term that refers to a group of symptoms involving motor movement characterized by tremors, rigidity, and bradykinesia.
10. **Answer: 3**
    RATIONALE: Carbidopa (Lodosyn) is classified as a dopaminergic agent that treats parkinsonism by supplementing the amount of dopamine in the brain.

11. **Answer: 1**
    RATIONALE: Entacapone (Comtan) is classified as a catechol-O-methyltransferase (COMT) inhibitor.
12. **Answer: 3**
    RATIONALE: Apomorphine (Apokyn) is classified as a nonergot dopamine receptor agonist.
13. **Answer: 4**
    RATIONALE: Benztropine (Cogentin) is classified as a cholinergic blocking drug used to treat Parkinson-like symptoms.

CHAPTER 28

SECTION I: ASSESSING YOUR UNDERSTANDING

Activity A FILL IN THE BLANKS

1. convulsion
2. seizure
3. Focal
4. depress
5. Status epilepticus

Activity B DOSAGE CALCULATION

1. 2 capsules
2. 2 capsules
3. 2 tablets
4. 4-mg tablets, will take 2 tablets each dose
5. 2 tablets

Activity C MATCHING

1. **1.** c   **2.** a   **3.** d   **4.** b
2. **1.** c   **2.** d   **3.** b   **4.** a

Activity D SHORT ANSWERS

1. The nurse should perform the following bedside assessments and document the responses using these questions:
   - "What is your name?"
   - "How are you feeling?"
   - Hold up two fingers and ask, "What do you see?"
   - "Where are you and where do you live?"
   - Ask the client to touch their left ear.
   - Show the client an item, like your pen, and ask, "What is this?"
2. When caring for a client on antiepileptic drug therapy, the nurse's role is to
   - Be prepared for changing orders that will adjust the dosage or type of antiepileptics based on client response to the therapy and the occurrence of adverse reactions during the initial treatment.
   - Monitor serum levels of antiepileptics on a regular basis for toxicity.
   - Document time of occurrence and duration of seizure, and psychic or motor activity occurring before, during, and after.
   - Assist primary health care provider in their evaluation of drug therapy.

Activity E CROSSWORD PUZZLE

SECTION II: APPLYING YOUR KNOWLEDGE

Activity F CASE STUDY

1. The nurse should obtain the following information from those who observed the seizure: description of the seizures (the motor or psychic activity occurring during the seizure), frequency of the seizures (approximate number per day), average length of a seizure, description of an aura if any has occurred (a subjective sensation preceding a seizure), description of the degree of impairment of consciousness, and description of what, if anything, appears to bring on the seizure.
2. Ms. Chase may be experiencing phenytoin toxicity. Signs of toxicity include slurred speech, ataxia, lethargy, dizziness, nausea, and vomiting.

SECTION III: PRACTICING FOR NCLEX

Activity G NCLEX-STYLE QUESTIONS

1. **Answer: 1**
   RATIONALE: While administering carbamazepine, the nurse should monitor for photosensitivity in the client.
2. **Answers: 2, 3, 5**
   RATIONALE: In the teaching plan of the client continuing hydantoin drug therapy, the nurse should include brushing and flossing teeth after each meal, since long-term administration of the hydantoins can cause gingivitis and gingival hyperplasia (overgrowth of gum tissue); avoiding consumption of discolored capsules; and taking medication with food. Notifying the health care provider if blurred vision occurs is included in the teaching plan when succinimides are taken.
3. **Answer: 3**
   RATIONALE: The nurse should immediately report to the primary health care provider the incidence of thrombocytopenia in the client. Sinus bradycardia, sinoatrial block, and Adams–Stokes syndrome are not hematologic changes but contraindications for phenytoin.
4. **Answer: 2**
   RATIONALE: A severe and potentially fatal rash can occur in clients taking lamotrigine. Should a rash occur, notify the primary health care provider immediately because the drug may be discontinued.
5. **Answer: 3**
   RATIONALE: The nurse should know that phenytoin is contraindicated in a client with hepatic abnormalities.
6. **Answer: 4**
   RATIONALE: The nurse should carefully observe for apnea and cardiac arrest in a client undergoing diazepam therapy. Apnea and cardiac arrest have occurred when diazepam is administered to older adults, very ill clients, and individuals with limited pulmonary reserve.
7. **Answer: 2**
   RATIONALE: The nurse should identify that phenytoin plasma levels are greater than 20 mcg/mL if the client exhibits signs of drug toxicity. Phenytoin plasma levels between 10 and 20 mcg/mL give the optimal anticonvulsant effect; less than 10 mcg/mL is not therapeutic.
8. **Answer: 3**
   RATIONALE: Simple seizures, motor seizures, and somatosensory seizures are classified as focal seizures.
9. **Answer: 1**
   RATIONALE: Tonic–clonic seizures and myoclonic seizures are classified as generalized seizures.
10. **Answer: 3**
    RATIONALE: Generalized seizures involve a loss of consciousness.
11. **Answer: 2**
    RATIONALE: Hydantoins like phenytoin (Dilantin) elicit their effects by stabilizing the hyperexcitability postsynaptically in the motor cortex of the brain.
12. **Answer: 1**
    RATIONALE: Carboxylic acid derivatives like valproic acid (Depakote) elicit their effects by increasing levels of gamma-aminobutyric (γ-aminobutyric) acid (GABA), which stabilizes cell membranes.

CHAPTER 29

SECTION I: ASSESSING YOUR UNDERSTANDING

Activity A FILL IN THE BLANKS

1. bisphosphonates
2. Allopurinol
3. immunosuppression
4. Gout
5. upright

Activity B DOSAGE CALCULATION

1. 1 tablet
2. 14 tablets
3. 2 tablets
4. 8:00 a.m.; client must wait at least 30 minutes before eating or drinking
5. 100 mL

Activity C MATCHING

1. **1.** c   **2.** d   **3.** a   **4.** b
2. **1.** b   **2.** a   **3.** d   **4.** c

Activity D SHORT ANSWERS

1. The preadministration assessments the nurse should conduct before administration of a bisphosphonate drug are as follows:
   - Obtain client's history of disorders, onset, symptoms, and current treatment or therapy.

- Appraise the client's physical condition and limitations, such as inability to carry out activities of daily living, including employment when applicable.
- Examine affected joints in extremities for appearance of skin over joint, evidence of joint deformity, and mobility of affected joint.
- Assess for pain in upper and lower back or hip.
- Document vital signs and weight.
- Perform laboratory tests and bone scans to measure bone density as ordered by the

primary health care provider including T-score and serum calcium level.

2. The ongoing assessments a nurse should perform when caring for a client administered a bisphosphonate drug are as follows:
- Evaluate periodically for musculoskeletal disorders.
- Inquire about pain relief and adverse reactions, especially heartburn or GI distress.
- Evaluate serum calcium levels and T-scores periodically.

Activity E CROSSWORD PUZZLE

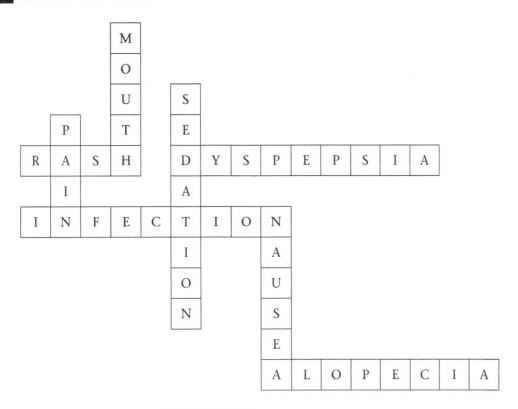

SECTION II: APPLYING YOUR KNOWLEDGE
Activity F CASE STUDY

1. The nurse examines the affected joints and notes the appearance of the skin over the joints and any joint enlargement prior to the primary health care provider examining the client.
2. During the pegloticase infusion, the client is closely monitored for the development of anaphylactic reactions.

SECTION III: PRACTICING FOR NCLEX
Activity G NCLEX-STYLE QUESTIONS

1. **Answer: 1**
   RATIONALE: Dyspepsia is the adverse reaction that the nurse should monitor for in the client. Sleepiness, lethargy, and constipation are the adverse reactions of the skeletal muscle relaxant diazepam.

2. **Answer: 2**
   RATIONALE: The use of alendronate is contraindicated in clients with hypocalcemia. The use of alendronate is not contraindicated in clients with hypertension, insomnia, or diabetes.
3. **Answer: 3**
   RATIONALE: The nurse should monitor for methotrexate toxicity in the client as an interaction of sulfa antibiotics with disease-modifying antirheumatic drugs.
4. **Answers: 1, 2, 3**
   RATIONALE: The nurse should monitor hematology, liver function, and renal function every 1–3 months in clients administered methotrexate. The primary care provider is notified of abnormal hematology, liver function, or kidney function findings.
5. **Answer: 4**
   RATIONALE: After administering DMARDs, the client should notify the primary health care

provider in the case of diarrhea. Administering drugs with food, drinking 10 glasses of water a day and avoiding driving or hazardous tasks in case of drowsiness are the instructions that a client should follow when administered drugs used to treat gout.

6. **Answer: 2**

   RATIONALE: The nurse should closely monitor the client for adverse reactions as an ongoing assessment for clients receiving bisphosphonates for osteoporosis. Obtaining the client's history of disorders, appraising the client's physical condition and limitations, and assessing for pain in the upper and lower back or hip are preadministration assessments for clients receiving drugs for musculoskeletal disorders.

7. **Answers: 1, 2, 5**

   RATIONALE: Nursing interventions include reporting adverse reactions (especially vision changes); being alert to reactions such as skin rash, fever, cough, or easy bruising; and being attentive to these clients as they often require emotional support, especially when their disorder is disabling and chronic.

8. **Answer: 4**

   RATIONALE: Infliximab (Remicade) should not be used in clients with cardiac disorders, specifically heart failure.

9. **Answer: 1**

   RATIONALE: Bisphosphonates are the class of medications used in the treatment of osteoporosis.

10. **Answer: 3**

    RATIONALE: Baclofen (Lioresal) is an example of a skeletal muscle relaxant.

11. **Answer: 1**

    RATIONALE: Zoledronic acid (Reclast) is a bisphosphonate administered once a year IV.

12. **Answer: 2**

    RATIONALE: Drowsiness is the most common adverse reaction to skeletal muscle relaxants like carisoprodol (Soma) that the nurse should discuss with the client.

CHAPTER 30

SECTION I: ASSESSING YOUR UNDERSTANDING

Activity A FILL IN THE BLANKS

1. inflammatory
2. expectorant
3. decongestant
4. vasoconstriction
5. respiratory

Activity B DOSAGE CALCULATION

1. 15 mL
2. 30 mg
3. 100 mcg
4. 10 mg
5. 60 mg

Activity C MATCHING

1. **1.** c   **2.** b   **3.** d   **4.** a
2. **1.** c   **2.** e   **3.** b   **4.** a   **5.** d

Activity D SHORT ANSWERS

1. The nurse should perform the following telephone assessments:
   - Ask about the type of cough (productive, nonproductive)
   - Ask the client to describe the color and amount of sputum present if any
   - Ask about self- or home remedies used already
   - Ask about vital signs, such as "Do you have a fever, are you breathing faster, or do you feel your heart beating faster?"

2. The decongestant used for sinusitis may be a topical or oral medication.
   - Assure the client that topical decongestants have minimal systemic effects.
   - Occasional adverse reactions seen with topical decongestants include nasal burning or stinging or dryness of the nasal mucosa.
   - Overuse of the topical form of decongestants can cause "rebound" nasal congestion. This means that the congestion becomes worse with the use of the drug.
   - When the topical form is used frequently or if the liquid is swallowed, it may produce adverse reactions similar to those seen with oral decongestants—tachycardia and other cardiac arrhythmias, nervousness, restlessness, insomnia, blurred vision, nausea, and vomiting.

Activity E WORD FIND PUZZLE

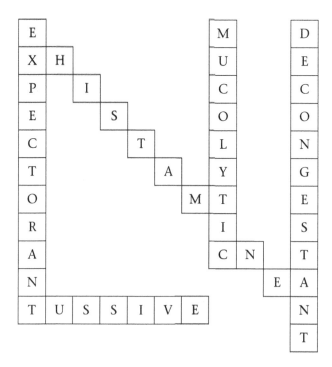

The drug class missing from the puzzle is intranasal steroids.

SECTION II: APPLYING YOUR KNOWLEDGE

Activity F CASE STUDY

1. The nurse should perform the following telephone assessments:
   - Ask about the type of cold symptoms.
   - Ask her to describe the color and amount of sputum present if any.
   - Ask about self- or home remedies used already, the current medication she is taking, and the frequency with which she is taking the medications.

2. Explain to Betty Peterson that overuse of the topical form of decongestants can cause "rebound" nasal congestion. This means that the congestion becomes worse with use of the drug. Although congestion may be relieved briefly after the drug is used, it recurs within a short time, which would prompt Betty to use the drug at more frequent intervals, perpetuating the rebound congestion. Remind Betty to take the drug exactly as prescribed. A simple but uncomfortable solution to rebound congestion is to withdraw completely from the topical medication. Ask if she would prefer the primary health care provider (PHCP) to recommend an oral decongestant. Explain homeopathic remedies if she is agreeable to their use.

SECTION III: PRACTICING FOR NCLEX

Activity G NCLEX-STYLE QUESTIONS

1. **Answers: 2, 3, 5**
   RATIONALE: When caring for a client who has been prescribed an expectorant for the treatment of a cough, the nurse should assess the respiratory status of the client, document the lung sounds of the client, and document the consistency of sputum.

2. **Answers: 2, 3, 5**
   RATIONALE: In the teaching plan for a client undergoing antitussive drug therapy, the nurse should include instructions to avoid irritants such as cigarette smoke, avoid drinking fluids for 30 minutes after taking the drug, and avoid chewing or breaking open the oral capsules.

3. **Answer: 4**
   RATIONALE: Although all the answers are correct instruction for use of a nasal decongestant, the priority instruction is to refrain from sharing the drug container with multiple users. Cross-contamination can happen and the infection can spread among the entire household.

4. **Answer: 4**
   RATIONALE: The nurse should know that antitussives are contraindicated in the client with hypersensitivity to the drug. Antitussives are not contraindicated in clients with cardiac problems, asthma, or liver dysfunction.

5. **Answers: 1, 2, 5**
   RATIONALE: The nurse should administer decongestants cautiously in clients with hypertension, hyperthyroidism, and glaucoma. No extra caution is required when the drug is used in conjunctivitis or nephropathy.

6. **Answer: 2**
   RATIONALE: The nurse should encourage fluid intake of up to 2000 mL per day, if this amount is not contraindicated by the client's condition or disease process, to promote effective airway clearance. There is no need to avoid juices or monitor fluid output, and antitussives are not recommended for a productive cough.

7. **Answer: 2**
   RATIONALE: Eucalyptus should not be used during pregnancy and lactation and in children younger than 2 years.

8. **Answer: 1**
   RATIONALE: The client should consult the PHCP if the cough lasts more than 10 days.

9. **Answer: 1**
   RATIONALE: Dornase alfa (Pulmozyme) is a mucolytic used specifically in the treatment of cystic fibrosis.

10. **Answer: 1**
    RATIONALE: Concurrent use of iodine products can increase the hypothyroid effects of antithyroid drugs.

11. **Answers: 1, 3**
    RATIONALE: The adverse effects of benzonatate include sedation, headache, dizziness, constipation, nausea, GI upset, pruritus, and nasal congestion. It is recommended that clients with cough drink plenty of fluids (1500–2000 mL daily) unless fluids are contraindicated due to another disease state. Benzonatate should not be crushed or chewed, as its local anesthetic effect could result in choking. Consumption of alcohol while taking benzonatate can increase CNS depression and increase sedation. The maximum daily dose of benzonatate is 600 mg daily.

12. **Answer: 1**
    RATIONALE: Thinning respiratory secretions is the mechanism of action for expectorants. Breaking down thick mucus in the lower lungs is the mechanism of action of mucolytics. Depressing the cough center in the brain is the mechanism of action for centrally acting antitussives. Anesthetizing stretch receptors in the respiratory passages is the mechanism of action for peripherally acting antitussives.

CHAPTER 31

SECTION I: ASSESSING YOUR UNDERSTANDING

Activity A FILL IN THE BLANKS

1. inflammatory
2. histamine
3. mucus
4. anxious
5. Bronchodilators

Activity B OUT IN THE COMMUNITY

1. Green zone peak flow is 280, yellow zone peak flow is 175–276/277, and red zone peak flow is below 175.
2. Asmanex 1 puff
3. 180 mcg

Activity E SUDOKU PUZZLE

PEV	ICS	DPI	LABA	SOB	MDI	EIB	SABA	COPD
SABA	LABA	EIB	DPI	COPD	ICS	PEV	SOB	MDI
COPD	SOB	MDI	PEV	EIB	SABA	DPI	LABA	ICS
DPI	EIB	ICS	SABA	LABA	SOB	MDI	COPD	PEV
MDI	PEV	SABA	EIB	ICS	COPD	LABA	DPI	SOB
LABA	COPD	SOB	MDI	PEV	DPI	ICS	EIB	SABA
ICS	DPI	PEV	SOB	SABA	EIB	COPD	MDI	LABA
EIB	SABA	LABA	COPD	MDI	PEV	SOB	ICS	DPI
SOB	MDI	COPD	ICS	DPI	LABA	SABA	PEV	EIB

SECTION II: APPLYING YOUR KNOWLEDGE

Activity F CASE STUDY

1. A client with step 3 persistent asthma should be treated daily with a low-dose inhaled corticosteroid plus a long-acting beta$_2$ (β_2) agonist (LABA) or medium-dose inhaled corticosteroid. She should also have a short-acting, inhaled beta$_2$ agonist (SABA) for rescue.
2. Environmental controls used to help control asthma include not smoking, not allowing smoking in the home, being aware of and avoiding asthma triggers (pollen, sulfites, etc.), washing bedding once a week in hot water, and wearing a scarf over the mouth and nose if cold air bothers the client.

Activity C MATCHING

1. 1. d   2. c   3. e   4. a   5. b
2. 1. b   2. e   3. a   4. c   5. d

Activity D SHORT ANSWERS

1. The long-term management of asthma uses a stepwise approach, meaning that medications and their frequency of administration are adjusted according to the severity of the client's asthma. Medications that reduce inflammation are the first-line (or step) intervention. Quick-relief medications include inhaled short-acting beta$_2$-adrenergic agonists (β_2-adrenergic agonists) (SABAs), and oral steroids are used as the steps progress.
2. Clients are encouraged to use asthma action plans for daily self-management and for the immediate management of acute respiratory exacerbations.

SECTION III: PRACTICING FOR NCLEX

Activity G NCLEX-STYLE QUESTIONS

1. **Answer: 2**
   RATIONALE: Xanthine derivatives are the drugs for clients with glaucoma. Long- and short-acting beta-adrenergic drugs (β-adrenergic drugs) as well as inhaled corticosteroids should be avoided in clients with glaucoma.

2. **Answer: 4**
   RATIONALE: The nurse should inform the client that beta blockers could increase the effects of aminophylline. Ketoconazole, rifampin, and loop diuretics decrease the effects of theophyllines, including aminophylline.

3. **Answer: 1**
   RATIONALE: The nurse should assess the electrocardiographic changes to check for the occurrence of adverse effects with aminophylline. Aminophylline belongs to the group theophylline, which causes electrocardiographic changes as adverse reactions. Changes in blood hemoglobin, fluid intake and output, and the consistency of stool are not associated with aminophylline.

4. **Answer: 2**
   RATIONALE: The nurse may observe anxiety as the client complains of dyspnea and wheezing, resulting in shortness of breath. Increased urination, decreased pulse rate, and decreased blood pressure are not indicators of asthma. During an asthmatic attack, there may be an increased pulse rate.

5. **Answer: 2**
   RATIONALE: When zafirlukast is given to a client on aspirin, there may be an increase in the plasma levels of zafirlukast. There is no decrease in the plasma levels or increase in the thrombolytic effects of aspirin due to such an interaction.

6. **Answers: 3, 4, 2, 5, 1**
   RATIONALE: In asthma, the mast cells release histamine. This causes increased mucous formation and edema of the airway, leading to bronchospasm and inflammation. This leads to narrowing of the airway along with clogging due to excessive mucus. When the airways are narrowed, there is decreased airflow to the lungs.

7. **Answers: 2, 3, 5**
   RATIONALE: Flunisolide, beclomethasone, and triamcinolone are inhalational corticosteroid agents used in the treatment of asthma. Cromolyn and ipratropium are not used in the chronic treatment of asthma. Cromolyn is a mast cell stabilizer. Ipratropium is an anticholinergic drug.

8. **Answer: 1**
   RATIONALE: The client is instructed to take montelukast orally only once in the evening. This drug should be taken even when there are no symptoms. The client should not take the drug more than once daily.

9. **Answer: 3**
   RATIONALE: Albuterol is a SABA. Formoterol, salmeterol, and arformoterol are long-acting beta$_2$ (β_2) agonists (LABAs).

10. **Answer: 1**
    RATIONALE: Long-acting beta$_2$ agonists have been shown in studies to increase the risk of asthma-related death.

11. **Answers: 1, 2, 5**
    RATIONALE: Worsening of cough, tachypnea, dyspnea, and generalized wheezing and chest tightness usually precede an asthma exacerbation.

12. **Answer: 2**
    RATIONALE: Stimulation of the central nervous system is the mechanism of action for xanthine derivatives.

CHAPTER 32

SECTION I: ASSESSING YOUR UNDERSTANDING

Activity A FILL IN THE BLANKS

1. edema
2. Carbonic
3. potassium
4. paresthesias
5. Dermatologic

Activity B DOSAGE CALCULATION

1. ½ tablet
2. 3 tablets
3. 10 mL
4. 2.5 tablets

Activity C MATCHING

1. 1. e   2. a   3. b   4. c   5. d
2. 1. c   2. a   3. d   4. b

Activity D SHORT ANSWERS

1. The nurse should perform the following preadministration assessments before the administration of a diuretic drug to a client:
   - The nurse should take the vital signs and weigh the client.
   - Current laboratory test results, especially the levels of serum electrolytes, should be carefully reviewed. (Clients with renal dysfunction should also have blood urea nitrogen [BUN] and creatinine clearance levels monitored.)
   - If the client has peripheral edema, the nurse should inspect the involved areas and record in the client's chart the degree and extent of edema.
   - If the client is to receive an osmotic diuretic, the focus of the assessment is on the client's disease or disorder and the symptoms being treated. For example, if the client has a low urinary output and the osmotic diuretic is given to increase urinary output, then the nurse should review the intake and output ratio and symptoms the client is experiencing.

2. The nurse should perform the following assessments after the administration of a diuretic drug:
   - During initial therapy, the nurse should observe the client for the effects of drug therapy. The type of assessment will depend on such factors as the reason for administration of the diuretic, type of diuretic administered, route of administration, and condition of the client.
   - The nurse should measure and record fluid intake and output, and report to the primary health care provider any marked decrease in the output.
   - During ongoing therapy, the nurse should weigh the client at the same time daily, making certain that the client is wearing the same amount or type of clothing.
   - Depending on the specific diuretic, frequent serum electrolyte, uric acid, and liver and kidney function tests

should be performed during the first few months of therapy, and periodically thereafter.

Activity E CROSSWORD PUZZLE

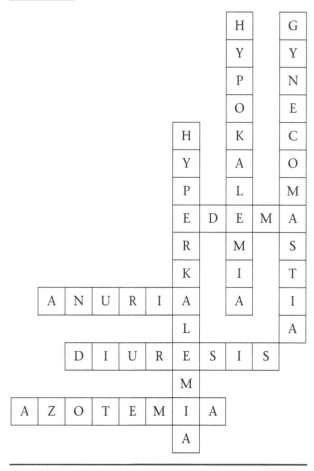

SECTION II: APPLYING YOUR KNOWLEDGE

Activity F CASE STUDY

1. The nurse will need to administer 3.4 mL to Mrs. Moore every 6 hours.

$$150 \text{ lb} \times 1 \text{ kg}/2.2 \text{ lb} = 68.2 \text{ kg}$$

$$68.2 \text{ kg} \times 1 \text{ mg}/\text{kg} = 68.2 \text{ mg}$$

$$68.2 \text{ mg} \times 1 \text{ mL}/20 \text{ mg} = 3.4 \text{ mL}$$

2. The adverse effects of furosemide (Lasix) include electrolyte and hematologic imbalances, anorexia, nausea, vomiting, dizziness, rash, photosensitivity, orthostatic hypotension, hypokalemia, and glycosuria.

SECTION III: PRACTICING FOR NCLEX

Activity G NCLEX-STYLE QUESTIONS

1. **Answers: 1, 3, 4**
   RATIONALE: The nurse should take a daily measurement and record the client's weight to monitor fluid loss. The nurse should measure fluid intake and output every 8 hours and assess respiratory rate (possible pulmonary edema) every 4 hours to assess that the client is achieving optimal response to therapy. The nurse need not check the pupil of the eye every 2 hours for dilation or check the client's response to light.

2. **Answer: 2**
   RATIONALE: When caring for a client receiving diuretics and experiencing GI upset, the nurse should instruct the client to take the drug with food or milk. The nurse need not instruct the client to take the drug on an empty stomach or avoid intake of fibrous food, as these are not appropriate interventions to reduce the symptoms or discomforts due to GI upset. The nurse should not instruct the client to reduce fluid intake to prevent discomfort associated with GI upset. Clients may exhibit anxiety with the frequent need to urinate as a result of the diuretic therapy, but the nurse should not reduce their fluid intake; the nurse should explain that the need to urinate frequently decreases after a few weeks of therapy.

3. **Answer: 2**
   RATIONALE: The nurse should monitor the client for an increased risk of hyperglycemia as an effect of interaction between the chlorothiazide and antidiabetic drug.

4. **Answers: 1, 3, 4**
   RATIONALE: Foods high in potassium include dried apricots, green beans, and molasses. Carrots are not a high-potassium food.

5. **Answer: 2**
   RATIONALE: The nurse should know that the client is experiencing an electrolyte imbalance. Warning signs of a fluid and electrolyte imbalance include dry mouth, thirst, weakness, lethargy, drowsiness, restlessness, muscle pains or cramps, confusion, gastrointestinal disturbances, hypotension, oliguria, tachycardia, and seizures.

6. **Answer: 3**
   RATIONALE: If the serum potassium levels in the client exceed 5.3 mEq/mL, the nurse should discontinue the drug and notify the primary health care provider immediately, since this could be a sign of hyperkalemia. The drug is not to be discontinued if the client experiences gout attacks, the urine tests positive for glucose, or excess fluid has been removed from the client's body.

7. **Answer: 1**
   RATIONALE: Furosemide is an example of a loop diuretic.

8. **Answer: 2**
   RATIONALE: Acetazolamide is a carbonic anhydrase inhibitor that exerts its effect by inhibiting the enzyme carbonic anhydrase.

9. **Answer: 1**
   RATIONALE: Mannitol is an osmotic diuretic that exerts its diuretic effects by increasing the density of the filtrate in the glomerulus.

10. **Answer: 1**
    RATIONALE: Spironolactone is a potassium-sparing diuretic that exerts its diuretic effect by antagonizing the action of aldosterone.

11. **Answer: 4**

   RATIONALE: Triamterene is a potassium-sparing diuretic that exerts its effect by depressing the reabsorption of sodium in the collecting tubules, thereby increasing sodium and water excretion.

12. **Answer: 1**

   RATIONALE: Hydrochlorothiazide is a thiazide diuretic that exerts its diuretic effect by inhibiting the reabsorption of sodium and chloride ions in the early distal tubule of the nephron.

CHAPTER 33

SECTION I: ASSESSING YOUR UNDERSTANDING

Activity A FILL IN THE BLANKS

1. Hyperlipidemia
2. lipid
3. liver
4. catalyst
5. Rhabdomyolysis

Activity B DOSAGE CALCULATION

1. 1 packet
2. 2 tablets
3. 2 tablets
4. 3 capsules
5. 2 tablets

Activity C MATCHING

1. **1.** d **2.** a **3.** b **4.** c
2. **1.** c **2.** a **3.** d **4.** b

Activity D SHORT ANSWERS

1. The nurse should perform the following assessments before administration of an antihyperlipidemic drug:
   - Documentation of serum cholesterol levels, liver functions tests, serum glucose, and HbA1c
   - Note of dietary history, focusing on the types of foods normally included in the diet
   - Recording of vital signs and weight
   - Childbearing status and possible pregnancy for selected drugs
   - If the hyperlipidemia is severe, inspection of skin and eyelids for evidence of xanthomas.

2. The nurse's role after an antihyperlipidemic drug is administered includes the following:
   - Frequent monitoring of blood cholesterol and triglyceride levels
   - Checking vital signs and assessing bowel functioning
   - Notifying the PHCP of change in serum trans-aminase levels.

Activity E CROSSWORD PUZZLE

Copyright © 2022 Wolters Kluwer

SECTION II: APPLYING YOUR KNOWLEDGE

Activity F CASE STUDY

1. Pravastatin is an HMG-CoA reductase inhibitor or statin drug. Mrs. Garcia should be told to take the pravastatin one tablet daily at bedtime and not to stop taking the medication even if she begins to feel better. Mrs. Garcia should be advised to contact her primary health care provider as soon as possible if muscle pain, tenderness, or weakness occurs. She should also be made aware of potential adverse reactions including headache, nausea, vomiting, and diarrhea.

2. Mrs. Garcia should be encouraged to stop smoking, decrease intake of saturated fat and cholesterol, increase intake of fiber, increase physical activity with the primary health care provider's permission, and maintain a healthy weight.

SECTION III: PRACTICING FOR NCLEX

Activity G NCLEX-STYLE QUESTIONS

1. **Answer: 1**
   RATIONALE: The nurse should instruct the client to take the drug 2 hours before cholestyramine, the bile acid sequestrant. The responses—a time gap of 1 hour when taking these drugs is too little, taking both the drugs 30 minutes before meals, and taking a bile acid sequestrant with warm water—are not the appropriate instructions.

2. **Answer: 4**
   RATIONALE: The nurse should monitor for arthralgia in the client. Vertigo, headache, and cholelithiasis are the adverse reactions to a different drug—gemfibrozil.

3. **Answer: 3**
   RATIONALE: The nurse should observe for enhanced effects of the anticoagulant in the client as the effect of the interaction of gemfibrozil with anticoagulants.

4. **Answers: 2, 3, 5**
   RATIONALE: The nurse should use HMG-CoA reductase inhibitors with caution in clients with a history of acute infection, visual disturbances, and endocrine disorders, as well as other conditions including alcoholism, hypotension, trauma, and myopathy.

5. **Answer: 1**
   RATIONALE: The nurse should tell the client who asks about garlic and who is on warfarin about bleeding risk.

6. **Answer: 1**
   RATIONALE: In case of a paradoxical elevation of blood lipid levels in the client receiving an antihyperlipidemic drug, the nurse should notify the PHCP for a different antihyperlipidemic drug. The nurse need not collect the blood samples for further examination, administer the next dose of the drug with milk, or record the fluid intake and output every hour, as these interventions will not help improve the client's condition.

7. **Answer: 3**
   RATIONALE: Red yeast naturally contains ingredients that help to control cholesterol levels; these include "healthy fats" and monacolin—the ingredient used in the drug lovastatin. Therefore, the supplement would have all the adverse reactions and drug interactions of the statin drugs. Taking this supplement with other antihyperlipidemic drugs can cause serious reactions, notably liver or muscle damage.

8. **Answers: 1, 2, 4**
   RATIONALE: The nurse should instruct the client to increase fluid intake, eat foods high in dietary fiber, and exercise daily to help prevent constipation. Taking oral vitamin K supplements or the drug 1 hour after meals will not help prevent constipation.

9. **Answer: 4**
   RATIONALE: Increased levels of LDL in combination with other risk factors can lead to the development of atherosclerotic heart disease.

10. **Answers: 2, 3**
    RATIONALE: The benefits of red yeast and garlic include lowering serum cholesterol and triglyceride levels.

11. **Answers: 1, 2, 3**
    RATIONALE: HMG-CoA reductase inhibitors, fibric acid derivatives, and bile acid resins are classes of medications used to treat hyperlipidemia. Calcium channel blockers and angiotensin II receptor blockers are used to treat hypertension.

12. **Answer: 2**
    RATIONALE: Bile acid resins can decrease the gastrointestinal absorption of several medications.

CHAPTER 34

SECTION I: ASSESSING YOUR UNDERSTANDING

Activity A FILL IN THE BLANKS

1. vasoconstrictor
2. diuretic
3. hypertensive
4. sodium
5. hyponatremia

Activity B DOSAGE CALCULATION

1. 2 tablets
2. 2 ampules
3. 2 tablets
4. 3 tablets
5. 2-mg tablet

Activity C MATCHING

1.	1. c	2. a	3. e	4. b	5. d
2.	1. b	2. d	3. e	4. a	5. c

Activity D SHORT ANSWERS

1. When caring for a client on captopril therapy, the nurse should perform the following assessments:
   - Monitor the blood pressure in the same arm in the same position every time. The blood pressure should be recorded every 15–30 minutes after the first dose of captopril is administered for at least 2 hours. This is to monitor for hypotension, which occurs with ACEIs. Notify the health care provider if there is an increase or decrease in blood pressure.
   - Weigh the client regularly during the initial period of the therapy. A weight gain of 2 lb or more per day should be reported.
   - Assess for edema of the extremities and also in the sacral area. If edema is present, the nurse should notify the health care provider.
2. When caring for a client taking antihypertensive drug therapy, the nurse should include the following points in the client teaching plan:
   - Take the drug regularly and do not discontinue or stop the drug on the client's own. The health care provider should be notified before doing so.
   - Have regular blood pressure checkups and record the readings.
   - Avoid over-the-counter drugs unless advised by the health care provider.
   - Avoid the consumption of alcohol, unless approved by the practitioner.
   - Learn ways to prevent dizziness or lightheadedness.
   - If drowsiness occurs, avoid performing hazardous tasks or tasks involving the need for alertness.
   - Learn about the adverse effects occurring with the therapy.
   - Contact the health care provider if adverse effects occur.
   - Implement diet recommendations given.

Activity E CROSSWORD PUZZLE

SECTION II: APPLYING YOUR KNOWLEDGE

Activity F CASE STUDY

1. Mr. Garcia's hypertension would be classified as stage 2 because his systolic blood pressure is greater than 140 mm Hg. He will most likely require a two-drug combination for control of his hypertension. Lopressor HCT is a combination of beta blocker and diuretic.

2. Mr. Garcia should be encouraged to follow the DASH diet, decrease salt intake, increase physical activity with the primary health care provider's permission, decrease stress, maintain a healthy weight, and take his medication every day, even if he begins to feel better.

SECTION III: PRACTICING FOR NCLEX

Activity G NCLEX-STYLE QUESTIONS

1. **Answer: 1**
   RATIONALE: Systolic pressure between 120 and 129 mm Hg is indicative of prehypertension. Prehypertension poses a risk for the development of hypertension. Individuals with such blood pressure changes should practice certain lifestyle changes.

2. **Answer: 2**
   RATIONALE: Captopril is an angiotensin-converting enzyme inhibitor (ACEI), which is contraindicated in clients with renal impairment. Hydralazine and minoxidil are vasodilating drugs used for hypertension management and are administered to clients with renal impairment after dose adjustments. Doxazosin is an alpha-adrenergic blocker (α-adrenergic blocker) used for the treatment of hypertension and may be administered with caution to clients with renal impairment.

3. **Answer: 4**
   RATIONALE: Nitroprusside is the drug that is to be administered in hypertensive emergencies. In hypertensive emergencies, nitroprusside, which is a potent vasodilator, should be given IV to bring down the blood pressure rapidly. If the blood pressure is not lowered, it results in damage to the kidneys, eyes, and heart. Amlodipine, acebutolol, and diltiazem are not the preferred drugs in case of hypertensive emergencies.

4. **Answers: 1, 4, 5**
   RATIONALE: The nurse should report changes such as swelling of the face, difficulty in breathing, and angina or severe indigestion to the primary health care provider in clients receiving minoxidil. Minoxidil causes a rapid rise in the heart rate. A rise in the heart rate of 20 beats per minute or more should be reported. Weight gain of 5 lb, and not 1 lb, or more should be reported.

5. **Answer: 1**
   RATIONALE: The nurse should ensure that captopril is taken 1 hour before or 2 hours after food; this is to enhance the absorption of captopril. Captopril should not be given along with food or an antacid. This will retard absorption. Rubbing the client's back prior to administration and engaging the client in exercise will not affect absorption.

6. **Answers: 1, 4, 5**
   RATIONALE: Orthostatic hypotension is common during the initial therapy with antihypertensives such as terazosin. The nurse should instruct the client to rise slowly from a sitting or lying position, to rest on the bed for 1 or 2 minutes before rising, and to stand still for a few minutes after rising for clients experiencing orthostatic hypotension. Increasing the fluid intake or applying a cool cloth on the forehead will not relieve the hypotensive condition.

7. **Answers: 1, 2, 4**
   RATIONALE: The nurse should inform the client that hypotension, sedation, and arrhythmia are the adverse effects seen with hawthorn use. Medical reports indicate a possible interaction with St. John's wort, used to relieve depression, causing a decrease in serum levels of calcium channel blockers. Due to a specific enzyme reaction, grapefruit or its juice should not be taken if a client is prescribed a calcium channel blocker.

8. **Answer: 1**
   RATIONALE: Prehypertension is defined as a systolic pressure between 120 and 129 mm Hg or a diastolic pressure at or below 80 mm Hg.

9. **Answer: 3**
   RATIONALE: Lisinopril, the angiotensin-converting enzyme inhibitors (ACEIs) act primarily to suppress the renin–angiotensin–aldosterone system. Verapamil and diltiazem are calcium channel blockers and furosemide is a diuretic.

10. **Answers: 1, 4**
    RATIONALE: Hypertension increases a person's risk for heart failure and kidney disease.

11. **Answer: 3**
    RATIONALE: Once primary hypertension develops, management of the disorder becomes a lifetime task.

12. **Answer: 2**
    RATIONALE: Among the known causes of secondary hypertension, kidney disease ranks first, with tumors or other abnormalities of the adrenal glands following.

CHAPTER 35

SECTION I: ASSESSING YOUR UNDERSTANDING

Activity A FILL IN THE BLANKS

1. coronary
2. calcium
3. smooth
4. dermatitis
5. erectile dysfunction

Activity B DOSAGE CALCULATION

1. 2 tablets
2. 2 tablets
3. 2.5 mL
4. 2 tablets

Activity C MATCHING

1. **1.** b   **2.** d   **3.** c   **4.** a
2. **1.** b   **2.** c   **3.** a

Activity D SHORT ANSWERS

1. The nurse should educate clients having anginal attacks about certain aspects of the disease and also about the use of antianginal drugs. The teaching plan should include the following:
   - Keep the medication in the original container.
   - You may take up to three pills in 15 minutes.
   - Notify the emergency response team if the pain worsens or if the pain is not relieved by the medication.
   - Avoid the consumption of alcohol, unless directed otherwise by the health care provider.
   - Keep an additional supply of the drug for events such as vacations and bad weather conditions.
   - Maintain a record of acute anginal attacks. This should include date, time of attack, and dose used to relieve pain.

2. The nurse should tell the adult child that the dose of sublingual nitroglycerin may be repeated every 5 minutes until pain is relieved or until the client has received three doses in a 15-minute period. The nurse should tell them to notify emergency response providers if the drug does not relieve pain or if pain becomes more intense despite use of this drug.

Activity E CROSSWORD PUZZLE

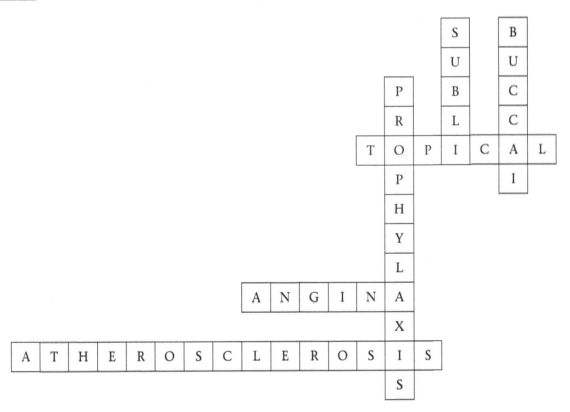

SECTION II: APPLYING YOUR KNOWLEDGE

Activity F CASE STUDY

1. Nitrates are used for the treatment of angina. It is taken for pains in your chest.
2. Mrs. Moore should be instructed to place one tablet under the tongue at the onset of chest pain, and not to swallow the tablet. The dose may be repeated every 5 minutes until chest pain is relieved or until three doses have been taken in a period of 15 minutes. If the pain is not relieved after the third dose, Mrs. Moore should be instructed to call the emergency responders in her area. Finally, she should be told to store the tablets in the original container away from heat and moisture.

Mapping—after listing her medications to this point you will find she is taking tolterodine (an anticholinergic) which is contraindicated when a client has heart failure.

SECTION III: PRACTICING FOR NCLEX

Activity G NCLEX-STYLE QUESTIONS

1. **Answer: 3**
   RATIONALE: Before preparing written teaching materials, the nurse should assess for language and reading level.
2. **Answer: 4**
   RATIONALE: Any activity that increases the workload of the heart, such as exercise or simply climbing stairs, can precipitate a painful angina attack.
3. **Answers: 2, 3, 5**
   RATIONALE: Calcium channel blockers affect the heart by:
   - Slowing the conduction velocity of the cardiac impulse
   - Depressing myocardial contractility
   - Dilating coronary arteries and arterioles, which in turn deliver more oxygen to cardiac muscle. Dilation of peripheral arteries reduces the workload of the heart. The end effect of these drugs is the same as that of the nitrates. An increased blood flow results in an increase in the oxygen supply to surrounding tissues.
4. **Answers: 4, 5**
   RATIONALE: The adverse effects occurring with diltiazem therapy include dizziness, peripheral edema, headache, and rhinitis. It also causes hypotension and bradycardia.
5. **Answer: 2**
   RATIONALE: When removing the system, fold the adhesive side onto itself to prevent adhesion to another person or pet.
6. **Answer: 3**
   RATIONALE: There is a correlation between the autoimmune disorder scleroderma and clients diagnosed with PAH.
7. **Answers: 1, 2, 3, 4, 5**
   RATIONALE: Nitrates are available in the following dosage forms for cardiac or chest pain: sublingual, translingual spray, transdermal, and parenteral. The rectal form of nitroglycerin is used for anal fissures
8. **Answer: 4**
   RATIONALE: Drugs used to treat PAH have teratogenic properties. All women who can possibly become pregnant need to be tested before drug treatment is started.
9. **Answers: 1, 2, 4**
   RATIONALE: Adverse reactions associated with antianginal medications include headache, dizziness, weakness, restlessness, hypotension, flushing, and rash.
10. **Answer: 1**
    RATIONALE: Nitrates are contraindicated in clients with known hypersensitivity, severe anemia, closed-angle glaucoma, head trauma, cerebral hemorrhage, and constrictive pericarditis.

CHAPTER 36

SECTION I: ASSESSING YOUR UNDERSTANDING

Activity A FILL IN THE BLANKS

1. Prothrombin
2. thrombus
3. Arterial
4. thrombolytics
5. extremities

Activity B DOSAGE CALCULATION

1. 0.4 mL
2. 3 tablets
3. 2 tablets
4. 4 tablets
5. 1 tablet

Activity C MATCHING

1. 1. d   2. c   3. a   4. b
2. 1. b   2. d   3. a   4. c

Activity D SHORT ANSWERS

1. The following factors should be considered by the nurse to determine the success of the treatment plan:
   - The therapeutic drug effect is achieved.
   - Adverse reactions are identified, reported to the primary health care provider, and managed successfully using appropriate nursing interventions.
   - The client demonstrates an understanding of the drug regimen.
   - The client verbalizes the importance of complying with the prescribed therapeutic regimen.
   - The client lists or describes early signs of bleeding.
2. Inspect the urine for a pink to red color and the stool for signs of GI bleeding (bright red to black stools). Visually check the catheter drainage every 2–4 hours and when the unit is emptied. A urinalysis may be necessary to determine if blood is in the urine.

Activity E CROSSWORD PUZZLE

SECTION II: APPLYING YOUR KNOWLEDGE

Activity F CASE STUDY

1. Initially a PT/INR will need to be drawn every 1–3 days. Once PT and INR are stable, they will need to be drawn at least every 4 weeks.
2. Signs of warfarin overdose include melena (blood in the stool), petechiae (pinpoint-sized red hemorrhagic spots on the skin), bleeding from the gums after teeth brushing, oozing from superficial injuries, and excessive menstrual bleeding (for women, not Mr. Phillip).

SECTION III: PRACTICING FOR NCLEX

Activity G NCLEX-STYLE QUESTIONS

1. **Answers: 1, 3, 4**
   RATIONALE: The nurse should monitor the client receiving alteplase for gingival bleeding, epistaxis, and ecchymosis. Thrombolytic drugs such as alteplase will dissolve most clots encountered, both occlusive and those repairing vessel leaks; hence, bleeding is a great concern when using these agents.

2. **Answer: 3**
   RATIONALE: The nurse should observe an increased risk of bleeding as the effect of the interaction of abciximab with aspirin in the client.

3. **Answer: 2**
   RATIONALE: All heparin-based products are derived from pork sources. Use of pork or porcine products is prohibited by some religious groups. Alert the primary health care provider if the client notes a Jewish or Muslim religious preference and is likely to undergo anticoagulant therapy. The drug fondaparinux (Arixtra) is artificially produced and does not contain pork products; this may be used as a substitute for one of the pork-derived heparin products.

4. **Answer: 1**
   RATIONALE: The nurse should instruct the client to use a soft toothbrush and to consult a dentist regarding routine oral hygiene, including the use of dental floss.

5. **Answer: 3**
   RATIONALE: The nurse should inspect for bright red to black stools, which are an indication of GI bleeding. Inspecting the urine for red-orange color is not a reliable indicator of bleeding when oral anticoagulants are taken. They may impart a red-orange color to alkaline urine, making it difficult to detect hematuria. In such conditions, a urinalysis would be necessary to detect hematuria.

6. **Answer: 4**
   RATIONALE: The nurse should avoid the intramuscular (IM) administration of heparin to avoid the possibility of the development of local irritation, pain, or hematoma. The application of firm pressure after injection helps to prevent hematoma formation. The nurse need not avoid administration sites such as the buttocks and lateral thighs, as these are also areas of heparin administration by the subcutaneous route. When heparin is given by the subcutaneous route, the nurse should avoid areas within 2 in. of the umbilicus because of the increased vascularity of that area.

7. **Answer: 3**
   RATIONALE: The nurse should observe the client for new evidence of bleeding if administration of the drug is necessary.

8. **Answers: 1, 2, 4, 5**
   RATIONALE: The nurse should observe for symptoms such as abdominal pain; coffee-ground emesis; black, tarry stools; hematuria; bleeding under the skin; joint pain; and spitting or coughing up blood in the client.

9. **Answer: 3**
   RATIONALE: Phytonadione (vitamin K) is indicated for the treatment of warfarin overdose.

10. **Answer: 1**
    RATIONALE: St. John's wort in combination with warfarin can result in an increased risk of bleeding.

11. **Answer: 4**
    RATIONALE: Clopidogrel (Plavix) 300 mg should only be administered as a single loading dose.

12. **Answers: 1, 2, 4**
    RATIONALE: The use of thrombolytic drugs is contraindicated in a client with known hypersensitivity to the medication, active bleeding, and a history of stroke, aneurysm, or recent intracranial surgery.

CHAPTER 37

SECTION I: ASSESSING YOUR UNDERSTANDING

Activity A FILL IN THE BLANKS

1. Left
2. proarrhythmic
3. action potential
4. digitalization

Activity B DOSAGE CALCULATION

1. 2 tablets
2. 1 ampule
3. 55 mg
4. 3 mL or 2 ampules (discard 1 mL of solution)
5. 195 mg

Activity C MATCHING

1. **1.** c   **2.** a   **3.** d   **4.** b
2. **1.** b   **2.** d   **3.** a   **4.** c

Activity D SHORT ANSWERS

1. Before starting digoxin, the nurse should make the following physical assessments:
   - Record the client's blood pressure, apical–radial pulse rate, and respiratory rate.
   - Measure the client's weight.
   - Check for distension of the jugular veins.
   - Examine for edema in the extremities.
   - Look for cyanosis, dyspnea, and mental changes.
   - Auscultate the lungs for any unusual sounds during inspiration or expiration.
   - Inspect any sputum expelled and note its appearance.

2. The nurse should include the following points in the teaching plan for clients taking digitalis:
   - Take the drug at the same time every day.
   - Remind caregivers to record the client's pulse before taking the drug. Withhold the drug and notify the primary health care provider (PHCP) if the pulse is less than 60 or more than 100 beats per minute.
   - Do not stop or discontinue the drug or take an extra dose without consulting the PHCP.
   - Report to the health care center if signs of digitalis toxicity such as nausea, vomiting, diarrhea, unusual fatigue, weakness, and vision changes occur.
   - Carry or wear a medical alert band.
   - Do not take over-the-counter drugs unless the health care provider approves them.
   - Keep the drug in its original container.

Activity E CROSSWORD PUZZLE

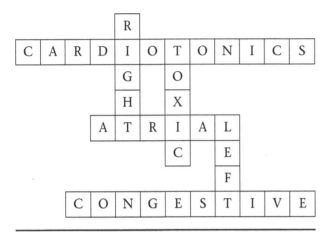

```
            R
C A R D I O T O N I C S
            G       O
            H       X
        A T R I A L
            C       E
                    F
    C O N G E S T I V E
```

SECTION II: APPLYING YOUR KNOWLEDGE

Activity F CASE STUDY

1. The nurse should prepare 1.5 mL for slow IV infusion: 0.75 mg × 1.0 mL/0.5 mg = 1.5 mL.
2. Prior to administering the IV digoxin, the nurse should complete a physical assessment of the client, which includes recording the blood pressure, apical–radial pulse, and respiratory rate; auscultating the lungs; examining the extremities for edema; checking for jugular vein distention; measuring weight; inspecting sputum if present; and looking for evidence of other problems (mental status changes, cyanosis, shortness of breath on exertion).

SECTION III: PRACTICING FOR NCLEX

Activity G NCLEX-STYLE QUESTIONS

1. **Answer: 1**
   RATIONALE: These signs and symptoms indicate that the client is experiencing heart failure. The symptoms of heart failure are cough, dyspnea, weakness, anorexia, and unusual fatigue. The signs of heart failure include pitting edema and distended jugular veins. There is also a reduced ejection fraction.
2. **Answer: 4**
   RATIONALE: A pulse rate of less than 60 beats per minute indicates the potential for digoxin toxicity. The nurse should withhold the drug and notify the PHCP. Increasing the infusion rate will augment the toxicity. Gastrointestinal suctioning causes hypokalemia, which sensitizes the heart to digoxin toxicity. Milrinone is given in unresponsive cases of heart failure, not in toxic states.
3. **Answers: 1, 4, 5**
   RATIONALE: The signs of digoxin toxicity include anorexia, blurred vision, and vomiting. Headache and weakness are the adverse effects of digoxin,

even at normal dosage, and do not signify digoxin toxicity.

4. **Answers: 1, 4, 5**
   RATIONALE: Weakness, arrhythmias, and lightheadedness are possible adverse effects of antiarrhythmic drugs. Another possible adverse effect is hypotension, and not hypertension. Somnolence, and not insomnia, may occur as another adverse effect associated with antiarrhythmic drugs.
5. **Answers: 2, 4, 5**
   RATIONALE: The appropriate intervention is to ensure that the client consumes small, frequent meals; restricts fluid intake at meals; and rinses the mouth after meals. These are techniques that help control nausea and vomiting. Fluid intake at meals will increase the feeling of nausea. Fluid intake should be avoided 1 hour before meals. Doubling the drug dosage will worsen the condition.
6. **Answers: 3, 4, 5**
   RATIONALE: The adverse effects of digitalis administration the nurse should assess for are drowsiness, vomiting, and arrhythmias.
7. **Answer: 4**
   RATIONALE: The nurse should notify the primary health care provider immediately when the pulse rate is below 60 beats per minute or above 120 beats per minute.
8. **Answers: 2, 3, 4, 1, 5**
   RATIONALE: The nurse should teach the steps involved in the calculation of the pulse. Place the nondominant arm on the table or arm of the chair. Place index and third fingers of the other hand on the wrist bone. Feel for a beating or pulsing sensation, which is the pulse. Record the number of times the pulse beats in a minute. If the pulse beats more than 100 beats per minute, notify the PHCP.
9. **Answer: 2**
   RATIONALE: Shortness of breath may be seen as a sign of heart failure in older clients on antiarrhythmic drug therapy. Other signs include an increase in weight and a decrease in urine output.
10. **Answers: 1, 2, 5**
    RATIONALE: The symptoms of right ventricular dysfunction include peripheral edema, neck vein distention, hepatic engorgement, weight gain, nausea, weakness, anorexia, and nocturia.
11. **Answers: 1, 2, 4**
    RATIONALE: ACEIs, beta blockers, and loop diuretics are currently first-line treatments for heart failure.
12. **Answer: 2**
    RATIONALE: Disopyramide is an example of a class IA antiarrhythmic drug.

CHAPTER 38

SECTION I: ASSESSING YOUR UNDERSTANDING

Activity A FILL IN THE BLANKS

1. gastrointestinal
2. esophagus
3. vomiting
4. Dronabinol
5. duodenal

Activity B DOSAGE CALCULATION

1. 6 capsules
2. 2 capsules
3. 1 tablet in each of the 4 doses
4. 2 tablets
5. 2 capsules

Activity C MATCHING

1. 1. c   2. e   3. a   4. b   5. d
2. 1. b   2. c   3. a   4. e   5. d

Activity D SHORT ANSWERS

1. The nurse should perform the following preadmission assessments:
   - Question the client regarding the type and intensity of symptoms.
   - Document the number of vomiting experiences and approximate amount of fluid lost.
   - Record vital signs and assess signs of fluid and electrolyte imbalances.
2. The nurse's role after the administration of the drug includes the following:
   - Monitor the client frequently for continued complaints of pain, sour taste, or spitting up of blood or coffee-ground–colored emesis.
   - Keep suction equipment available in case the need for insertion of a nasogastric tube or suctioning is warranted to prevent aspiration of the emesis.
   - Monitor vital signs and observe the client for signs and symptoms of electrolyte imbalance if vomiting is severe.
   - Carefully measure intake and output until vomiting ceases.
   - Document on the chart each case of vomiting.
   - Notify the PHCP if there is blood in the emesis or if vomiting suddenly becomes more severe.
   - In those with prolonged and repeated episodes of vomiting, measure the client's weight.

Activity E LABELING

1. Mouth or oral cavity
2. Throat
3. Trachea
4. Esophagus
5. Diaphragm
6. Stomach
7. Liver
8. Gallbladder
9. Pancreas
10. Small intestine
11. Appendix
12. Large intestine
13. Rectum
14. Anus

SECTION II: APPLYING YOUR KNOWLEDGE

Activity F CASE STUDY

1. The following drugs may be utilized in the prevention of motion sickness: promethazine, dimenhydrinate (Dramamine), diphenhydramine (Benadryl), meclizine (Antivert), and scopolamine (Transderm Scop).
2. The nurse should teach Janna about the following when using the scopolamine patch:
   - One patch is applied behind the ear approximately 4 hours before the antiemetic effect is needed.
   - Discard any disk that becomes detached and replace it with a fresh disk applied behind the opposite ear.
   - Wash hands thoroughly after patch application and removal to avoid drug coming in contact with the eyes.
   - The disk will last about 3 days, at which time Janna may remove the disk and apply another, if needed.
   - Only use one disk at a time.
   - Stress the importance of observing caution when driving or performing hazardous tasks while using the medication.

SECTION III: PRACTICING FOR NCLEX

Activity G NCLEX-STYLE QUESTIONS

1. **Answer: 3**
   RATIONALE: The nurse should teach the client to monitor for euphoria, which is an adverse reaction to dronabinol.
2. **Answer: 1**
   RATIONALE: The nurse should observe for a decrease in pain relief since the aspirin will be excreted faster when taken with an antacid.
3. **Answers: 1, 2, 4**
   RATIONALE: The nurse should administer promethazine with caution to clients with hypertension, sleep apnea, or epilepsy.
4. **Answer: 4**
   RATIONALE: The main concern with motion sickness drugs is drowsiness. The nurse should instruct the client to avoid driving or performing other detailed tasks when taking the drug, because drowsiness may occur with use.

5. **Answer: 1**
   RATIONALE: The nurse should monitor the client for rate of infusion at frequent intervals during administration through IV because too rapid an infusion may induce cardiac arrhythmias.
6. **Answer: 4**
   RATIONALE: The nurse should record the fluid intake and output of the client who experiences diarrhea after taking the antacid drug as a measure to monitor dehydration. Changing to a different antacid will usually alleviate the problem if it is a magnesium-based antacid, but this would require an order from the PHCP and is not an independent nursing action.
7. **Answer: 3**
   RATIONALE: The nurse should remove items with a strong smell and odor to prevent vomiting and to enhance the client's appetite. Suggesting that the client consume milk products or perform physical exercises will not help the client improve his appetite. The nurse should give frequent oral rinses to the client to remove the disagreeable taste that accompanies vomiting.
8. **Answer: 3**
   RATIONALE: Magaldrate (Riopan) is a combination product that contains magnesium and aluminate. Magaldrate (Riopan) treats heartburn by neutralizing stomach acidity and by combining with hydrochloric acid (HCl) and increasing the pH of the stomach acid.
9. **Answer: 1**
   RATIONALE: The nurse should warn a client taking magnesium- and sodium-containing antacids concerning the risk of diarrhea associated with taking products containing either medication.
10. **Answer: 4**
    RATIONALE: The nurse should warn a client taking aluminum- and calcium-containing antacids concerning the risk of constipation associated with taking products containing either medication.
11. **Answer: 1**
    RATIONALE: Sodium bicarbonate is the antacid that is contraindicated in clients with cardiovascular problems such as hypertension and congestive heart failure and those on sodium-restricted diets, as sodium bicarbonate can alter the body's sodium–water balance and cause fluid retention.

12. **Answer: 2**
    RATIONALE: Administering an antacid to a client taking digoxin will decrease the absorption of digoxin and result in a decreased digoxin effect.

CHAPTER 39

SECTION I: ASSESSING YOUR UNDERSTANDING

Activity A FILL IN THE BLANKS

1. diarrhea
2. chamomile
3. laxative
4. pruritus
5. aminosalicylates

Activity B DOSAGE CALCULATION

1. 21 capsules
2. 1 tablet
3. 25 mg
4. Two 15-mL containers
5. 2 tablets

Activity C MATCHING

1. 1. c   2. a   3. d   4. b
2. 1. d   2. b   3. a   4. c

Activity D SHORT ANSWERS

1. The nurse should perform the following preadministration assessment:
   - Question the client regarding the type and intensity of symptoms such as pain, discomfort, diarrhea, or constipation.
   - Listen to the bowel sounds and palpate the abdomen.
   - Monitor the client for signs of guarding or discomfort.
2. The nurse's role after the administration of the drug to the client includes:
   - Assessing the client for relief of symptoms such as diarrhea, pain, or constipation
   - Notifying the primary health care provider if the drug fails to relieve symptoms
   - Monitoring vital signs
   - Observing the client for adverse drug reactions
   - Evaluating the effectiveness of the drug and the client's response to therapy.

Activity E CROSSWORD PUZZLE

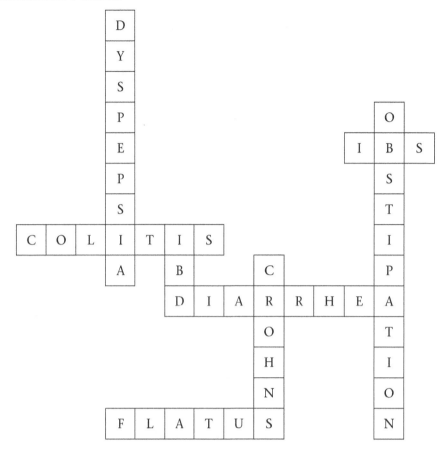

SECTION II: APPLYING YOUR KNOWLEDGE

Activity F CASE STUDY

1. The amitriptyline and ferrous sulfate may be contributing to the constipation. The following medications may cause constipation in clients: anticholinergics, antihistamines, phenothiazines, tricyclic antidepressants, opioids, non–potassium-sparing diuretics, iron preparations, barium, clonidine, and antacids containing calcium or aluminum.

2. The nurse could recommend the following nonpharmacologic treatments to Ms. Peterson to help with constipation: increase daily fluid and fiber intake and if possible increase physical activity.

SECTION III: PRACTICING FOR NCLEX

Activity G NCLEX-STYLE QUESTIONS

1. **Answer: 1**
   RATIONALE: The nurse should monitor for decreased blood glucose level in the client as a result of the interaction between mesalamine and antidiabetic drugs.

2. **Answer: 2**
   RATIONALE: The nurse should monitor for signs of constipation or dehydration—dry skin and mucous membranes, nausea, and lightheadedness—on administering loperamide to a client with acute diarrhea.

3. **Answer: 1**
   RATIONALE: These drugs are contraindicated in clients whose diarrhea is associated with organisms that can harm the intestinal mucosa (*Escherichia coli, Salmonella,* and *Shigella* spp.). Severe diarrhea, IBD, and IBS are conditions treated with an antidiarrheal.

4. **Answer: 2**
   RATIONALE: The nurse should instruct the client to chew the drug thoroughly because complete particle dispersion enhances antiflatulent action.

5. **Answer: 1**
   RATIONALE: The nurse should encourage the client with chronic diarrhea to drink extra fluids. When diarrhea is severe, the client should use commercial electrolytes. The nurse should

encourage clients with constipation to eat foods high in fiber and to exercise often.

6. **Answer: 4**
   RATIONALE: The nurse should instruct the client to take mineral oil in the evening on an empty stomach for optimal response to therapy.

7. **Answer: 2**
   RATIONALE: The nurse should monitor for serious electrolyte imbalances in the client, an effect of the prolonged use of laxatives.

8. **Answer: 3**
   RATIONALE: Antidiarrheals are contraindicated in clients with obstructive jaundice, pseudomembranous colitis, and abdominal pain of unknown origin. Constipation, nausea, and abdominal distention are adverse reactions associated with the administration of antidiarrheals.

9. **Answer: 3**
   RATIONALE: Clients with a sulfonamide allergy should avoid the use of aminosalicylates such as mesalamine to treat an ulcerative colitis flare.

10. **Answer: 1**
    RATIONALE: Chamomile is a herbal product that has been used to treat digestive upset and stomach ulcers.

11. **Answer: 3**
    RATIONALE: Diphenoxylate (Lomotil) is chemically related to opioid drugs and treats diarrhea by decreasing intestinal peristalsis.

12. **Answer: 2**
    RATIONALE: Simethicone (Mylicon) is an OTC drug used to treat flatulence.

CHAPTER 40

SECTION I: ASSESSING YOUR UNDERSTANDING

Activity A FILL IN THE BLANKS

1. insulin
2. polyuria
3. hyperglycemia
4. hemoglobin
5. ketoacidosis

Activity B DOSAGE CALCULATION

1. 2 tablets
2. 45 units total of insulin
3. 1 tablet
4. 1 tablet
5. 1 tablet

Activity C MATCHING

1. **1.** b   **2.** c   **3.** a
2. **1.** c   **2.** d   **3.** a   **4.** b

Activity D SHORT ANSWERS

1. The nurse should consider the following factors when evaluating the success of the treatment plan:
   - The therapeutic drug effect is achieved, and normal or near-normal blood glucose levels are maintained.
   - Hypoglycemic reactions are identified, reported to the primary health care provider, and managed successfully.
   - Anxiety is reduced.

2. An effective teaching program helps the client master the skills of self-care. Use principles of adult learning to start with small, obtainable goals. You may begin with blood sugar monitoring, then the skill of injection before discussing long-term complications. Success in small increments can help these clients gradually accept the diagnosis and begin to understand their feelings. In turn, this empowers the client and reduces uncertainty that leads to anxiety. The client in this situation gains confidence and then is able to talk about the disorder, express concerns, and ask questions.

Activity E CROSSWORD PUZZLE

Across: POLYDIPSIA; GLUCOMETER; POLYPHAGIA

Down: HYPOGLYCEMIA; GLUCAGON; LIPODYSTROPHY; HYPERGLYCEMIA; POLYURIA

SECTION II: APPLYING YOUR KNOWLEDGE

Activity F CASE STUDY

1. The nurse should evaluate Mrs. Arthur's and Betty's basic understanding of blood glucose monitoring, which should include the following points:
   - Does she understand the manufacturer's instructions?
   - Is the finger properly prepared by cleansing with warm, soapy water; rinsing with warm water; and drying well?
   - Does she close the container to prevent damage to the remaining strips when one is removed?
   - Does she perform a finger stick on the side of a finger (not the tip), where there are fewer nerve endings and more capillaries?
   - Is she able to produce a large, hanging drop of blood?
   - Is she able to drop the blood sample on the test strip and read the number on the meter?
   - Can she record the time and test results in the record-keeping book?
   - Does she understand the importance of cleaning and calibrating the device?

2. The nurse should tell Mrs. Arthur the following about the medications she is taking: the diuretic in the drug Hyzaar can cause hyperglycemia, which could cause a higher reading on the blood glucose monitor. If she had been taking the medication before hospitalization, then those readings would have seen that rise already and it would not be new.

SECTION III: PRACTICING FOR NCLEX

Activity G NCLEX-STYLE QUESTIONS

1. Answer: 1
   RATIONALE: Pioglitazone is a thiazolidinedione. Thiazolidinediones are contraindicated for clients with symptomatic heart failure.

2. **Answer: 3**
   RATIONALE: The nurse informs the client that the need for insulin is greatest during the third trimester of pregnancy. Insulin requirements usually decrease in the first trimester, increase during the second and third trimesters, and decrease rapidly after delivery. Insulin is not required before conception, as gestational diabetes occurs during pregnancy.

3. **Answer: 2**
   RATIONALE: The nurse should administer regular insulin to the client 30–60 minutes before a meal to achieve optimal results.

4. **Answer: 2**
   RATIONALE: When preparing an insulin mixture, the nurse should draw up lispro (a rapid-acting insulin analog) first in the syringe and then draw the long-acting insulin.

5. **Answer: 3**
   RATIONALE: The nurse should instruct the client receiving alpha-glucosidase inhibitors to keep a source of glucose ready for signs of low blood glucose.

6. **Answer: 4**
   RATIONALE: The insulin pump method is used for the client who has undergone renal transplantation and pregnant women with diabetes with early long-term complications, since it attempts to mimic the body's normal pancreatic function.

7. **Answer: 1**
   RATIONALE: Before insulin administration, the nurse should make sure that air bubbles are eliminated from the syringe barrel and the hub of the needle.

8. **Answer: 4**
   RATIONALE: Glycosylated hemoglobin (HbA1C) measures glucose control over the past 3–4 months.

9. **Answer: 1**
   RATIONALE: Insulin is produced by the pancreas.

10. **Answer: 1**
    RATIONALE: Lispro (Humalog), an insulin analog, is an example of rapid-acting insulin product.

11. **Answer: 2**
    RATIONALE: Glargine (Lantus) is an example of long-acting insulin product.

12. **Answer: 1**
    RATIONALE: Aspart (Apidra) is given immediately before a meal or within 5 10 minutes of beginning a meal.

CHAPTER 41

SECTION I: ASSESSING YOUR UNDERSTANDING

Activity A FILL IN THE BLANKS

1. corticosteroids
2. prolactin
3. gonadotropins
4. feedback
5. vasopressin, oxytocin

Activity B DOSAGE CALCULATION

1. 2 mL
2. 2 tablets
3. 2 mL
4. 13 tablets
5. 2 tablets

Activity C MATCHING

1. **1.** b   **2.** a   **3.** d   **4.** c
2. **1.** c   **2.** d   **3.** b   **4.** a

Activity D SHORT ANSWERS

1. The nurse should teach the following steps of injection of the growth hormone therapy:
   - Swirl the vial containing the hormone; do not shake it.
   - Do not administer the solution if it is cloudy.
   - Give the drug at bedtime to closely adhere to the body's natural release of the hormone.

2. The nurse's role in educating the client and the family includes the following:
   - Answer questions about the therapeutic regimen for increasing the growth of the child.
   - Instruct on the proper injection technique.
   - Encourage parents and child to keep all clinic or office visits.
   - Explain that the child may experience sudden growth and increase in appetite.
   - Instruct the parents to report lack of growth; symptoms of diabetes such as increased hunger, increased thirst, or frequent voiding; or symptoms of hypothyroidism such as fatigue, dry skin, and intolerance to cold.

CROSSWORD PUZZLE

```
C R Y P T O R C H I S M
                Y
      V A S O P R E S S I N
                E
                R
                S
                T
                I         G     A
                M         O     N
          C U S H I N G O I D
                L         I     A     V
                A         R     D     U
                T         S     S     L
                I         U           A
                O         T           T
                N         I           O
                          S           R
                          M           Y
```

SECTION II: APPLYING YOUR KNOWLEDGE

Activity F CASE STUDY

1. Items the students can do include:
   - Be sure she is wearing her medical identification.
   - Remind her to carry a sports drink bottle to be sure she has liquids available at all times.
   - Remind her to carry extra doses of the drug when out for extended periods of time.
   - Should she get hurt, tell the EMS responders about her condition.
2. Adverse reactions of desmopressin (DDAVP) include headache, nausea, nasal congestion, abdominal cramps, and water intoxication.

SECTION III: PRACTICING FOR NCLEX

Activity G NCLEX-STYLE QUESTIONS

1. **Answer: 4**
   RATIONALE: The nurse should anticipate a decrease in the antidiuretic effect due to the effect of the interaction between vasopressin and oral anticoagulants.
2. **Answer: 2**
   RATIONALE: The nurse should monitor for a rise in blood glucose level in a client receiving glucocorticoids for thyroiditis. An increase in blood sugar is an adverse reaction that can be seen in a client with latent diabetes.

3. **Answer: 2**
   RATIONALE: The nurse should inform the client to not overuse the injected joint, even if the pain is gone.
4. **Answer: 3**
   RATIONALE: When administering fludrocortisone, check the client's blood pressure at frequent intervals. Hypotension may indicate insufficient dosage.
5. **Answer: 1**
   RATIONALE: The nurse should tell the client to discontinue the drug therapy if visual disturbances occur. This could be an emergent situation and the client should be referred to an ophthalmologist.
6. **Answer: 3**
   RATIONALE: The most appropriate nursing diagnosis for a client receiving glucocorticoids for systemic lupus erythematosus would include disturbed body image related to adverse reactions. The glucocorticoids can cause cushingoid symptoms, such as redistribution of body fat.
7. **Answer: 1**
   RATIONALE: The nurse should give an enema before administering the first dose of vasopressin to the client undergoing abdominal roentgenography. The drug is then administered before abdominal roentgenography, two injections of 10 units each.
8. **Answers: 2, 4**
   RATIONALE: The nurse is likely to observe buffalo hump and moon face. Other reactions include oily skin and acne, osteoporosis, purple striae on the abdomen and hips, altered skin pigmentation, and weight gain in the client with cushingoid syndrome from long-term glucocorticoid therapy.
9. **Answer: 1**
   RATIONALE: Vasopressin is a hormone secreted by the posterior pituitary gland.
10. **Answer: 3**
    RATIONALE: Diabetes insipidus is treated with replacement of vasopressin.
11. **Answer: 1**
    RATIONALE: Vasopressin is the hormone responsible for the regulation of reabsorption of water by the kidneys.
12. **Answer: 1**
    RATIONALE: Clomiphene (Clomid) is the medication that binds to estrogen receptors, decreasing the amount of available estrogen receptors and causing the anterior pituitary to increase secretion of FSH and LH.

CHAPTER 42

SECTION I: ASSESSING YOUR UNDERSTANDING

Activity A FILL IN THE BLANKS

1. Hyperthyroidism
2. hypothyroid
3. Iodine
4. euthyroid
5. Antithyroid

Activity B DOSAGE CALCULATION

1. 2 tablets
2. 2 tablets
3. 1 tablet
4. 2 tablets
5. 20 mcg

Activity C MATCHING

1. **1.** b **2.** c **3.** a
2. **1.** c **2.** a **3.** d **4.** b

Activity D SHORT ANSWERS

1. The nurse should provide the following information to the client and family, emphasizing the importance of taking the thyroid hormone replacement therapy:
   - Replacement therapy is for life, with the exception of transient hypothyroidism seen in those with thyroiditis.
   - Do not increase, decrease, or skip a dose unless advised to do so by the primary health care provider.
   - Notify the primary health care provider if any of the following occur: headache, nervousness, palpitations, diarrhea, excessive sweating, heat intolerance, chest pain, increased pulse rate, or any unusual physical changes or events.
   - Weigh yourself weekly and report any significant weight gain or loss to the primary health care provider.
2. The nurse should consider the following factors to determine the success of the therapy:
   - The therapeutic effect is achieved.
   - Adverse reactions are identified and reported to the primary health care provider.
   - The client verbalizes the importance of complying with the prescribed treatment regimen.
   - The client verbalizes an understanding of the treatment modalities and importance of continued follow-up care.
   - The client and family demonstrate an understanding of the drug regimen.

Activity E CROSSWORD PUZZLE

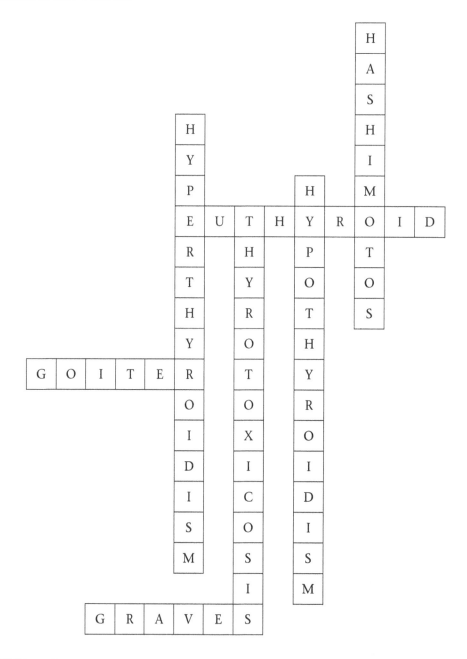

SECTION II: APPLYING YOUR KNOWLEDGE

Activity F CASE STUDY

1. The nurse should instruct Mrs. Wong to take the levothyroxine (Synthroid) in the morning before breakfast to ensure better drug absorption.
2. Early effects of levothyroxine (Synthroid) treatment can occur in as few as 48 hours; however, the full effects of thyroid hormone replacement may not be apparent for several weeks.

SECTION III: PRACTICING FOR NCLEX

Activity G NCLEX-STYLE QUESTIONS

1. **Answer: 2**
   RATIONALE: Agranulocytosis is the primary adverse reaction to report to the primary health care provider because of the greater risk for infection.
2. **Answer: 1**
   RATIONALE: The nurse should observe for decreased effectiveness of the cardiac drug when the thyroid hormones are administered with digoxin to the client.

3. **Answer: 3**
   RATIONALE: The nurse should monitor for mild diuresis as a sign of therapeutic response after the thyroid hormone is administered to the client. Agranulocytosis, headache, and loss of hair are the adverse reactions to antithyroid preparations.

4. **Answer: 2**
   RATIONALE: Development of chest pain in the client is a symptom that would indicate the dosage of the thyroid hormone can be reduced.

5. **Answer: 4**
   RATIONALE: Altered mental status, along with high fever and extreme tachycardia are the signs of an impending thyroid storm.

6. **Answer: 2**
   RATIONALE: Thyroid hormones are contraindicated in clients with known hypersensitivity to the drug, an uncorrected adrenal cortical insufficiency, or thyrotoxicosis.

7. **Answers: 1, 3, 4**
   RATIONALE: The nurse should report signs of hyperthyroidism such as moist skin, moderate hypertension, and increased appetite to the primary health care provider before the next dose is due because it may be necessary to decrease the daily dosage.

8. **Answer: 2**
   RATIONALE: Hashimoto thyroiditis is an inflammatory disease causing hypothyroidism.

9. **Answer: 3**
   RATIONALE: Levothyroxine (Synthroid) is the drug of choice for hypothyroidism because it is relatively inexpensive, requires once-a-day dosing, and has a more uniform potency than do other thyroid hormone replacement drugs.

10. **Answer: 1**
    RATIONALE: A nurse should be cautious not to administer levothyroxine (Synthroid) to a client who has recently had a myocardial infarction.

11. **Answer: 1**
    RATIONALE: Levothyroxine (Synthroid) is in pregnancy category A, and it is safe to use during pregnancy.

CHAPTER 43

SECTION I: ASSESSING YOUR UNDERSTANDING

Activity A FILL IN THE BLANKS

1. menarche
2. endogenous
3. Catabolism
4. secondary sex characteristics
5. androgens

Activity B DOSAGE CALCULATION

1. 1 tablet
2. 3 tablets
3. 2 tablets
4. 1.5 tablets
5. 2 capsules

Activity C MATCHING

1. **1.** c   **2.** a   **3.** d   **4.** b
2. **1.** b   **2.** c   **3.** d   **4.** a

Activity D SHORT ANSWERS

1. Treatment with androgens may lead to an increase in fluid volume. When a nurse is monitoring clients on androgen therapy, the following assessments should be made:
   - The nurse should observe the client for any signs of edema as a result of sodium and water retention making the client edematous. She should also make a note of any puffiness of the eyelids. If the client is ambulatory, there may be dependent swelling of the hands or feet. If the client is nonambulatory, the nurse may need to look for swelling of the sacral area.
   - The client's weight should be noted prior to androgen therapy, to be used as a guide. As part of the ongoing assessment, the nurse needs to compare the client's weight with the preadministration weight on a daily basis.
   - The nurse needs to monitor daily fluid intake and output to calculate the fluid balance. The nurse should be aware that older adults with heart and kidney diseases pose a greater risk, as they are at an increased risk of developing sodium and water retention.

2. The nurse should include the following points in the teaching plan when educating a client about oral contraceptives:
   - Read the package insert carefully. Discuss any questions with the health care provider.
   - Take the first dose as directed by the instructions or by the primary health care provider.
   - The drug should be taken at intervals not exceeding once every 24 hours. It is best taken with the evening meal or at bedtime. The dose schedule has to be followed for proper efficacy of the drug. Failure to comply may lead to pregnancy.
   - Until the first week of the next cycle, an additional birth control method should be used.
   - If 1 day's dose is missed, the missed dose should be taken as soon as remembered, or two tablets taken the next day.
   - If 2 days are missed, then two tablets need to be taken for the next 2 days and then the normal dosing schedule should be continued. Another form of birth control must be used until the cycle is completed and a new cycle has begun.
   - If 3 days in a row or more are missed, the drug should be discontinued. Another form of birth control may be used until a new cycle can begin. Before restarting the regimen, absence of pregnancy, due to a break in the regimen, needs to be confirmed.
   - If unsure what to do about a missed dose, contact the primary health care provider.
   - Both active and passive smoking should be avoided while taking oral contraceptives.

■ Any adverse reactions such as fluid retention or edema to the extremities; weight gain; pain, swelling, or tenderness in the legs; blurred vision; chest pain; yellowed skin or eyes; dark urine; or abnormal vaginal bleeding should be reported.

■ Periodic examinations by the primary health care provider and laboratory tests are needed during the therapy.

Activity E CROSSWORD PUZZLE

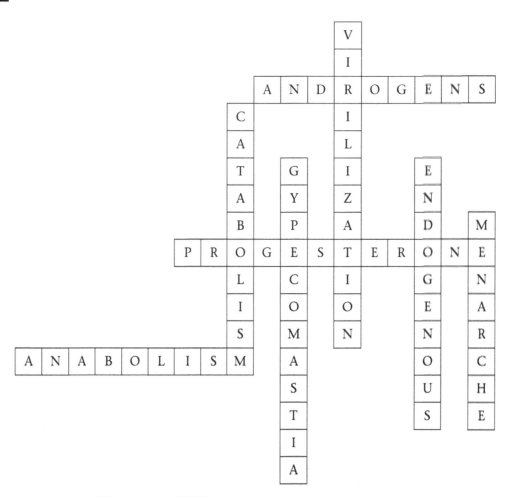

SECTION II: APPLYING YOUR KNOWLEDGE

Activity F CASE STUDY

1. High-dose levonorgestrel (Plan B) should be given within 72 hours after unprotected intercourse or contraceptive failure.
2. Levonorgestrel (Plan B) should be taken the following way: first dose within 72 hours of event and a second dose 12 hours later. If vomiting occurs within 1 hour after taking either dose, the physician should be notified.

SECTION III: PRACTICING FOR NCLEX

Activity G NCLEX-STYLE QUESTIONS

1. **Answer: 2**
   RATIONALE: Androgen therapy may be prescribed for testosterone deficiency. The male hormone testosterone and its derivatives are collectively called *androgens*. Thus, androgen therapy may be prescribed for testosterone deficiency. Symptoms of benign prostatic hypertrophy are treated by androgen hormone inhibitors, and not by androgen therapy. Male pattern baldness occurs due to androgens, and androgen hormone inhibitors are used for its prevention.

2. **Answer: 4**
   RATIONALE: Anabolic steroids may be used to promote weight gain following profound weight loss due to surgery, trauma, or infections. Anabolic steroids are not intended for increase in muscle mass and strength in young, healthy individuals.

3. **Answer: 1**
   RATIONALE: Increased antidiuretic effects may be seen when androgens or androgen hormone inhibitors are used in a client on oral anticoagulant therapy.

4. Answer: 2

RATIONALE: Gynecomastia or enlargement of the breast is a complication of androgen therapy seen among male clients. Testicular atrophy, and not enlargement of testes, may be seen as another side effect of androgen therapy. Virilization is the appearance of male secondary sexual characteristics in females and is seen as a side effect of androgen therapy in females, and not males. Water retention, and not frequent urination, is seen in clients on androgen therapy.

5. Answers: 1, 4, 5

RATIONALE: Androgens aid in the development and maintenance of male secondary sex characteristics: facial hair, deep voice, body hair, body fat distribution, and muscle development.

6. Answer: 2

RATIONALE: Severe mental changes, such as uncontrolled rage (called "roid rage"), severe depression, suicidal tendencies, inability to concentrate, and personality changes, are not uncommon.

7. Answer: 4

RATIONALE: If a woman has missed 1 day's dose of an oral contraceptive, she should be advised to take the missed dose as soon as remembered or to take two tablets the next day. Discontinuing the drug and using another form of birth control until the next cycle is needed when the doses for 3 days in a row or more have been missed, not when only 1 day's dose is missed. Remembering to take one tablet the next day and forgetting about the missed dose does not help, as it may reduce the contraceptive effectiveness and lead to pregnancy.

8. Answer: 4

RATIONALE: The female hormone estropipate is a synthetic estrogen. Estropipate is not produced endogenously and must be obtained from outside as a drug. Estradiol, estrone, and estriol are estrogens that are produced endogenously in the body.

9. Answer: 2

RATIONALE: If hair loss occurs, suggest wearing head coverings such hats, scarves, or a wig; mild skin pigmentation may be covered with makeup, but severe and widespread pigmented areas and acne are often difficult to conceal.

10. Answer: 1

RATIONALE: Fluoxymesterone is an androgen that can be used to treat hypogonadism.

11. Answer: 2

RATIONALE: Oxymetholone is an anabolic steroid that can be used to treat anemia.

12. Answer: 1

RATIONALE: Nandrolone is an example of an anabolic steroid.

CHAPTER 44

SECTION I: ASSESSING YOUR UNDERSTANDING

Activity A FILL IN THE BLANKS

1. contractions
2. posterior
3. eclampsia
4. tocolysis
5. antidiuretic

Activity B DOSAGE CALCULATION

1. 1 mL
2. 2 tablets
3. 1 tablet
4. 10 mL
5. 0.25 mL
6. 0.5 mL

Activity C MATCHING

1.	1. c	2. b	3. a	4. e	5. d
2.	1. b	2. c	3. a	4. e	5. d

Activity D SHORT ANSWERS

1. The nurse should immediately discontinue the oxytocin infusion if any of these changes are noted:
   - A significant change in the FHR or rhythm
   - A marked change in the frequency, rate, or rhythm of uterine contractions
   - A marked increase or decrease in the client's blood pressure or pulse or any significant change in the client's general condition.
2. During the ongoing assessment of a client receiving a tocolytic drug, the role of the nurse includes:
   - Recording blood pressure, pulse, and respiratory rate
   - Monitoring FHR
   - Checking the IV infusion rate
   - Examining the area around the IV needle insertion site for signs of infiltration
   - Monitoring uterine contractions (frequency, intensity, length) or lack of contractions
   - Measuring maternal intake and output.

Activity E CROSSWORD PUZZLE

				P		O			T				
				R		X			O				
				E		Y			C				
				E		T			O				
E				C		O			L				
C				L		C			Y				
L				A		I			S				
A	L	B	U	M	I	N	U	R	I	A			
M				P					S				
P				S									
S				I									
I				A	N	T	E	P	A	R	T	U	M
A													

SECTION II: APPLYING YOUR KNOWLEDGE

Activity F CASE STUDY

1. The nurse should obtain the following information during the preadministration assessment of Stella: obstetric history (parity, gravidity, previous obstetric problems, type of labor, stillbirths, abortions, live-birth infant abnormalities) and a general health history. Immediately before starting the IV infusion of oxytocin (Pitocin), the nurse assesses the fetal heart rate and the client's blood pressure, pulse, and respiratory rate.

2. The adverse effects of oxytocin (Pitocin) include fetal bradycardia, uterine rupture, uterine hypertonicity, nausea, vomiting, cardiac arrhythmias, anaphylactic reactions, and water intoxication.

SECTION III: PRACTICING FOR NCLEX

Activity G NCLEX-STYLE QUESTIONS

1. **Answer: 3**
   RATIONALE: Drugs may be used to induce an early vaginal delivery when there are fetal or maternal problems, such as a client with diabetes and a large fetus.

2. **Answer: 2**
   RATIONALE: Methylergonovine is usually given IM at the time of the delivery of the anterior shoulder or after the delivery of the placenta.

3. **Answer: 4**
   RATIONALE: Magnesium at one time was one of the most commonly used drugs to decrease uterine muscle contractions and is used for seizure control with eclampsia.

4. **Answer: 3**
   RATIONALE: Corticosteroids are administered to the fetus in utero to enhance organ maturity.

5. **Answer: 4**
   RATIONALE: Carboprost is an oxytocic drug that can be given to clients whom are hypertensive.

6. **Answers: 1, 3, 4**
   RATIONALE: When administering methylergonovine for controlling postpartum bleeding, the nurse should monitor the vital signs at least every 4 hours and should note the character and amount of vaginal bleeding. The nurse should immediately notify the primary health care provider when abdominal cramping is moderate to severe.

7. **Answer: 1**
   RATIONALE: When oxytocin is administered IV, there is a danger of excessive fluid volume (water intoxication) because oxytocin has an antidiuretic effect.

8. **Answer: 1**
   RATIONALE: Magnesium sulfate is used to manage preterm labor in pregnancies of greater than 27 weeks' gestation. It is a calcium antagonist and works to decrease the force of uterine contractions.

9. **Answer: 1**
   RATIONALE: Oxytocin is used antepartum to induce uterine contractions.
10. **Answer: 2**
    RATIONALE: Oxytocin is an endogenous hormone produced by the posterior pituitary gland.
11. **Answer: 1**
    RATIONALE: Oxytocin (Pitocin) intranasally is known to stimulate the milk ejection reflex.
12. **Answer: 1**
    RATIONALE: A nurse should monitor a client receiving oxytocin (Pitocin) for the following adverse effects: cardiac arrhythmias, fetal bradycardia, uterine rupture, uterine hypertonicity, nausea, vomiting, and anaphylactic reactions.

CHAPTER 45

SECTION I: ASSESSING YOUR UNDERSTANDING

Activity A FILL IN THE BLANKS

1. menopause
2. heart
3. stress
4. testes
5. prostate

Activity B DOSAGE CALCULATION

1. 2 tablets
2. 2 tablets
3. 3 days, plus 1 tablet left
4. 2 capsules
5. 2 tablets in a day

Activity C MATCHING

1. 1. c   2. a   3. b
2. 1. b   2. c   3. d   4. a

Activity D SHORT ANSWERS

1. Studies question the effectiveness of ERT for postmenopausal women and the increased risk of cardiovascular disease. Encourage the client to ask questions about her therapy. Inaccurate information is clarified before starting therapy. Refer questions that cannot or should not be answered by a nurse to the primary health care provider.
2. The nurse should include the following points in the teaching plan when educating a client about transdermal estrogen:
   - Be sure to read the package insert carefully. Some systems are applied twice weekly; others are applied every 7 days.
   - Apply the system immediately after opening the pouch, with the adhesive side down. Apply to clean, dry skin of the trunk, buttocks, abdomen, upper inner thigh, or upper arm. Do not apply to breasts, waistline, or a site exposed to sunlight. The area should not be oily or irritated. Be careful with heat sources such as an electric blanket that can increase the rate of absorption.
   - Press the system firmly in place with the palm of the hand for about 10 seconds. The application site is rotated, with at least 1-week intervals between applications to a particular site.
   - Avoid areas that may be exposed to rubbing or where clothing may rub the system off or loosen the edges.
   - Remove the old system before applying a new system. Rotate application sites to prevent skin irritation.
   - Follow the directions of the primary health care provider regarding application of the system (e.g., continuous, 3 weeks' use followed by 1 week off, changed weekly, or applied twice weekly).
   - If the system falls off, reapply it or apply a new system. Continue the original treatment schedule.

Activity E SUDOKU PUZZLE

BPH	GU	DHT	ED	OBS	AHI	ERT	UTI	HRT
HRT	OBS	AHI	UTI	GU	ERT	BPH	ED	DHT
ERT	UTI	ED	BPH	HRT	DHT	GU	AHI	OBS
AHI	HRT	GU	DHT	ED	UTI	OBS	BPH	ERT
ED	DHT	UTI	OBS	ERT	BPH	HRT	GU	AHI
OBS	BPH	ERT	HRT	AHI	GU	ED	DHT	UTI
UTI	AHI	HRT	GU	BPH	OBS	DHT	ERT	ED
DHT	ED	BPH	ERT	UTI	HRT	AHI	OBS	GU
GU	ERT	OBS	AHI	DHT	ED	UTI	HRT	BPH

SECTION II: APPLYING YOUR KNOWLEDGE

Activity F CASE STUDY

1. Finasteride is an androgen hormone inhibitor. Women who are pregnant or of the age that they may become pregnant should not handle this medication.
2. Finasteride is also used for male pattern baldness. Mr. Phillip's hair may be growing as an added effect of the medication.

SECTION III: PRACTICING FOR NCLEX

Activity G NCLEX-STYLE QUESTIONS

1. Answer: 1
   RATIONALE: When caring for a client experiencing dry mouth, the nurse should instruct the client to suck on sugarless lozenges. Sucking on hard candy can also bring relief to clients with dry mouth, and so the nurse need not instruct the client to refrain from consuming them.

2. Answer: 2
   RATIONALE: The nurse should monitor for dry eyes in the client taking the drug solifenacin. Dry eyes, blurred vision, and dry mouth are common adverse reactions to antispasmodic drugs.

3. Answer: 3
   RATIONALE: Androgen hormone inhibitors are prescribed for benign prostatic hypertrophy and male pattern baldness.

4. Answer: 3
   RATIONALE: The nurse should know that antispasmodics are contraindicated in clients with myasthenia gravis.

5. Answer: 3
   RATIONALE: Impaired vision may occur as an adverse effect of the herb black cohosh. It may cause high, and not low, blood pressure. It does not cause ringing in the ears, but rather is used to treat this symptom seen during menopause. The herb causes weight gain, and not weight loss.

6. Answer: 1
   RATIONALE: The nurse should instruct the client to increase the intake of fluids to alleviate the effect of constipation due to flavoxate. Increasing the client's intake of citrus fruits, decreasing the client's consumption of milk products, or administering the drug with tepid water will not help alleviate the effect of constipation.

7. Answer: 4
   RATIONALE: Increased time for sexual arousal is needed as fat atrophies and hormonal changes occur in the aging female reproductive system. Additionally, the pelvic floor muscles weaken; the vaginal pH changes to an alkaline environment, making it susceptible to yeast infections; and the walls shorten and become less elastic.

8. Answer: 2
   RATIONALE: The estradiol transdermal system is used after removal of the ovaries in premenopausal women (female castration) and primary ovarian failure. It provides a more continual source of the medication.

9. Answer: 3
   RATIONALE: Changes in kidney size and blood flow to the kidney reduce renal function by almost 50% in older individuals.

10. Answer: 1
   RATIONALE: Dutasteride (Avodart) is an example of an androgen hormone inhibitor used to treat clients with benign prostatic hypertrophy.

11. Answer: 2
   RATIONALE: Flutamide is a drug used for advanced prostatic cancer.

12. Answer: 3
   RATIONALE: When the need to void is sudden and urgent and there may be a loss of urine, this type of incontinence is called urge incontinence and can be treated with drugs called antispasmodics. Stress incontinence occurs when the urinary sphincter becomes less flexible and is less able to close tightly, resulting in urine leakage. This type of incontinence is typically treated with surgical or behavioral interventions.

CHAPTER 46

SECTION I: ASSESSING YOUR UNDERSTANDING

Activity A FILL IN THE BLANKS

1. bladder
2. urethra
3. cystitis
4. bacteriostatic
5. bactericidal

Activity B DOSAGE CALCULATION

1. 1 capsule
2. 2 packets
3. 6 tablets
4. 10 mL

Activity C MATCHING

1. **1.** b   **2.** a   **3.** c

Activity D SHORT ANSWERS

1. The nurse can instruct the group that because the female urethra is considerably shorter than the male urethra, women are affected by UTIs much more frequently than men.

2. The nurse should include the following teaching points for the group of young mothers:
   - Wipe front to back when changing diapers.
   - Avoid tight clothing or prolonged wet diapers.
   - Avoid "overcleaning" and irritating the skin.
   - Increase fluid intake, gauging the amount by the color of the baby's urine (it should be pale yellow during the day).

Activity E LABELING

1. Peritoneal lining
2. Adrenal gland
3. Kidney
4. Ureter
5. Bladder
6. Prostate gland
7. Urethra
8. Descending aorta
9. Inferior vena cava

SECTION II: APPLYING YOUR KNOWLEDGE

Activity F CASE STUDY

1. Prior to leaving the office, the nurse should discuss the following adverse reactions to nitrofurantoin (Macrobid) with Janna: nausea, anorexia, peripheral neuropathy, headache, and bacterial/fungal superinfection precautions.

2. The nurse should recommend the following nonpharmacologic measures to Janna:
   - Learn ways to reduce UTIs, such as how to wipe front to back after going to the bathroom.
   - Avoid tight clothing, prolonged wearing of pantyhose, tight pants, or wet bathing suits.
   - Shower instead of bathing, rinsing well, and avoid "overcleaning" and irritating the skin.
   - Use tampons for menstrual periods instead of pads; make a habit of voiding every 4 hours and changing the tampon.
   - Increase fluid intake, gauging the amount you drink to the color of your urine (it should be pale yellow during the day).
   - Vitamin C supplements and cranberry juice help maintain an acid environment in the bladder.
   - Be sure to drink fluids and void regularly when cycling or horseback riding.

SECTION III: PRACTICING FOR NCLEX

Activity G NCLEX-STYLE QUESTIONS

1. **Answer: 2**
   RATIONALE: They are primarily excreted by the kidneys and exert their major antibacterial effects in the urine as it travels through the bladder.

2. **Answer: 1**
   RATIONALE: Nitrofurantoin has been known to cause acute and chronic pulmonary reactions.

3. **Answer: 1**
   RATIONALE: The nurse should monitor the client for an increased risk of bleeding when sulfamethoxazole is administered with oral anticoagulants.

4. **Answer: 3**
   RATIONALE: The nurse should administer the urinary tract anti-infective with cranberry juice to the client. Even other fluids, preferably water, are encouraged during drug administration, although the nurse need not administer the drug strictly with warm water.

5. **Answer: 3**
   RATIONALE: The nurse should avoid administration of phenazopyridine for more than 2 days when the client is also receiving an antibacterial drug for the UTI. When used for more than 2 days, the drug may mask the symptoms of a more serious disorder.

6. **Answer: 2**
   RATIONALE: The nurse should administer the drug with milk to prevent irritation in the stomach of the client receiving a nitrofurantoin urinary tract anti-infective.

7. **Answers: 1, 2, 3**
   RATIONALE: During preadministration assessment, the nurse should question the client regarding symptoms of infection before instituting therapy, take and record the client's vital signs, and record the color and appearance of the urine. The nurse also assesses for and documents pain, urinary frequency, bladder distension, or other symptoms associated with the urinary system.

8. **Answer: 3**
   RATIONALE: Some drugs used in the treatment of UTIs, such as nitrofurantoin, do not belong to the antibiotic or sulfonamide groups of drugs.

9. **Answer: 1**
   RATIONALE: Phenazopyridine is a dye that exerts a topical analgesic effect on the lining of the urinary tract.

10. **Answer: 3**
    RATIONALE: The use of nitrofurantoin has been known to cause acute and chronic reactions in the respiratory system.

11. **Answer: 1**
    RATIONALE: Cranberry juice inhibits bacteria from attaching to the walls of the urinary tract and prevents certain bacteria from forming dental plaque in the mouth.

12. **Answer: 2**
    RATIONALE: Clients who are allergic to tartrazine should not be administered methenamine because it contains tartrazine dye and an allergic reaction may result.

CHAPTER 47

SECTION I: ASSESSING YOUR UNDERSTANDING

Activity A FILL IN THE BLANKS

1. Reye
2. Artificially
3. Booster
4. Immunity
5. Cell

Activity B DOSAGE CALCULATION

1. 0.3 mL
2. 6 clients
3. 3 mL
4. 1.5 mL
5. 8 injections

Activity C MATCHING

1. 1. e   2. a   3. d   4. b   5. c

Activity D SHORT ANSWERS

1. Did you find any variation with other students and the recommended vaccinations?
2. Try taking the quiz with the assumption that you are not a student in a health care field—are the recommended immunizations different? What if you decided to go on an overseas medical mission—what would be the recommendation?

Activity E SUDOKU PUZZLE

HEP B	DTaP	FLU	CMI	MMR	CDC	IgA	IPV	IGIV
IGIV	MMR	CDC	IPV	DTaP	IgA	HEP B	CMI	FLU
IgA	IPV	CMI	HEP B	IGIV	FLU	DTaP	CDC	MMR
CDC	IGIV	DTaP	FLU	CMI	IPV	MMR	HEP B	IgA
CMI	FLU	IPV	MMR	IgA	HEP B	IGIV	DTaP	CDC
MMR	HEP B	IgA	IGIV	CDC	DTaP	CMI	FLU	IPV
IPV	CDC	IGIV	DTaP	HEP B	MMR	FLU	IgA	CMI
FLU	CMI	HEP B	IgA	IPV	IGIV	CDC	MMR	DTaP
DTaP	IgA	MMR	CDC	FLU	CMI	IPV	IGIV	HEP B

SECTION II: APPLYING YOUR KNOWLEDGE

Activity F CASE STUDY

1. For the 2021 schedule Jimmy is due for second doses of RV, DTaP, Hib, PCV13, and IPV.
2. Four months of age is before the catch-up period for the hepatitis B (Hep B). The *Haemophilus influenzae* vaccine can be given at 6 months; you would need to find out if it was the PedvaxHIB or Comvax because then it would be only two doses and not three before the age of 6 months.

SECTION III: PRACTICING FOR NCLEX

Activity G NCLEX-STYLE QUESTIONS

1. **Answer: 3**
   RATIONALE: Humoral immunity protects the body against bacterial and viral infections. Special lymphocytes (white blood cells), called B lymphocytes, produce circulating antibodies to act against a foreign substance.

2. **Answer: 2**
   RATIONALE: Vaccine is defined as a substance containing either weakened or killed antigens developed for the purpose of creating resistance to disease.

3. **Answer: 3**
   RATIONALE: Lymphocytes play a major role in providing cellular and humoral immunity. Immunity refers to the ability of the body to identify and resist potentially harmful microorganisms. This ability enables the body to inhibit tissue and organ damage. T lymphocytes play a major role in maintaining cellular immunity, and B lymphocytes in maintaining humoral immunity. Neutrophils, basophils, and eosinophils do not play a major role in humoral immunity.

4. **Answers: 1, 2, 4**
   RATIONALE: Vaccines are used in routine immunization of infants and children, immunization of adults against tetanus, adults at high risk for certain diseases (e.g., pneumococcal

and influenza vaccines), and children or adults at risk for exposure to a particular disease (e.g., hepatitis A for those going to endemic areas). The rubella vaccine is never given to pregnant women as it might lead to infection. It is given for immunization of nonpregnant women of childbearing age. Vaccines and toxoids are contraindicated in leukemia.

5. **Answer: 3**
   RATIONALE: Antivenins should be administered within 4 hours of exposure to yield the most effective response. Antivenins are used for passive, transient protection from the toxic effects of bites by spiders (black widow and similar spiders) and snakes (rattlesnakes, copperhead, cottonmouth, and coral). The nurse should know that the most effective response is obtained when the drug is administered within 4 hours after exposure. If the drug is administered beyond 4 hours, it might lessen the therapeutic value and its action against the venom.

6. **Answer: 3**
   RATIONALE: Chickenpox can cause herpes zoster (shingles), which is a painful condition, later in life.

7. **Answer: 1**
   RATIONALE: In lactation, vaccines are to be used with caution. Contraindications for the use of vaccines include acute febrile illnesses, leukemia, lymphoma, immunosuppressive illness, drug therapy, and nonlocalized cancer.

8. **Answer: 3**
   RATIONALE: Cell-mediated immunity depends on the actions of T lymphocytes.

9. **Answer: 4**
   RATIONALE: T lymphocytes are responsible for a delayed-type immune response seen in cell-mediated immunity.

10. **Answer: 1**
    RATIONALE: Immunizations are a form of artificial active immunity.

11. **Answer: 3**
    RATIONALE: The administration of immune globulins or antivenins is a form of passive immunity.

12. **Answer: 1**
    RATIONALE: The nurse must administer toxoids and vaccines to a client prior to exposure to the disease-causing organism in order for the client to be protected against the disease.

CHAPTER 48

SECTION I: ASSESSING YOUR UNDERSTANDING

Activity A FILL IN THE BLANKS

1. Cytokines
2. Erythropoiesis
3. Anemia
4. Erythrocytes or red blood cells

Activity B DOSAGE CALCULATION

1. 300 mcg
2. 0.77 mL (dose = 232 mcg)
3. 14 tablets
4. 2 mL
5. 0.75 mL

Activity C MATCHING

1. **1.** d **2.** c **3.** b **4.** a
2. **1.** d **2.** c **3.** b **4.** a

Activity D SHORT ANSWERS

1. Before administering the first dose of ferrous gluconate, the nurse should perform the following assessments in the client:
   - Obtain a general health history and ask about the symptoms of anemia (fatigue, shortness of breath, sore tongue, headache, pallor).
   - Take vital signs to provide a baseline during therapy.
   - Other physical assessments may include the client's general appearance and, in the severely anemic, an evaluation of the client's ability to carry out the activities of daily living.
   - Track and record the client's weight and hemoglobin levels.

2. The nurse should instruct the client on a balanced diet with an emphasis on foods that are high in iron:
   - Lean red meats
   - Cereals
   - Dried beans
   - Leafy green vegetables.

Activity E WORD FIND PUZZLE

			L	Y	M	P	H	O	C	Y	T	E
				L							T	O
			N	A						Y		S
			T	E					C			I
		E			U			O			B	N
	L				T	Y				A	O
E				R	R				S	P
T				A			O		O	H
		K					P		P	I
		A						H	H	L
	G							I
R	E	D	B	L	O	O	D	C	E	L	L	L
M	O	N	O	C	Y	T	E					

SECTION II: APPLYING YOUR KNOWLEDGE

Activity F CASE STUDY

1. The WBC, known as the neutrophil, is one of the major cells in the line of defense from infection. Because of its rapid growth cycle, the neutrophil is a target of the cancer chemotherapy drugs, as well as the cancer cells themselves. Chemotherapy-induced neutropenia is a major reason that cancer treatments may be delayed or canceled. When this happens, the client is at a greater risk for continued growth of the cancer or illness from the treatment. Colony-stimulating factors (CSFs) are drugs used to stimulate the growth and production of WBCs to help fight off infection.

2. Filgrastim (Neupogen) should be used cautiously in clients with hypothyroidism and is contraindicated in clients with known hypersensitivity to the drug or any of its components.

SECTION III: PRACTICING FOR NCLEX

Activity G NCLEX-STYLE QUESTIONS

1. **Answer: 2**
   RATIONALE: The nurse should monitor the client administered a folic acid injection for allergic hypersensitivity. There are few if any other adverse reactions.

2. **Answer: 3**
   RATIONALE: Clients with vitamin B_{12} anemia are treated with vitamin B_{12} IM administered weekly. The parenteral route is used because the vitamin is ineffective orally, owing to the absence of the intrinsic factor in the stomach, which is necessary for utilization of vitamin B_{12}.

3. **Answer: 3**
   RATIONALE: When a client is administered iron supplements along with methyldopa, the client should be monitored for the decreased effect of the Parkinson's medication, which would result in an increase of the Parkinson disease symptoms.

4. **Answer: 3**
   RATIONALE: People with a strict vegetarian (vegan) lifestyle need to supplement their diets to fulfill their nutritional needs and prevent a deficiency of vitamin B_{12}.

5. **Answer: 2**
   RATIONALE: In the teaching plan, the nurse should instruct the client receiving ferrous tablets that the drug may be taken with food or meals if the client experiences gastrointestinal upset, although it is preferred that they be taken on an empty stomach.

6. **Answers: 1, 2, 5**
   RATIONALE: The nurse should monitor for adverse reactions such as bone pain, hypertension, nausea, vomiting, alopecia, and hypersensitive reactions when a client is administered a CSF for neutropenia.

7. **Answer: 1**
   RATIONALE: When teaching a client receiving oral iron supplements about adverse reactions, the nurse should inform the client that the color of their stools will turn black.

8. **Answer: 1**
   RATIONALE: The nurse should instruct clients receiving iron supplements to avoid milk, which interferes with iron absorption.

9. **Answer: 3**
   RATIONALE: Red blood cells, also known as erythrocytes, supply cells with oxygen from the lungs.

10. **Answer: 1**
    RATIONALE: Megakaryocytes divide into platelets that control the bleeding from microscopic or major tears in our tissues.

11. **Answer: 4**
    RATIONALE: Infection is likely to occur when a client is neutropenic.

12. **Answer: 3**
    RATIONALE: Anemia can also cause decreased platelet production.

13. **Answer: 1**
    RATIONALE: Hematopoiesis is the process by which the body is stimulated to make more of a specific type of blood cell.

CHAPTER 49

SECTION I: ASSESSING YOUR UNDERSTANDING

Activity A FILL IN THE BLANKS

1. Cell-mediated
2. antibody
3. multiple
4. Immunosuppressant
5. momab

Activity B DOSAGE CALCULATION

1. 2 syringes. Prefilled syringes hold one 300 mg/2 mL. Two doses every month.
2. 71 kilograms
3. 710 milligrams of drug
4. 1 capsule per dose
5. 28 capsules are needed for the 14 days

Activity C MATCHING

1. d   2. e   3. c   4. b   5. a

Activity D SHORT ANSWERS

1. This reaction is due to the sensitivity of the client to the tissue of origin of the mAb. Mouse and human tissues are used to make the drugs. mAbs composed of more mouse tissue than human tissue is more likely to cause a hypersensitive reaction than those mAbs with more mouse tissue.

2. Hypersensitive infusion reactions can be somewhat lessened by premedication. Reassure the client that the medications administered before the immunotherapy will help to ease the adverse reactions. Often, a combination of acetaminophen and diphenhydramine (with or without a steroid) are given 30 minutes before the infusion. Warm blankets should be provided for client comfort. If clients react again, they most likely will be stopped and another treatment considered.

Activity E EXPLAIN THE DRUG NAME

1, 3 —use exclusively human tissue
2 —uses a combination of human and animal tissue, but primarily human
4, 5 —use a combination of human and animal tissue

SECTION II: APPLYING YOUR KNOWLEDGE

Activity F CASE STUDY

Companies find going directly to consumers is still making them money.

https://www.fiercepharma.com/marketing/pharma-tv-ad-spenders-blow-up-december-spendiest-month-2020-by-top-10-brands

https://www.psychologytoday.com/us/blog/animal-emotions/201910/were-being-bombarded-ads-drugs

https://www.npr.org/sections/health-shots/2017/04/29/525877472/those-tv-drug-ads-distract-us-from-the-medical-care-we-need

https://www.nytimes.com/2017/12/24/business/media/prescription-drugs-advertising-tv.html

SECTION III: PRACTICING FOR NCLEX

Activity G NCLEX-STYLE QUESTIONS

1. Answer: 3
RATIONALE: Immunosuppressant drugs are used in transplant clients to intentionally suppress the production and activity of immune cells—the immune system; as a result, they do not recognize, and attack the new organ.

2. Answer: 3, 4
RATIONALE: History of travel to areas of infectious diseases (requires immunization) or having had an infectious disease are important to know because the immunotherapy can create a flare reaction.

3. Answer: 4
RATIONALE: The skin rash adverse reaction when mAbs are administered is an inflammatory reaction. The other options can potentiate the reaction

4. Answer: 1
RATIONALE: Hypersensitive infusion reactions can be somewhat lessened by premedication. Often, a combination of acetaminophen and diphenhydramine (with or without a steroid) are given 30 minutes before the infusion.

5. Answer: 3
RATIONALE: Clients with relapsing MS may be prescribed glatiramer for self-administration. It comes in a 20 mg/mL formula used daily or 40 mg/mL taken three times weekly. These products are not interchangeable; the 40 mg formula cannot be used for daily dosing.

6. Answer: 2
RATIONALE: Passive immunity requires multiple doses to provide ongoing protection. They can be administered by different routes, daily or less.

7. Answer: 3
RATIONALE: Encourage clients to balance activity with rest periods to reduce fatigue. Although it may sound counterintuitive, exercise helps reduce fatigue; encourage clients to take small walks or participate in yoga.

8. Answer: 3
RATIONALE: Antibodies are the proteins produced by the immune system in response to foreign antigens. They are Y-shaped molecules that bind to antigens on a pathogenic cell, acting as a flag to the immune system to attack and destroy the cell

9. Answer: 1, 2, 4
RATIONALE: Immunosuppressant drug actions include inhibition of the inflammatory response, inhibition of the activation of T cells, and reduction of antibody formation. They do not involve B cells.

10. Answer: 1
RATIONALE: Monoclonal antibodies create an immune response, similar to having influenza. The following are the classic "flu-like" symptoms and include chills, cough, fever, headache, and malaise. Clients may experience the many other symptoms with treatment such as GI disturbances, pain, or edema.

11. Answer: 1
RATIONALE: A generalized inflammatory response may occur, which is initially supported with nursing interventions. Should the inflammation advance, steroids may be added to adverse reaction interventions.

12. Answer: 2
RATIONALE: The FDA recommends that biosimilars have an addition suffix of four randomly generated letters included in the name.

CHAPTER 50

SECTION I: ASSESSING YOUR UNDERSTANDING

Activity A FILL IN THE BLANKS

1. chemotherapy
2. myelosuppression
3. neutropenia
4. metastasis
5. Chemoprotective

Activity B SEQUENCING

1. 4   5   3   1   2

Activity C MATCHING

1. **1.** b   **2.** e   **3.** a   **4.** c   **5.** d
2. **1.** c   **2.** a   **3.** d   **4.** b

Activity D SHORT ANSWERS

1. Some drugs leave the body relatively unchanged; therefore, to prevent exposure to others in the home:
   - Men should avoid using urinals or standing at the toilet.
   - Sit to urinate for at least 48 hours following the last dose of the drug.
   - Toilets should be double flushed with the lid down to prevent spray in the bathroom.
2. The nurse should explain the following guidelines when a client is transferred to another facility to receive chemotherapeutic drugs:
   - It is to ensure the drugs are prescribed by a provider trained specifically in the care of oncology clients.
   - There are specific policies established for preparation and administration of the drugs that not all facilities can offer.
   - The staff has the ability to increase the frequency of assessments if the client's condition changes.
   - Nurses are given specific training for the handling and administration of the traditional chemotherapy drugs.

Activity E CROSSWORD PUZZLE

	A	N	T	I	B	I	O	T	I	C	S	
					I							
			A		O							
			L		L							
			K		O							
			A		G							
			L		I							
		V	I	N	C	A						
			N									
I	N	T	E	R	F	E	R	E				

SECTION II: APPLYING YOUR KNOWLEDGE

Activity F CASE STUDY

1. Vincristine is a plant alkaloid that interferes with amino acid production in the S phase and formation of microtubules in the M phase.

2. The steps the client can take to promote good oral hygiene and reduce the effects of vincristine include the following:
   - Inspect the oral cavity for increased irritation, knowing that 5–7 days after chemotherapy is started stomatitis typically presents.
   - Avoid any foods or products that are irritating to the mouth, such as alcoholic beverages, spices, alcohol-based mouthwash, or toothpaste.
   - Report any white patches on the tongue (possible candidiasis fungal infection), throat, or gums; any burning sensation; and bleeding from the mouth or gums.
   - Perform mouth care every 4 hours, including a rinse with normal saline solution.
   - Avoid lemon/glycerin swabs because they tend to irritate the oral mucosa and complicate stomatitis.
   - The oncology health care provider may order a topical viscous anesthetic, such as lidocaine viscous, to decrease discomfort.

SECTION III: PRACTICING FOR NCLEX

Activity G NCLEX-STYLE QUESTIONS

1. **Answers: 1, 4, 5**
   RATIONALE: Chemotherapy is administered in a series of cycles to allow for the recovery of the normal cells, to destroy more of the malignant cells, and to allow normal cells that rapidly divide and reproduce to grow back. Chemotherapy is administered at the time the cell population is dividing as part of a strategy to optimize cell death.
2. **Answers: 1, 2, 4, 5**
   RATIONALE: The nurse informs the client that drinking green tea can cause nervousness, insomnia, restlessness, and GI upset.
3. **Answer: 2**
   RATIONALE: The nurse should explain that an antimetabolite is cell cycle specific and incorporates itself into the cellular components during the S phase of cell division, thus interfering with the synthesis of RNA and DNA.
4. **Answer: 2**
   RATIONALE: When preparing a nursing care plan for ongoing assessment of the client, the general condition should be used, especially with an older client, to determine what specific assessments should be conducted on an ongoing basis.
5. **Answer: 1**
   RATIONALE: When administering a subcutaneous injection, the nurse should use no more than 1 mL of the drug.
6. **Answer: 3**
   RATIONALE: The nurse should provide the client small, frequent meals, which are better tolerated than three large meals.

7. **Answer: 4**
   RATIONALE: The nurse should offer consistent and empathetic care to the client and the family, as treatment is spread over time and provides the nurse with several opportunities to help relieve their anxiety.
8. **Answer: 2**
   RATIONALE: The nurse should inform the client to take the drug as directed on the prescription.
9. **Answer: 3**
   RATIONALE: The part of cell growth that entails RNA and protein synthesis preparing for division is known as the G_2 phase.
10. **Answer: 4**
    RATIONALE: Green tea is the herbal product thought to have the benefits of overall sense of well-being, cancer prevention, dental health, and maintenance of heart and liver health.
11. **Answer: 2**
    RATIONALE: The vinca alkaloids, like vinblastine, are the class of antineoplastic drugs that interfere with amino acid production in the S phase and the formation of microtubules in the M phase.
12. **Answer: 1**
    RATIONALE: Podophyllotoxins are the class of antineoplastic drugs that stop cells in the S and G_2 phase, thereby causing cell division to cease.

CHAPTER 51

SECTION I: ASSESSING YOUR UNDERSTANDING

Activity A FILL IN THE BLANKS

1. Adaptive
2. angiogenesis
3. Cytotoxic
4. proteins
5. immune

Activity B SEQUENCING

1. 3   2   4   1

Activity C MATCHING

1. **1.** b   **2.** e   **3.** a   **4.** d   **5.** c

Activity D SHORT ANSWERS

1. Pseudoprogression is a delayed clinical response where the tumor may appear to continue to grow up until about the 16th week. Clients need to be made aware of this happening, and to assure them that the fear of lack of tumor response despite treatment is a normal feeling at this time.
2. Because GI issues can progress quickly from loose stools to colitis, clients and caregivers are taught to immediately inform the HCP of bowel habit changes—abdominal pain, nausea, cramping, and blood, mucous, or tarry stools. When the client is an inpatient, inspect stools for blood or mucus.

Stool should be sent to rule out *C. difficile* or other pathogens.

Activity E EXPLAIN THE DRUG NAME

1, 4 —use exclusively human tissue
2, 3 —use a combination of human and animal tissue, but primarily human
5 —uses a combination of human and animal tissue

SECTION II: APPLYING YOUR KNOWLEDGE

Activity F CASE STUDY

1. Herceptin is a monoclonal antibody—trastuzumab, whereas Enhertu is both a trastuzumab biosimilar and another drug biosimilar—deruxtecan-nxki.
2. Much like trade drugs versus generic drugs, a biosimilar is like the original biologic, only some of the inactive portions may be different. You can tell biologics from biosimilars because biosimilars have an addition suffix of four randomly generated letters included in the name.

SECTION III: PRACTICING FOR NCLEX

Activity G NCLEX-STYLE QUESTIONS

1. **Answer: 2**
   RATIONALE: Food may exacerbate the skin rash of erlotinib if taken with food. For mAbs taken orally, there are no special precautions for handling, yet it is important to take it at the same time daily to support effectiveness. There are no specific fluid requirements for taking the oral drug.
2. **Answer: 3**
   RATIONALE: Infusion reactions tend to be more pronounced when the mAb is produced from mouse tissue or a combination of tissues.
3. **Answer: 1**
   RATIONALE: Diarrhea may be a gastrointestinal adverse reaction to immunotherapy, typically the inhibitors. It is due to the inflammatory response and is seen more frequently when treating GI tumors.
4. **Answer: 2**
   RATIONALE: Clients should be taught before the drug is given that an infusion reaction is anticipated and may be uncomfortable. Warm blankets should be provided for client comfort.
5. **Answer: 2**
   RATIONALE: The importance of taking the drug at the same time each day to maintain a consistent body level is emphasized. A calendar or automated medication box indicating the doses to take and dates the drug is to be taken is often helpful for the client.
6. **Answer: 3**
   RATIONALE: Encourage clients to balance activity with rest periods to reduce fatigue. Although it may sound counterintuitive, exercise helps reduce

fatigue; encourage clients to take small walks or participate in yoga.

7. Answer: 4

RATIONALE: Drugs that offer passive immunity target foreign objects but do not remember the invader. Therefore, these therapies must be repeated for ongoing protection.

8. Answer: 3

RATIONALE: Over 500 TAAs have been identified for cancers specifically.

9. Answer: 4

RATIONALE: Cancer vaccines are designed for treatment not prevention. They develop antibodies and are capable of memory to fight ongoing disease—active immunity. Cytokines (interferons) and mAbs work by passive immunity.

10. Answer: 1

RATIONALE: Cytokines create an immune response, similar to having influenza. The following are the classic "flu-like" symptoms and include chills, cough, fever, headache, and malaise. Clients may experience the many other symptoms with treatment such as GI disturbances, pain, or edema.

11. Answer: 2

RATIONALE: Immunotherapy drugs tend to have less adverse reactions than traditional chemotherapy because they do not interfere with healthy cells.

12. Answer: 3

RATIONALE: Checkpoint inhibitors are a subclass of monoclonal antibodies.

CHAPTER 52

SECTION I: ASSESSING YOUR UNDERSTANDING

Activity A FILL IN THE BLANKS

1. superinfection
2. antipsoriatics
3. hypersensitivity
4. antiseptic
5. germicide

Activity B DOSAGE CALCULATION

1. 2 bottles
2. 20 treatments
3. 42 applications
4. 2 cups

Activity C MATCHING

1. 1. b   2. d   3. a   4. c
2. 1. d   2. a   3. b   4. c

Activity D SHORT ANSWERS

1. The preadministration assessment involves a visual inspection and palpation of the involved area(s). The nurse should carefully record the areas of involvement, including size, color, and appearance. A specific description is important so that changes can be readily identified, indicating worsening or improvement of the lesions. The nurse should note the presence of scales, crusting, or drainage or any complaint of itching. Some agencies may provide a figure on which the lesions can be drawn, indicating the shape and distribution of the involved areas.

2. At the time of each application, the nurse inspects the affected area for changes (e.g., signs of improvement or worsening of the infection) and for adverse reactions such as redness or rash. The nurse contacts the primary health care provider and the drug is not applied if these or other changes are noted, or if the client reports new problems such as itching, pain, or soreness at the site.

Activity E CROSSWORD PUZZLE

		C	O	R	P	O	R	I	S
	A		N						
	N		Y		V				
	T		C		E				
	I		H		S		P		
	S		O		I		E		
G	E	R	M	I	C	I	D	E	
	P		Y		O		I		
	T		C		L		S		
	I		O		O				
	C		S		R				
			I						
C	R	U	R	I	S				

SECTION II: APPLYING YOUR KNOWLEDGE

Activity F CASE STUDY

1. Common adverse reactions seen with the use of a topical antifungal are rash, itching, urticaria (hives), dermatitis, irritation, or redness, which may indicate a hypersensitivity (allergic) reaction to the drug.

2. Prolonged use of topical antibiotic preparations may result in a superficial superinfection (an overgrowth of bacterial or fungal microorganisms not affected by the antibiotic being administered).

SECTION III: PRACTICING FOR NCLEX

Activity G NCLEX-STYLE QUESTIONS

1. **Answer: 3**
   RATIONALE: Topical corticosteroids are contraindicated as monotherapy for plaque psoriasis.

2. **Answer: 2**
   RATIONALE: Proteolysis is the enzymatic action that helps remove dead soft tissues by reducing proteins to simpler substances.

3. **Answer: 3**
   RATIONALE: Benzocaine is a topical anesthetic, and topical anesthetics are used cautiously in clients receiving class I antiarrhythmic drugs such as tocainide and mexiletine because the toxic effects are additive and potentially synergistic.

4. **Answer: 1**
   RATIONALE: Alclometasone dipropionate is a topical corticosteroid, and with the use of topical corticosteroids, systemic reactions may occur with hypothalamic–pituitary–adrenal axis suppression, such as Cushing syndrome, hyperglycemia, and glycosuria.

5. **Answer: 2**
   RATIONALE: Numbness and dermatitis and mild and transient pains are the adverse reactions to the application of collagenase.

6. **Answer: 3**
   RATIONALE: Salicylic acid is a keratolytic drug, which is well tolerated; a flu-like syndrome is an infrequent adverse reaction to keratolytic drugs.

7. **Answer: 2**
   RATIONALE: Topical antiseptics and germicides are used for washing the hands before and after caring for clients, as a surgical scrub, and as a preoperative skin cleanser.

8. **Answer: 1**
   RATIONALE: Aklief, a retinoid drug, might be used topically by a client with acne vulgaris.

9. **Answer: 3**
   RATIONALE: Terbinafine (Lamisil) is a topical antifungal drug that might be used to treat onychomycosis (a nail fungus).

10. **Answer: 3**
    RATIONALE: If for any reason it becomes necessary to inactivate collagenase, this can be accomplished by washing the area with povidone–iodine.

11. **Answer: 1**
    RATIONALE: Docosanol (Abreva) is available over the counter and can be recommended for clients with HSV.

CHAPTER 53

SECTION I: ASSESSING YOUR UNDERSTANDING

Activity A FILL IN THE BLANKS

1. otic
2. otitis media

3. cerumen or wax
4. Glaucoma
5. Cycloplegia

Activity B DOSAGE CALCULATION

1. Every 6 hours
2. 5 drops
3. Yes, the total dose will be 1.5 mL
4. 5 drops
5. 10 drops (doses)

Activity C MATCHING

1. **1.** b   **2.** d   **3.** a   **4.** c
2. **1.** c   **2.** a   **3.** b

Activity D SHORT ANSWERS

1. The nurse may be responsible for examining the outer structures of the ear—namely, the earlobe and skin around the ear. The nurse should document a description of any drainage or impacted cerumen and check with the primary health care provider before administering an otic preparation to a client with a perforated eardrum.

2. The nurse assesses the client's response to therapy by confirming whether a decrease in pain or inflammation has occurred. The nurse should examine the outer ear and ear canal for any local redness or irritation that may indicate sensitivity to the drug.

Activity E LABELING

1 = Outer ear;   2 = Middle ear;   3 = Inner ear

SECTION II: APPLYING YOUR KNOWLEDGE

Activity F CASE STUDY

1. When assessing the infant, look for pulling, grabbing, or tugging at his ears. Because infants cannot tell you about pain, this may be a sign that the child's ear hurts. Additional signs include a change in behavior, crying, fussiness or irritability, or a fever. The nurse should validate this behavior with the parent.

2. The nurse should advise the mother that before instillation of otic preparations, she should hold the container in her hand for a few minutes to warm it to body temperature. Cold and too warm (above body temperature) preparations may cause dizziness or other sensations after being instilled into the ear. To keep solutions in the ear when instilling ear drops, the mother should have the child lie on his side with the affected ear up toward the ceiling. When administering an otic drug, the ear canal should be straightened. In children younger than 3 years, the ear canal is straighter and needs less manipulation. The mother should gently pull the outer ear down (instead of up) and back and drop the solution into the ear canal, being sure to never insert the dropper or applicator tip into the ear canal.

SECTION III: PRACTICING FOR NCLEX
Activity G NCLEX-STYLE QUESTIONS

1. **Answer: 1**
   RATIONALE: Prolonged use of otic preparations containing an antibiotic such as ofloxacin may result in a superinfection, due to an overgrowth of bacterial or fungal microorganisms not affected by the antibiotic being administered.

2. **Answer: 2**
   RATIONALE: Ofloxacin is considered a pregnancy category C drug, and although no interactions have been reported with otic use, it should be administered in pregnancy only if the potential benefit justifies the risk to the fetus.

3. **Answer: 3**
   RATIONALE: Before instilling an otic solution, the nurse informs the client that while the solution remains in the ear canal, a feeling of fullness may be felt in the ear and that hearing in the treated ear may be temporarily impaired.

4. **Answer: 1**
   RATIONALE: When instilling ear drops, the nurse has the client lie on their side with the ear toward the ceiling. If the client wishes to remain in an upright position, the head is tilted toward the untreated side with the ear toward the ceiling. To straighten the ear canal in adults and children ages 3 years and older, the cartilaginous portion of the outer ear is gently pulled up and back. The dropper or applicator tip should never be inserted into the ear canal.

5. **Answer: 3**
   RATIONALE: The nurse should stop using Cerumenex if ear drainage, discharge, pain, or irritation occurs. Also, Cerumenex should not be used for more than 4 days. If excessive cerumen remains, the primary health care provider should be consulted.

6. **Answer: 2**
   RATIONALE: Being a sympathomimetic drug, dipivefrin may cause transient local reactions such as brow ache, headache, burning and stinging, eye pain, allergic lip reactions, and ocular irritation.

7. **Answer: 4**
   RATIONALE: Dapiprazole, being an alpha-adrenergic (α-adrenergic blocker) blocker, may cause local effects such as ptosis (drooping of the upper eyelid), burning in the eye, eyelid edema, itching, corneal edema, brow ache, dryness of the eye, tearing, and blurred vision.

8. **Answer: 1**
   RATIONALE: Echothiophate iodide is a cholinesterase inhibitor ophthalmic preparation; therefore, the ophthalmic solution is less likely to be systemic, instead local adverse reactions could include eyelid muscle twitching, iris cysts, burning, lacrimation, conjunctivitis, ciliary redness, brow ache, and headache. Abdominal cramps, cardiac irregularities, and urinary incontinence are systemic adverse reactions to oral cholinesterase inhibitors.

9. **Answer: 3**
   RATIONALE: Antipyrine is used as an analgesic in otic preparations.

10. **Answer: 1**
    RATIONALE: The nurse can recommend carbamide peroxide to aid in the removal of cerumen from the ear canal.

11. **Answer: 2**
    RATIONALE: Cerumenex should not be allowed to stay in the ear canal for more than 30 minutes before irrigation.

12. **Answer: 1**
    RATIONALE: A client should not use over-the-counter ear wax removal products for more than 4 days; if excessive cerumen remains, the client should consult a physician.

CHAPTER 54

SECTION I: ASSESSING YOUR UNDERSTANDING
Activity A FILL IN THE BLANKS

1. electrolyte
2. alkaline
3. overload
4. Lactated Ringer's
5. morphine

Activity B DOSAGE CALCULATION

1. 100 mL/hour
2. 10 mL
3. 2 tablets

Activity C MATCHING

1. **1.** c   **2.** a   **3.** d   **4.** b

Activity D SHORT ANSWERS

1. The nurse should consider the following factors when evaluating the intravenous replacement solution therapy to determine its effectiveness:
   - The therapeutic effect of the drug is achieved.
   - The fluid volume deficit is corrected.
   - The nutrition deficit is corrected.
   - The client and family demonstrate an understanding of the procedure.

2. The nurse should include the following points for the intake of oral potassium supplement in a client teaching plan:
   - Take the drug exactly as directed on the prescription container. Do not increase, decrease, or omit doses of the drug unless advised to do so by the primary health care provider.
   - Take the drug immediately after meals or with food and a full glass of water.

- Avoid the use of nonprescription drugs and salt substitutes (many contain potassium) unless use of a specific drug or product has been approved by the primary health care provider.
- Contact the primary health care provider if tingling of the hands or feet, a feeling of heaviness in the legs, vomiting, nausea, abdominal pain, or black stools should occur.
- If the tablet has a coating (an enteric-coated tablet), swallow it whole. Do not chew or crush the tablet

- If effervescent tablets are prescribed, place the tablet in 4–8 ounces of cold water or juice. Wait until the fizzing stops before drinking. Sip the liquid during a period of 5–10 minutes.
- If an oral liquid or a powder is prescribed, add the dose to 4–8 ounces of cold water or juice and sip slowly during a period of 5–10 minutes. Measure the dose accurately.

Activity E CROSSWORD PUZZLE

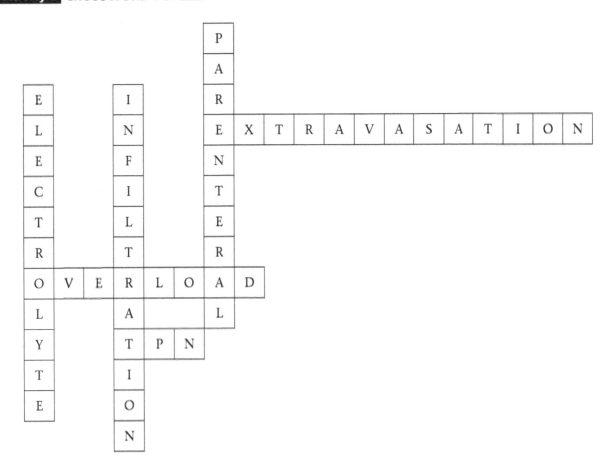

SECTION II: APPLYING YOUR KNOWLEDGE

Activity F CASE STUDY

1. The drip rate would be 42 drops/minute.

1000 mL/4 hours = 250 mL/hour
250 mL/hour × 1 hour/60 minutes = 4.2 mL/minute
4.2 mL/minute × 10 drops/mL = 42 drops/minute

2. Signs and symptoms a client with fluid overload might exhibit include headache, weakness, blurred vision, behavioral changes (confusion, disorientation, delirium, drowsiness), weight gain, isolated muscle twitching, hyponatremia, rapid breathing, wheezing, coughing, rise in blood pressure, distended neck veins, elevated central venous pressure, and convulsions.

SECTION III: PRACTICING FOR NCLEX

Activity G NCLEX-STYLE QUESTIONS

1. **Answer: 2**
   RATIONALE: When caring for a client who needs to be administered magnesium, the nurse should confirm that the client does not have a heart block or myocardial damage because presence of these conditions contraindicates the use of magnesium.

2. **Answers: 3, 4**
   RATIONALE: When caring for a client who is being administered potassium orally and experiencing

GI distress, the nurse ensures that the supplement is given immediately after meals or with food and a full glass of water. Potassium in the form of effervescent tablets, powder, or liquid must be thoroughly mixed with 4–8 ounces of cold water, juice, or other beverage. Offering smaller meals and giving antacids will not diminish the distress and may hamper drug absorption. Monitoring for signs and symptoms of nausea is an assessment, not an intervention.

3. **Answer: 1**

   RATIONALE: When caring for a client who is being administered plasma protein fractions, the nurse should monitor for adverse reactions such as urticaria. Other adverse reactions may include nausea, chills, fever, and hypotensive episodes.

4. **Answers: 1, 3**

   RATIONALE: To maintain the patency of the lock, a solution of saline or dilute heparin may be ordered for injection into the heparin lock before and after the administration of a drug administered via IV route.

5. **Answer: 2**

   RATIONALE: If the client has heart failure, bicarbonate may be given cautiously. Bicarbonate is contraindicated in clients with metabolic or respiratory alkalosis, hypocalcemia, or severe abdominal pain of unknown cause.

6. **Answer: 3**

   RATIONALE: Calculations for conversion use a chart to determine the amount of drug compared to morphine, the gold standard discussed in Chapter 15.

7. **Answer: 3**

   RATIONALE: One week or up to 7 days. Peripheral TPN is used for relatively short periods (no more than 5–7 days) and when the central venous route is not possible or necessary.

8. **Answer: 2**

   RATIONALE: Depending on clinical judgment, two unsuccessful venipuncture attempts on the same client warrant having a more skilled individual attempt the procedure.

9. **Answer: 1**

   RATIONALE: Potassium and magnesium are the major intracellular fluid electrolytes.

10. **Answer: 4**

    RATIONALE: Sodium and calcium are the major extracellular fluid electrolytes.

11. **Answer: 2**

    RATIONALE: Potassium is the electrolyte necessary for the transmission of impulses and the contraction of smooth, cardiac, and skeletal muscles.

12. **Answer: 2**

    RATIONALE: Every 1–2 hours when the client is critical or unable to respond or tell the nurse about an issue with the infusion.

Templates: Concept (Mind) Mapping

INTRODUCTION

Concept (or sometimes called mind) mapping is used to pictorially organize data. In this section, we show you how to use boxes, lines, and diagraming to map out important concepts involved in pharmacology. This tool is helpful in understanding the complex and interwoven medical problems of today's health care. Here are the step-by-step instructions for using these templates to create concept maps and increase your pharmacologic knowledge.

ABOUT THE MAPS

In Chapter 5 of *Introductory Clinical Pharmacology,* you are introduced to seven case study clients and given background information about each one. Their stories in each subsequent chapter of the textbook then challenge you to use clinical reasoning skills to add to the map.

Activities in the *Study Guide to Accompany Introductory Clinical Pharmacology* further build upon the real-life case studies by providing concept-mapping exercises using the clients and situations illustrated in the text, which help you to

- learn how medication action reduces symptoms
- interact with one another
- complicate existing client problems.

Seven templates are provided on the following pages—one template for each of the clients introduced in Chapter 5 of the textbook. The templates are also provided as part of the student resources of *Introductory Clinical Pharmacology* at thePoint.

WHERE TO FIND MAPPING DATA

As with any client you encounter in the clinical setting, oftentimes very little information is provided at first interaction. An introduction, similar to that first interaction, is provided for you in Chapter 5 of the textbook. You will find on the templates in this appendix that we have used the Chapter 5 information to begin to visualize (draw) each client's introductory medical problems, symptoms, or client history.

Look for the section at the beginning of each chapter of the textbook called *Pharmacology in Practice.* This section will tell you which of the seven clients is featured in the chapter and gives you information to add on the select concept map. At the end of each chapter, the *Pharmacology in Practice: Clinical Reasoning* section provides more information about the client scenario presented earlier.

Then, add data to the concept map as you complete the activities in Section II, *Applying Your Knowledge,* of this study guide. As you complete the map, you will discover and be able to anticipate side effects, drug–drug interactions, and other pharmacologic issues.

Keep in mind that there may be more than one way to complete a concept map. The novel feature about these exercises is that you can keep adding information to your client maps regardless of which unit of the textbook you start with or read. As the client stories evolve, you will uncover more and more data. For example, if you are asked to read about cardiac drugs (Unit 8) before you learn about anti-infectives (Unit 2), or the first unit studied is pain management (Unit 3), it does not matter. You may come to find the same conclusions about these clients as if you studied the units in sequence. This is because as you obtain information about the clients and their conditions, you build the client care map as you go. These discoveries help you solidify your knowledge about pharmacologic interactions—a vital part of today's nursing practice.

STEP-BY-STEP INSTRUCTIONS

To begin making your first pharmacology concept map, this example uses the template provided for Mrs. Moore and additions to the map come from the information in Unit 2, Chapter 6. Let us explain how this works.

STEP 1: LOCATE THE TEMPLATE

Take out (best to copy or download a copy) Mrs. Moore's template, here in the study guide. You will find that the introductory information from Chapter 5 of the textbook about her mental status (the symptoms of forgetfulness and confusion) and the medical condition (heart failure) is already included on the template.

STEP 2: ADD THE DATA FROM THE TEXTBOOK CASE STUDY

Return to Chapter 6 of the textbook (Antibacterial Drugs: Sulfonamides). Using similar lines and boxes to make linkages, add the data facts found in the section *Pharmacology in Practice* at the beginning of Chapter 6.

- Add a box with the new medical diagnosis: urinary tract infection (UTI). Your map should now have three boxes linked to Mrs. Moore: (1) UTI, (2) mental status, and (3) heart failure.
- Add a box labeled *Sulfonamide* that is linked to the UTI box. You may want to add the drugs used to treat different medical conditions. This will help you later to see the linkages to interactions, precautions, and contraindications when various drugs are added to the client's map.

STEP 3: ADD NEW INFORMATION LEARNED IN THE TEXTBOOK

The readings from the section *Nursing Process* in Chapter 6 state that in elders, forgetfulness and confusion may be symptoms of a UTI. Using this information, draw a dotted line from the UTI box to the boxes with mental status information. *You made the first connection between problem and symptom!*

STEP 4: ADD INFORMATION FROM CLINICAL REASONING SUMMARY SECTION

As you gain drug knowledge from reading each chapter, continue to add information to each client's concept map. In the summary of Chapter 6 (*Pharmacology in Practice: Clinical Reasoning*), Mrs. Moore's urinalysis did have bacteria in the sample. Add these data to your concept map in the UTI box. Now you have a good picture of the symptoms, which indicated treatment with a sulfonamide was warranted in this situation with Mrs. Moore.

STEP 5: WHAT HAPPENED TO THE CLIENT IN THE STUDY GUIDE

Look for extra data to add from the study guide Section II, *Applying Your Knowledge*. In the study guide, Mrs. Moore is the same client, with reinforced information to begin building maps. In most chapters of the study guide, additional data for mapping will be included for the same or a different client than the one in the corresponding chapter of the textbook. This helps you reinforce pharmacologic concepts of the textbook.

As you learn from your textbook and study guide, continue to add information from the other chapters that feature Mrs. Moore. Do the same for the other six clients featured. By following these easy steps and building these concept maps, you will learn to analyze real client situations long before you see similar ones in your clinical practice. Once again helping you to become the best client care provider and advocate as you assume your professional practice role.

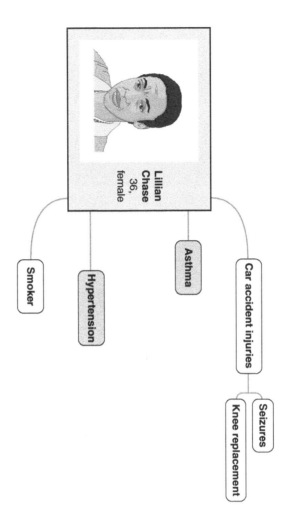

Lillian Chase
36, female

Smoker

Hypertension

Asthma

Car accident injuries

Seizures

Knee replacement

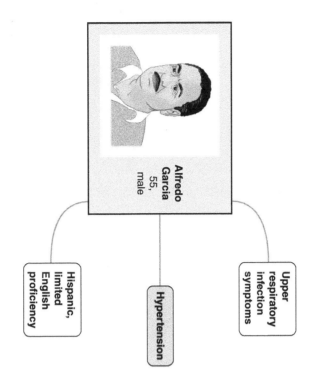

Alfredo Garcia
55, male

Hispanic, limited English proficiency

Hypertension

Upper respiratory infection symptoms

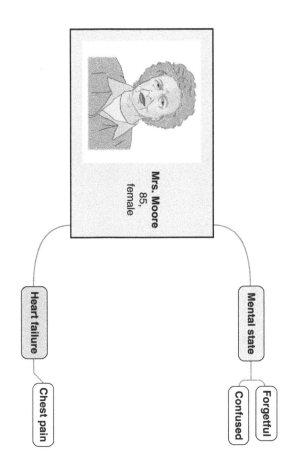

Mrs. Moore
85, female

Heart failure

Chest pain

Mental state

Forgetful

Confused

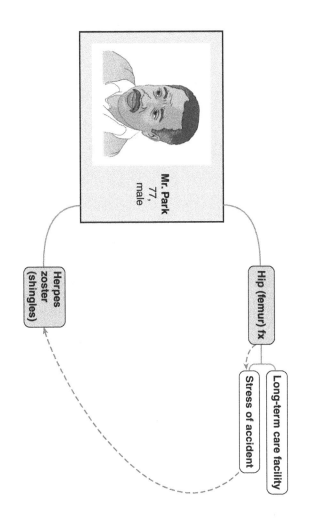

Mr. Park
77,
male

Herpes
zoster
(shingles)

Hip (femur) fx

Stress of accident

Long-term care facility

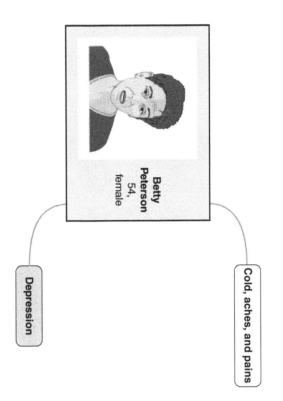

Betty Peterson
54, female

Depression

Cold, aches, and pains

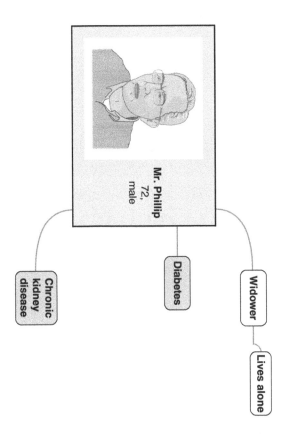

Mr. Phillip
72,
male

Chronic kidney disease

Diabetes

Widower

Lives alone

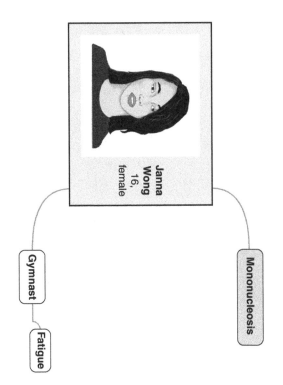

Janna
Wong
16,
female

Gymnast

Fatigue

Mononucleosis